Key Concepts of Atherogenesis

Key Concepts of Atherogenesis

Edited by **Ashton Goldberg**

FOSTER
ACADEMICS

New Jersey

Published by Foster Academics,
61 Van Reypen Street,
Jersey City, NJ 07306, USA
www.fosteracademics.com

Key Concepts of Atherogenesis
Edited by Ashton Goldberg

International Standard Book Number: 978-1-63242-252-1 (Hardback)

Printed in the United States of America.

Contents

Preface

Important concepts related to atherogenesis are provided in this book. The book also presents current developments in the dynamics of cholesterol transport. It discusses topics related to the various concepts and models of atherosclerosis. This book will be of significance for students, researchers and clinicians who are interested in the varied aspects of this disease.

The information shared in this book is based on empirical researches made by veterans in this field of study. The elaborative information provided in this book will help the readers further their scope of knowledge leading to advancements in this field.

Finally, I would like to thank my fellow researchers who gave constructive feedback and my family members who supported me at every step of my research.

Editor

Atherosclerosis-Models and Concepts

Illuminating Atherogenesis Through Mathematical Modeling

L. R. Ritter[1], Akif Ibragimov[2], Jay R. Walton[3]
and Catherine J. McNeal[4]

[1]*Department of Mathematics, Southern Polytechnic State University*
[2]*Department of Mathematics & Statistics, Texas Tech University*
[3]*Department of Mathematics, Texas A & M University*
[4]*Department of Internal Medicine, Division of Cardiology and Department of Pediatrics,*
Division of Endocrinology, Scott & White Hospital
USA

1. Introduction

Mathematical Medicine is a relatively new and expanding area of Applied Mathematics research with a growing number of mathematicians, experimentalist, biomedical engineers, and research physicians involved in collaborative efforts on a global scale. Mathematical models are playing an increasing role in our understanding of such complex biological processes as the onset, progression, and mitigation of various diseases. The cardiovascular system is particularly intricate, and the formulation and analysis of mathematical models presents a myriad of challenges to the investigator. (See (Quarteroni, 2001) for a survey on the subject.) Mathematical studies of the cardiovascular system have included continuum mechanical models of vascular soft tissue (Holzapfel et al., 2000; Humphery & Rajagopal, 2002; Taylor & Humphrey, 2009), fluid dynamical models of the interaction between blood flow and vessel walls (Baek et al., 2007; Quarteroni, 2001; Veneziani, 1998), and mathematical models, such as that of the present work, of biochemical characteristics of the vasculature (Ibragimov et al., 2005; Neumann et al., 1990; Saidel et al., 1987). The disease of atherosclerosis, and its initiation atherogenesis, involves a complex interplay between mechanical, genetic, pathogenic, and biochemical processes. A comprehensive view of atherosclerosis will ultimately require integration of these various modeling perspectives. Herein, we focus on the inflammatory component of atherogenesis, in particular the role of immune cells–primarily macrophages–in the presence of oxidatively modified low density lipoproteins (LDL cholesterol) within the intimal layer of large muscular arteries. We present a mathematical model of the key inflammatory spiral that characterizes the initiation of atherosclerosis, and perform some analyses of this model.

It is well accepted that atherosclerosis is marked by chronic inflammation (Creager & Braunwald , eds.; Fan & Watanabe, 2003; Ross, 1995; 1999; Wilson , ed.). Changes in the permeability of the endothelial layer and subsequent deposition of lipids in the intima cause an up-regulation of chemoattractants such as monocyte chemotactic protein 1, interleukin-8 and macrophage colony-stimulating factor that are secreted by the endothelial and other cells. In addition, LDL molecules become trapped in the subendothelial intima where they are subject to oxidative modification by reactive oxygen species. Macrophages begin to accumulate in the region where they assume a pro-inflammatory phenotype. The stimulation of macrophages may be due to the presence of inflammatory extra-cellular matrix fragments. In addition, oxidized LDL is recognized by a macrophage scavenger receptor with some degree of interindividual variation (Boullier et al., 2001; Martín-Fuentes et al., 2007; Mosser & Edwards, 2008; Podrez et al., 2002). Macrophages attempting to internalize these particles may become engorged with cholesterol and transform into foam cells. In this state, these immune cells are incapable of performing the customary immune function and become part of a developing atherosclerotic lesion. The immune response is mediated by those chemical signals emitted by endothelial cell, immune cells, and immune cell derived foam cells. The *corruption* [1] of the immune process caused by ingestion of oxidized LDL can trigger an inflammatory response which results in increased immune cell migration to the site, possible further corruption, and ultimately accumulation of debris (necrotic, apoptotic, and lipid laden cells) characterizing plaque onset. This inflammatory spiral facilitated by chemotaxis, the process modeled herein, is a hallmark of atherogenesis.

It will become evident that our model incorporates many parameters characterizing such things as the rate at which macrophages move within the intimal tissue (independent of and in response to chemokines), rates of phenotype changes for macrophages, rates of phagocytosis and uptake of lipids by immune cells, degratation rates of various chemicals, chemical reaction rates and so forth. Some of these have value ranges that are known *in vitro* or *in vivo*, but many are unknown. The analytical techniques employed at present are linear stability studies. This allows us to obtain criteria based on the *relative* values of parameters and to interpret these criteria in terms of the propensity for a lesion to initiate—or not. These criteria will take the form of various inequalities in section 4.

In the next section, we lay out the disease paradigm and the assumptions upon which the mathematical model is constructed. This is followed by a presentation of the general model in the form of a system of nonlinear, primarily parabolic partial differential equations with mixed third type boundary conditions. In section 4, we perform stability analyses of the model under two different assumptions regarding the source of inflammatory components. Two stability theorems are given along with a bio-medical interpretation of the criteria derived. Also included is a discussion of the existence of unstable equilibria with a focus on the role of an antioxidant presence and the competing processes of macrophage motility (unrelated to chemotaxis) and chemotaxis. The chapter closes with a brief conclusion.

2. The disease paradigm and model basis

The large muscular arteries most vulnerable to atherosclerotic lesions can be considered as thick walled tubes consisting of three distinct layers. The outermost layer, called the adventitia, provides structural integrity through a strong collagen network. The middle layer, the media, provides flexibility and adaptability through layers of smooth muscle cells enmeshed in an elastin and collagen network. And the thin, innermost layer, called the intima, is where the atherosclerotic lesions begin to develop. A monolayer of endothelial cells forms an interface between the intima and the lumen through which blood flows. These endothelial cells are highly active in the circulatory process providing a smooth surface for fluid flow,

---

[1] The term "corruption" refers to the formation of foam cells due to the failure of the scavenger receptor to down regulate in response to excess cellular cholesterol content (Steinberg, 2002), and to the ability of C-reactive protein and oxLDL to increase the inflammatory properties of monocytes (Zhang & Wahl, 2006).

secreting anticoagulant, procoagulant, and inflammatory factors and regulating the exchange of cells and molecules between the blood and arterial wall. Insult to the endothelium and so called endothelial dysfunction is a precursor to atherosclerosis. A number of pathological conditions, genetic factors, and behavioral practices may result in endothelial dysfunction (Davignon & Ganz, 2004). This process appears to be characterized by a change in the permeability of the endothelial layer that allows lipids to migrate into the subendothelial layer followed by an influx of the cells that comprise the immune response. Following endothelial dysfunction and migration of lipoproteins and immune cells, we identify two significant steps to atherogenesis. These are oxidative modification of LDL, and the initiation of an inflammatory spiral.

2.1 Lipoprotein oxidation

Lipoproteins are micellar particles which contain regulatory proteins that direct the blood trafficking of cholesterol and other lipids to various cells in the body.. There are four major classes of lipoprotein–chylomicrons, very low-density lipoproteins (VLDL), low-density lipoproteins, and high-density lipoproteins (HDL)—but the bulk of cholesterol is contained in the latter two. Low density lipoproteins consist of a lipid core, a surface protein and a number of antioxidant defenses. LDLs deposit cholesterol in the tissues for cell metabolism. High density lipoproteins contain most of the remaining cholesterol in the body. These particles take excess lipids from tissues and return them to the liver for processing—the process referred to as reverse transport. Elevated plasma levels of LDL indicate a high risk of disease primarily because of their susceptibility to becoming trapped within the intima and subsequently attacked by radical oxygen species. The inflammation of atherosclerotic lesions occurs in areas of intimal thickening enriched by deposits of oxidized LDL.

The modification of LDL is a complicated process that has been the subject of several studies, and the reader is directed to the articles (Parthasarathy et al., 1992; Steinberg, 1997) and the review (Young & McEneny, 2001) and the references therein for a more complete and detailed description. Cobbold, Sherratt and Maxwell provided a mathematical model of the *in vitro* cascade of oxidation of LDL cholesterol in 2002 formulated according to a linear chemical reaction process (Cobbold et al., 2002). This model is adapted and included in the present model of atherogenesis. In brief, the mechanics of the process can be described as follows: In the tissue, where the concentration of reactive oxygen species (ROS) may be relatively high and external antioxidant defenses low, each interaction of an ROS and an LDL molecule will result in oxidizing one of the vitamin E molecules on the lipid surface. It is also possible that an oxidized vitamin E molecule (α-tocopherol radical) may be reduced back to a vitamin E molecule by an antioxidant present (Niki et al., 1984; Watanabe et al., 1999). If, through a finite sequence of oxidation of vitamin E molecules, an LDL molecule losses all of its innate defense against free radical attack, it is susceptible to peroxidation of its lipid core. Once fully modified, the oxidized LDL is both attractive to macrophages and unable to leave the intima (unlike oxidized HDL particles (Tall, 1998)).

2.2 The inflammatory response

Accompanying the permeability changes to the endothelium and the influx of lipids is the immune response. Various white blood cells (monocytes, T-lymphocytes, neutrophils) migrate into tissues in response to chemical signals. Once in the subendothelial intima, monocytes differentiate into macrophages. Under normal healthy conditions, these immune cells aid in the degradation of apoptotic cells as well as the removal of foreign agents such as bacteria or viruses through phagocytosis. As stated, macrophages have a high affinity for oxidized LDL. However, attempts to take up the modified lipids by the process of phagocytosis are unsuccessful, and the lipid laden macrophages transform into foam cells (Goldstein et al., 1977; Podrez et al., 2002; Steinberg, 1997). Unable to perform their normal immune function, these lipid-laden cells signal other immune cells to the site precipitating accumulation of fatty tissue and the progression toward plaque growth. Additional chemical signals secreted by the foam cells and endothelial cells summon more immune cells to the site. Additional macrophages migrate to the localized site of inflammation. The chemical mediators of inflammation can increase binding of oxidized LDL to cells in the arterial wall (Hajjar & Haberland, 1997). Hence, the new macrophages become engorged with oxidized LDL and the cycle of chemical signaling continues.

The role of macrophages in initiation of an atherosclerotic lesion is complicated and far from singular. [2] In addition to foam cells, apoptotic macrophages are regularly found in lesions. Apoptosis of cells (macrophage and others) within a plaque is found to have both stabilizing as well as destabilizing affects (Cui et al., 2007; Tabas, 2004). Phagocytosis of apoptotic cells (not necessarily macrophages) may induce resistance to foam cell formation among macrophages. This occurs when during phagocytosis, the macrophage takes in high levels of membrane-derived cholesterol as opposed to lipoprotein-derived cholesterol. In Cui *et al.* , the authors report that ingestion of apoptotic cells induced a survival response in the macrophages in their experiments (Cui et al., 2007). It is also known that macrophages appear in different phenotypes that are non-static in the sense that they may change types—a process that is reversible (Kadl et al., 2010; Mosser & Edwards, 2008; Stout et al., 2005), and that the different types serve opposing functions (e.g. inflammatory versus anti-inflammatory). Moreover, the sources of additional immune cells include transport across the endothelium as well as migration via the vasa vasorum that provides blood to the artery wall. The mathematical model is constructed to allow for the diverse functions of the immune cells. (For a mathematical study similar to that presented here that focuses primarily on the competing role of inflammatory and anti-inflammatory macrophages, we direct you to the article (Ibragimov et al., 2008).)

3. The mathematical model

We begin by identifying the key chemical and cellular species involved in atherogenesis. For each species, an evolution equation is derived through the classical approach of imposing a mass balance in an arbitrary control volume and subsequent reduction to a pointwise statement. We do not consider here the volume of a lesion but rather the concentration of each species at any point.

Our model consists of five classes of generalized species–two cellular and three chemical–that have critical roles in the initiation of an atherosclerotic lesion. These classes are labeled and denoted as follows:

$\mathcal{I}$ Immune cells: These are primarily monocyte derived macrophages but may include other white blood cells (T-cells and perhaps neutrophils).

$\mathcal{D}$ Debris: This is the bulk of a forming lesion consisting of apoptotic cells, macrophage derived foam cells, and potentially necrotic tissue . Our use of the term *debris* is unconventional in the sense that we do not intend to suggest that these are inert cells

---

[2] The reader is directed to the article Mosser & Edwards (2008) for an excellent review of the array of macrophage phenotypes and functions.

or simply a byproduct of some process and merely occupy space. As will be seen in the mathematics to follow, this species type plays a pivotal role in the inflammatory feedback.

$\mathcal{C}$ Chemoattractant: This chemical species represents any of a number of cytokines and chemotactic molecules including macrophage colony stimulating factor, monocyte chemotactic protein-1, and various interleukin proteins. Any chemical that is used in the regulation of the immune response primarily through inducing chemotaxis is included in this species type.

$\mathcal{L}$ & $\mathcal{L}_{ox}$ Low density lipoproteins: The LDL species consists of two major sub-types, those in a native (un-oxidized) state, and those molecules that have undergone full peroxidation of the lipid core.

$\mathcal{R}$ Reactive oxygen species: These are free radical molecules that induce oxidative damage to the lipoproteins present. This species is a byproduct of various metabolic processes within the arterial wall.

Also included in the model are several input parameters. Of particular interest are the parameters A_{ox}, that is a level of antioxidants such as vitamins C, E, and beta-carotene, and $\mathcal{L}_B$ representing the serum concentration of LDL.

Each of the representative variables here is a vector with each component representing a specific member of the class. For example,

$$\mathcal{I} = (\mathcal{I}_1, \mathcal{I}_2, \ldots, \mathcal{I}_{N_I})^T$$

where each component $\mathcal{I}_i$, $i = 1, \ldots, N_I$ may be a different specific white blood cell, a different phenotype, or may represent cells in different roles. We allow for $\mathcal{I}$ to have N_I components, $\mathcal{D}$ to have N_D, $\mathcal{C}$ to have N_C, $\mathcal{L}$ to have $N_L + 1$[3], and each of $\mathcal{L}_{ox}$ and $\mathcal{R}$ are scalar valued. If we isolate any representative variable u from this list, we construct an equation of the form

$$\frac{\partial u}{\partial t} = -\nabla \cdot \mathbf{J}_u + Q_u$$

that equates the evolution of the concentration of species u to a spatial flux field $\mathbf{J}_u$ and any net source Q_u due to cellular interactions, chemical secretion or uptake, chemical reactions, and the like. The flux fields and source terms are outline below for each variable.

3.1 Governing equations

The equations governing these species and based upon the disease paradigm outlined in section 2 are

$$\frac{\partial}{\partial t}\mathcal{I}_i = \mu_{I_i}\nabla^2\mathcal{I}_i - \nabla \cdot \left(\sum_{k=1}^{N_C} \chi_{ik}(\mathcal{C}_k, \mathcal{I}_i)\nabla\mathcal{C}_k \right) -$$

$$- \sum_{k=1}^{N_D} a_{ik}\mathcal{D}_k\mathcal{I}_i - \sum_{k=1,k\neq i}^{N_I} b_{ik}\mathcal{I}_k\mathcal{I}_i - c_i\mathcal{I}_i\mathcal{L}_{ox} - d_{1i}\mathcal{I}_i, \qquad (3.1)$$

---

[3] The model of LDL oxidation presented by Cobbold, Sherratt and Maxwell includes LDL molecules in a fully native state containing N_L vitamin E molecules. Studies show the number of such antioxidant defenses is on average 6 per LDL molecule but may vary from 3 to 15 (Esterbauer et al., 1992; Stocker, 1999). We then consider $\mathcal{L}_i$ to contain i vitamin E molecules where $\mathcal{L}_0$ represents LDL molecules completely depleted of native vitamin E that has yet to undergo full oxidation of its core.

$$\frac{\partial}{\partial t}\mathcal{D}_i = \mu_{D_i}\nabla^2\mathcal{D}_i + \tau_i\sum_{k=1}^{N_I}(c_k + f_k)\mathcal{I}_k\mathcal{L}_{ox} - \sum_{k=1}^{N_I}\hat{a}_{ik}\mathcal{I}_k\mathcal{D}_i - d_{2i}\mathcal{D}_i,\tag{3.2}$$

$$\frac{\partial}{\partial t}\mathcal{C}_i = \mu_{C_i}\nabla^2\mathcal{C}_i + \sum_{k=1}^{N_D}p_{ik}\mathcal{D}_k\mathcal{C}_i - \sum_{k=1}^{N_I}e_{ik}\mathcal{I}_k\mathcal{C}_i - d_{3i}\mathcal{C}_i,\tag{3.3}$$

$$\frac{\partial}{\partial t}\mathcal{L}_{N_L} = \mu_{L_{N_L}}\nabla^2\mathcal{L}_{N_L} - k_R\mathcal{R}\mathcal{L}_{N_L} + k_A A_{ox}\mathcal{L}_{N_L-1} - d_{4N_L}\mathcal{L}_{N_L},\tag{3.4}$$

$$\frac{\partial}{\partial t}\mathcal{L}_i = \mu_{L_i}\nabla^2\mathcal{L}_i + k_R\mathcal{R}(\mathcal{L}_{i+1} - \mathcal{L}_i) - k_A A_{ox}(\mathcal{L}_i - \mathcal{L}_{i-1}) - \\ - d_{4i}\mathcal{L}_i, \quad 1 \leq i \leq N_L - 1\tag{3.5}$$

$$\frac{\partial}{\partial t}\mathcal{L}_0 = \mu_{L_0}\nabla^2\mathcal{L}_0 + k_R\mathcal{R}\mathcal{L}_1 - k_A A_{ox}\mathcal{L}_0 - k_{Ro}\mathcal{R}\mathcal{L}_0 - d_{40}\mathcal{L}_0,\tag{3.6}$$

$$\frac{\partial}{\partial t}\mathcal{L}_{ox} = \mu_{L_{ox}}\nabla^2\mathcal{L}_{ox} + k_{Ro}\mathcal{R}\mathcal{L}_0 - \sum_{k=1}^{N_I}f_k\mathcal{I}_k\mathcal{L}_{ox},\tag{3.7}$$

$$\frac{\partial}{\partial t}\mathcal{R} = \mu_R\nabla^2\mathcal{R} - \sum_{k=1}^{N_L}k_R\mathcal{R}\mathcal{L}_k - k_{Ro}\mathcal{R}\mathcal{L}_0 - hA_{ox}\mathcal{R} + \mathbf{p}_R.\tag{3.8}$$

The various parameters appearing in (3.1)–(3.8) require explanation; a succint description of each is given in table 1. Each species is subject to diffusion, or diffusive motility in the case of immune cells, and this is reflected in the flux terms $\mu_u\nabla^2 u$ (u represents any of the various state variables $\mathcal{I}$–$\mathcal{R}$) with the coefficient μ with a subscript a measure of the motility or diffusive capability of the respective species.

χ_{ik}	chemotactic sensitivity of immune species i to chemical stimulant k
$a_{ik}, \hat{a}_{ik}$	binding of immune cells to the lesion for removal
b_{ik}	measure of subspecies interaction for immune cells
c_i, f_i	rates of foam cell formation
d_{ni}	cell turn over or chemical degradation rate
p_{ik}	rate of chemical attractant production due to the lesion presence
e_{ik}	uptake of chemoattractant during chemotaxis
k_R, k_{R_0}, k_A	rate of oxidation, peroxidation, and reverse (anti-oxidation), respectively
d_{ni}	cell turn over or chemical degradation rate
p_{ik}	rate of chemical attractant production due to the lesion presence
e_{ik}	uptake of chemoattractant during chemotaxis
τ_i, h	efficiency factors
p_R	production of free-radicals due to normal metabolism

Table 1. Bio-physiological Interpretation of Parameters

The terms $\chi_{ik}(\mathcal{C}_k, \mathcal{I}_i)\nabla\mathcal{C}_k$ are the contribution to the flux field for macrophages due to chemotaxis. The coefficient $\chi_{ik}(\mathcal{C}_k, \mathcal{I}_i)$ is the chemo-tactic sensitivity of immune cell i to chemoattractant k. This is the classic Keller-Segel model of chemotaxis (Keller & Segel, 1971). The dependence of χ_{ik} on the immune cells is generally taken to be linear, however there is no present need to specify a particular form for these functions. Each of the immune cells, debris, chemoattractants, and native LDL species may undergo natural turnover or chemical degradation represented by the last terms in equations (3.1)–(3.6).

The immune cell equations contain three significant cross interaction terms. The terms $a_{ik}\mathcal{D}_k\mathcal{I}_i$ capture binding of macrophages with debris—in particular, these and the analogous terms $\hat{a}_{ik}\mathcal{I}_k\mathcal{D}_i$ in (3.2), account for phagocytosis of debris by healthy macrophages and removal for future processing in the liver. We also allow for inter-species interactions via the terms $b_{ik}\mathcal{I}_k\mathcal{I}_i$

in (3.1). This accounts, for example, for potential change of phenotype of macrophages during the inflammatory process. Recent studies have demonstrated that such changes may occur (reversibly) in vitro and in animal models (Kadl et al., 2010; Stout et al., 2005). Finally, the formation of foam cells through binding with oxidized LDL appears in equations (3.1) and (3.7) in the removal terms $c_i \mathcal{I}_i \mathcal{L}_{ox}$ and $f_k \mathcal{I}_k \mathcal{L}_{ox}$. This foam cell formation appears as a source term in equation (3.2) as $\tau_i \sum_{k=1}^{N_I} (c_k + f_k) \mathcal{I}_k \mathcal{L}_{ox}$, where $0 \le \tau_i \le 1$, $\sum_{i=1}^{N_D} \tau_i = 1$. The parameter τ_i allows us to catagorize different contributions to the lesion—different types of *debris*.

The equation for the chemoattractants includes (in addition to those terms already mentioned) a source term reflecting production of these chemicals in response to the presence of debris $p_{ik} \mathcal{D}_k \mathcal{C}_i$. The removal terms $e_{ik} \mathcal{I}_k \mathcal{C}_i$ represent the reduction of the chemoattractant concentration by binding with macrophages during chemotaxis.

As stated, the equations governing the lipid oxidation reactions (3.4)–(3.8) are a modification of the model of lipoprotein oxidation presented by Cobbold, Sherratt and Maxwell in 2002 (Cobbold et al., 2002). The chemical kinetics are assumed to be a linear reaction model in which an LDL molecule containing i vitamin E particles reacts with a reactive oxygen species, with reaction rate k_R to produce an LDL molecule with $i - 1$ vitamin E molecules. This model also allows for the reverse oxidation reaction in that an LDL molecule with $i < N_L$ vitamin E molecules may react with the antioxidant species A_{ox}, with reaction rate k_A, to produce an LDL molecule with $i + 1$ vitamin E defenses. Any LDL molecule that has been completely depleted of its native antioxidant defenses contributes to the concentration $\mathcal{L}_0$. A subsequent reaction of an $\mathcal{L}_0$ molecule with an ROS (with reaction rate k_{R_0}) results in peroxidation of the lipid core and a fully modified LDL particle. The ROS is depleted through these reactions and through direct reaction with the anti-oxidant species–the latter occurring with the rate of reaction h appearing in equation (3.8). The primary source of ROS is as a byproduct of metabolic processes within the intima. The term $\mathbf{p}_R$ represents this source. The reader is encouraged to see (Cobbold et al., 2002) for a detailed construction of the model.

The modifications of Cobbold-Sherratt-Maxwell model presented here are two fold. First, we allow for spatial variation through a standard Fickian diffusion. More significant to the study of atherogenesis, we include the uptake of modified LDL by macrophages leading to foam cell formation and subsequent inflammation. The terms $f_k \mathcal{I}_k \mathcal{L}_{ox}$ represent removal of oxidized LDL through macrophage binding and the contribution to the forming lesion as seen in (3.2), (3.7) and (3.8).

3.2 Domain and boundary conditions

The system (3.1)–(3.8) can be considered in two or three spatial dimensions. In (Ibragimov et al., 2005), the current authors performed numerical simulations of a simplified model accounting only for immune cells, debris, chemoattractant, and later smooth muscle cells (a species not considered here as we are interested only with the earliest onset of cellular aggregation). Such simulations were performed in a two dimensional annular domain, and demonstrated the ability of the model to produce such features as localization of immune cells during inflammation and localized aggregation. The subsequent focus has been on illuminating the interplay of the various parameters by considering the initiation of inflammation as due to an instability in an equilibrium state. The general spatial regime considered is a deformed annulus (in two dimensions) or a deformed annular tube (in three spatial dimensions). In either case, the mathematical domain Ω is intended to represent the tunica intima, the innermost subendothelial layer of an arterial wall. The annulus, or annular tube, has an inner and outer boundary denoted by Γ_I and Γ_O, respectively. The inner boundary Γ_I corresponds to the monolayer of endothelial cells that form the interface between the arterial wall and the lumen, while the boundary Γ_O represents the inner elastic lamina that separates the intima from the media. In the following analyses, we will assume that there is no transport of any species across the boundary Γ_O. While there may well be some transport across this elastic lamina—in particular of free radicals due to metabolic processes within the media—we will assume here that any such contribution is negligible relative to production, consumption, and inter-species reactions within the intima.

Influx through the inner boundary Γ_I is for some species a significant source in the model. In particular, the chemoattractant and native LDL are subject to a third type boundary condition on Γ_I modeling transport in response to a chemical potential across the endothelial cells. This corresponds mathematically to the conditions

$$-\mu_{C_i}\frac{\partial C_i}{\partial \mathbf{n}} = \alpha_{C,i}(C_i - C_*), \quad \text{and} \tag{3.9}$$

$$-\mu_{L_{N_L}}\frac{\partial \mathcal{L}_{N_L}}{\partial \mathbf{n}} = \alpha_L(\mathcal{L}_{N_L} - \mathcal{L}_B). \tag{3.10}$$

Here, $\mathbf{n}$ is the outward unit normal to Γ_I, C_* is a baseline level of chemoattractant present at the endothelium, and $\mathcal{L}_B$ is the serum level of LDL. The parameters $\alpha_{C,i}$ are assumed to be non-negative. However, the sign of α_L is not specified so that (3.10) may correspond with either forward transport of native LDL into the subendothelial intima or reverse transport of native LDL into the blood. We assume here that LDL in the blood stream is fully native (has undergone no free radical attack) so that only native LDL is capable of either forward or reverse transport.

The immune cells are also subject to transport across the endothelium. The mechanism here is a chemo-tactic sensitivity regulated by the level of chemoattractant at the endothelium. The boundary condition is therefore a mixed third type condition with the flux of immune cells dependent on the chemoattractant species.

$$-\mu_{I_i}\frac{\partial \mathcal{I}_i}{\partial \mathbf{n}} = -\alpha_{I,i}(\mathcal{C}). \tag{3.11}$$

Each function $\alpha_{I,i}(\mathcal{C})$, $i = 1,\ldots,N_I$ is a nonnegative monotone function of the vector $\mathcal{C}$ of chemoattractants [4].

The remaining boundary conditions are

$$\frac{\partial Y}{\partial \mathbf{n}} = 0, \quad Y = \mathcal{D}, \mathcal{L}_i, \mathcal{L}_{ox}, \mathcal{R} \quad i = 0,\ldots,N_L - 1, \quad \text{on} \quad \Gamma_I$$

$$\frac{\partial Y}{\partial \mathbf{n}} = 0, \quad Y = \mathcal{I}, \mathcal{C}, \mathcal{D}, \mathcal{L}, \mathcal{L}_{ox}, \mathcal{R} \quad \text{on} \quad \Gamma_O. \tag{3.12}$$

This is the mathematical representation of the previous statement that no transport of any species across the inner elastic lamina separating the intima and the media is considered significant relative to the interactions within the intima, and that only fully native LDL,

---

[4] We can state the boundary condition for the immune cells in the more general form

$$\mathbf{J}_{I_i} \cdot \mathbf{n} = -\tilde{\alpha}_{I,i}(\mathcal{C})$$

where $\mathbf{J}_{I_i} = -\left(\mu_{I_i}\nabla\mathcal{I}_i - \sum_{k=1}^{N_c}\chi_{ik}(\mathcal{C}_k,\mathcal{I}_i)\nabla\mathcal{C}_k\right)$ is the flux field for the ith immune cell species, and $\tilde{\alpha}_{I,i}$ is a corresponding reformulation of the right hand side of (3.11).

immune cells and chemoattractant enter into the system via the endothelial layer. We may further consider the completely homogeneous Neumann conditions under the conditions that $\alpha_{C,i} = \alpha_L = \alpha_{I,i} = 0$. This closed system requires a modification of (3.1) to include a source term. This may be interpreted as modeling the vasa vasorum as the sole source of immune cells contributing to the inflammatory process. In reality, supply both via the vasa vasorum and via transport across the endothelium occur simultaneously. Study of the two extreme cases considered here is done to illuminate both the biological and mathematical differences these two delivery mechanisms make in the modeling and analysis.

4. Mathematical analysis of the model

There are several approaches to analyzing a particular mathematical model including numerical simulations, asymptotic and perturbation methods, and stability analyses. As suggested, the last of these, stability analyses, is particularly applicable under the present circumstances since we do not have experimental data from which to glean relevant ranges for many of the parameters. A classical approach to mathematical models of biological phenomena—especially those characterized by pattern formation, morphogenesis, and aggregation (Keller & Segel, 1971; Murray, 2002; Turing, 1952), is to consider significant state changes as resulting from a mathematical instability. This will result in the criteria based on relative parameter ranges. The inequalities will depend not only on the relationships between parameter ranges, but also on the source of inflammatory factors, and on the size of the domain (intimal thickness).

We present stability analyses of the system (3.1)–(3.8) under some specified conditions. The system considered throughout this section will be simplified to account for one of each of the species types $\mathcal{I}, \mathcal{D}, \mathcal{C}$, one native LDL species (which may be considered an averaging over each of $\mathcal{L}_i$), an oxidized LDL species, and free-radicals. The system of equations is

$$\frac{\partial \mathcal{I}}{\partial t} = \mu_I \nabla^2 \mathcal{I} - \nabla \cdot (\chi(\mathcal{I}, C)\nabla C) - d_1 \mathcal{I} - c\mathcal{I}\mathcal{L}_{ox} - a\mathcal{I}\mathcal{D} + M\phi_0 \tag{4.1}$$

$$\frac{\partial \mathcal{D}}{\partial t} = \mu_D \nabla^2 \mathcal{D} + \hat{c}\mathcal{I}\mathcal{L}_{ox} - \hat{a}\mathcal{I}\mathcal{D} - d_2 \mathcal{D} \tag{4.2}$$

$$\frac{\partial \mathcal{C}}{\partial t} = \mu_C \nabla^2 \mathcal{C} + p\mathcal{D} - e\mathcal{C}\mathcal{I} - d_3 \mathcal{C} \tag{4.3}$$

$$\frac{\partial \mathcal{L}}{\partial t} = \mu_L \nabla^2 \mathcal{L} - k_R \mathcal{L}\mathcal{R} + k_A A_{ox} r \mathcal{L}_{ox} - d_4 \mathcal{L} \tag{4.4}$$

$$\frac{\partial \mathcal{L}_{ox}}{\partial t} = \mu_{L_{ox}} \nabla^2 \mathcal{L}_{ox} + k_{R_0} \mathcal{L}\mathcal{R} - A_{ox} r \mathcal{L}_{ox} - f\mathcal{I}\mathcal{L}_{ox} \tag{4.5}$$

$$\frac{\partial \mathcal{R}}{\partial t} = \mu_R \nabla^2 \mathcal{R} - k_R \mathcal{L}\mathcal{R} - h A_{ox} \mathcal{R} + p_{\mathcal{R}}. \tag{4.6}$$

The modification to (3.1) appearing in (4.1) includes the source term of macrophages via the vasa vasorum as previously indicated (which may be set to zero if appropriate.) Since we are considering only one native LDL species, we also modify the equations to allow for reverse oxidation of oxidized LDL and allow for an efficiency factor r for such reactions. Subscripts have been eliminated where they are no longer needed. For ease of notation $\hat{c} = c + f$.

Our analysis of (4.1)–(4.6) consists of a linear stability analysis using an energy estimate—i.e. Lyapunov functional—approach. That is, we consider certain equilibrium solutions of this system as characterizing a *healthy* state free from certain inflammatory markers. We then ask whether such equilibria are linearly, asymptotically stable.

4.1 Stability with zero transport across the endothelium

We consider a uniform, *healthy* equilibrium solution of (4.1)–(4.6) subject to the boundary conditions (3.9), (3.10), (3.11), and (3.12) in the special case that $\alpha_C = \alpha_L = \alpha_I = 0$. We label this equilibrium solution $(\mathcal{I}_e, \mathcal{D}_e, \mathcal{C}_e, \mathcal{L}_e, \mathcal{L}_{oxe}, \mathcal{R}_e)$, and introduce the perturbation variables u, v, w, z, y, s which are defined by

$$\mathcal{I} = \mathcal{I}_e + u, \quad \mathcal{D} = \mathcal{D}_e + v, \quad \mathcal{C} = \mathcal{C}_e + w,$$

$$\mathcal{L} = \mathcal{L}_e + z, \quad \mathcal{L}_{ox} = \mathcal{L}_{oxe} + y, \quad \text{and} \quad \mathcal{R} = \mathcal{R}_e + s.$$

Substituting the assumed form for $\mathcal{I}$–$\mathcal{R}$ into (4.1)–(4.6) and keeping only terms that are linear in the perturbation variables results in the system of equations

$$\frac{\partial u}{\partial t} = \mu_I \nabla^2 u - \nabla \cdot (\chi \nabla w) - Au - Bu - Cu - Dv - Ey \tag{4.7}$$

$$\frac{\partial v}{\partial t} = \mu_D \nabla^2 v + Fu - Gu - Hv - Iv + Jy \tag{4.8}$$

$$\frac{\partial w}{\partial t} = \mu_C \nabla^2 w - Ku + Lv - Mw - Nw \tag{4.9}$$

$$\frac{\partial z}{\partial t} = \mu_L \nabla^2 z - P_1 z + P_2 y - P_3 s \tag{4.10}$$

$$\frac{\partial y}{\partial t} = \mu_{L_{ox}} \nabla^2 y - Q_1 u + Q_2 z - Q_3 y - Q_4 y + Q_5 s \tag{4.11}$$

$$\frac{\partial s}{\partial t} = \mu_R \nabla^2 s - R_1 z - R_2 s - R_3 s \tag{4.12}$$

with the boundary conditions

$$\frac{\partial u}{\partial n} = \frac{\partial v}{\partial n} = \frac{\partial w}{\partial n} = \frac{\partial z}{\partial n} = \frac{\partial y}{\partial n} = \frac{\partial s}{\partial n} = 0 \quad \text{on} \quad \Gamma_I \cup \Gamma_O. \tag{4.13}$$

The various parameters appearing here are the rates at equilibrium given by

$$A = d_1, \quad B = c\mathcal{L}_{oxe}, \quad C = a\mathcal{D}_e, \quad D = a\mathcal{I}_e, \quad E = c\mathcal{I}_e,$$

$$F = c_{15}\mathcal{L}_{oxe}, \quad G = \hat{a}\mathcal{D}_e, \quad H = \hat{a}\mathcal{I}_e, \quad I = d_2, \quad J = \hat{c}\mathcal{I}_e,$$

$$K = e\mathcal{C}_e, \quad L = p, \quad M = e\mathcal{I}_e, \quad N = d_3, \quad P_1 = k_R\mathcal{R}_e + d_4, \quad P_2 = k_A A_{ox} r,$$

$$P_3 = k_R \mathcal{L}_e, \quad Q_1 = f\mathcal{L}_{oxe}, \quad Q_2 = k_{R_0}\mathcal{R}_e, \quad Q_3 = A_{ox} r, \quad Q_4 = f\mathcal{I}_e,$$

$$Q_5 = k_{R_0}\mathcal{L}_e, \quad R_1 = k_R\mathcal{R}_e, \quad R_2 = k_R\mathcal{L}_e, \quad R_3 = hA_{ox},$$

and $\chi = \chi(\mathcal{I}_e, \mathcal{C}_e)$. Each of these constants is assumed to be nonnegative, and due to balance of mass $F = B + Q_1$, $J = E + Q_4$, $Q_2 = (P_1 - d_4) + R_1$, and $Q_5 = P_3 + R_2$. Let $\mathbf{U} = (u, v, w, z, y, s)$. Before proceeding, we define stability in the following way:

Definition 4.1. *The equilibrium state is called asymptotically stable if every solution of the linearized initial boundary value problem (4.7)–(4.13) for the perturbation variables vanishes at infinity in the sense that there exists a positive functional*

$$\mathcal{F}(\mathbf{U}) = \Phi(t) \quad \text{such that} \quad \lim_{t \to \infty} \Phi(t) = 0.$$

Our study of (4.7)–(4.13) requires the construction of an appropriate functional $\mathcal{F}$, and this construction gives rise to the inequalities involving the parameters including intimal thickness. In the interest of brevity, much of the computational details are omitted here. The main results are stated with a discussion.

We begin by assuming that the product terms uv and uw are nonnegative within Ω. Physically, this can be interpreted as saying that an increase in debris ($v > 0$) and an increase in chemoattractant ($w > 0$) results in an increase in immune cells ($u > 0$). Likewise a decrease in debris and chemoattractant ($v < 0$, $w < 0$) is met with a decrease in immune cells ($u < 0$). This is a rather minor and biologically reasonable condition. However it can be dropped, and a weaker stability theorem obtained (Ibragimov et al., 2010a).

The transition matrix characterizing the species interactions associated with the system (4.7)–(4.12) is

$$\Lambda = \begin{bmatrix} -(A+B+C) & -D & 0 & 0 & -E & 0 \\ F-G & -(H+I) & 0 & 0 & J & 0 \\ -K & L & -(M+N) & 0 & 0 & 0 \\ 0 & 0 & 0 & -P_1 & P_2 & -P_3 \\ Q_1 & 0 & 0 & Q_2 & -(Q_3+Q_4) & Q_5 \\ 0 & 0 & 0 & -R_1 & 0 & -(R_2+R_3) \end{bmatrix}$$

We will assume that the eigenvalues of Λ have negative real part. (The implication of this and other imposed conditions will be discussed later.) In the following construction, this ensures that integrals of the form $\int_\Omega U_i \to 0$ as $t \to \infty$ for $U_i = u, v, w, z, y$, or s. This follows from Green's theorem and the homogeneous Neumann boundary conditions. This constraint does not guarantee stability of the system or even point-wise boundedness of each U_i. We will also assume here that $\mu_D = 0$ which is consistent with the immobile nature of the lesion core.

A sequence of inequalities is obtained by multiplying (4.7) by u (4.8) by v, and so forth and integrating over the domain Ω to secure bounds on the rate of change of the total energy of the perturbations. In so doing, we introduce consideration of the geometry and size of the domain through use of the Poincaré inequality

$$\text{(Poincaré)} \quad \int_\Omega u^2 \le \frac{1}{|\Omega|} \left(\int_\Omega u \right)^2 + C_p \int_\Omega |\nabla u|^2.$$

Here, $|\Omega|$ is the volume of the domain, and the parameter C_p is dependent on the geometry of the domain [5].

For ease of notation, we set

$$A_1 = A + B + C, \quad G_1 = G - F, \quad H_1 = H + I, \quad \text{and} \quad M_1 = M + N.$$

And in addition to the condition imposed upon the matrix Λ, suppose that

[Condition 4.1.1] $E < 1$, [Condition 4.1.2] $\dfrac{\chi L}{2\mu_C} < \dfrac{1}{4}$, [Condition 4.1.3] $\dfrac{\chi K}{2M_1\mu_C} < \dfrac{1}{8}$,

[Condition 4.1.4] $L < 1$, [Condition 4.1.5] $G_1 > 0$, and [Condition 4.1.6] $J < 1$.

---

[5] When an L^2 norm is considered, C_p is related to the inverse of the first positive eigenfrequency of a free membrane (Acosta & Durán, 2003).

Following a systematic construction of integral inequalities from the equations (4.7)–(4.12) we arrive at the principal inequality essential to the present analysis.

$$\frac{d}{dt}\int_\Omega\left[\left(\frac{1}{2}+\frac{\chi K}{2\mu_C D}+\frac{A_1}{2C}\right)u^2+\left(\frac{1}{2}+\frac{H_1}{2G_1}\right)v^2+\left(\frac{1}{2}+\frac{\chi M_1^2}{2K\mu_C D}\right)w^2\right.$$

$$+\frac{1}{2}z^2+\frac{1}{2}y^2+\frac{1}{2}s^2+(uv)+\frac{\chi M_1}{\mu_C D}(uw)+\frac{\mu_I}{2D}|\nabla u|^2+\left.\frac{\chi M_1}{2KD}|\nabla w|^2\right]\le$$

$$-\int_\Omega\left[C_u u^2+C_v v^2+C_w w^2+C_z z^2+C_y y^2+C_s s^2+\right.$$

$$\left. C_{uv}(uv)+C_{uw}(uw)+C_{\nabla u}|\nabla u|^2+C_{\nabla w}|\nabla w|^2\right]. \tag{4.14}$$

The coefficients on the right hand side of the inequality (4.14) are

$$\begin{aligned}
C_u &= A_1+\frac{C_p}{2}\left(\mu_I-\frac{\chi}{2}\right)-\frac{D+E+Q_1}{2}, &\qquad C_s &= R_2+R_3+\mu_R C_p-\frac{P_3+Q_5+R_1}{2},\\
C_v &= H_1-\frac{D+J+L}{2}-\frac{\chi L}{2\mu_C D}-\frac{\chi M_1 L}{2K\mu_C D}, &\qquad C_{uv} &= G_1,\\
C_w &= M_1+\frac{C_p}{2}\left(\mu_C-\frac{\chi}{2}\right)-\frac{L}{2}, &\qquad C_{uw} &= K,\\
C_z &= P_1+\mu_L C_p-\frac{P_2+P_3+Q_2+R_1}{2}, &\qquad C_{\nabla u} &= \frac{1}{2}\left(\mu_I-\frac{\chi}{2}\right),\\
C_y &= Q_3+Q_4+\mu_{Lox} C_p-\frac{P_2+Q_1+Q_2+Q_5+E+J}{2}-\frac{E}{2D}-\frac{J}{2G_1}, &\qquad C_{\nabla w} &= \frac{1}{2}\left(\mu_C-\frac{\chi}{2}\right).
\end{aligned}$$

$$\tag{4.15}$$

We are now able to state our first major result.

Theorem 4.1. *The equilibrium solution $(\mathcal{I}_e,\mathcal{D}_e,\mathcal{C}_e,\mathcal{L}_e,\mathcal{L}_{oxe},\mathcal{R}_e)$ of (4.1)–(4.6) subject to the homogeneous Neumann boundary conditions is asymptotically stable provided*

(i) $\int_\Omega uv>0$ and $\int_\Omega uw>0$

(ii) all eigenvalues of Λ have negative real part,

(iii) Conditions 4.1.1–4.1.6 hold, and

(iv) $M=min\{C_u,C_v,C_w,C_z,C_y,C_s,C_{uv},C_{uw},C_{\nabla u},C_{\nabla w}\}>0$

The proof requires a definition of the functional as the obvious modification of the left hand side of (4.14). Of interest are the physical interpretations of the sufficiency conditions stated here. The meaning of the conditions on the products uv and uw has already been given. It can also be noted that each of the coefficients appearing in the array (4.15) is written as a positive term minus a non-negative term to highlight the relationships necessary between the parameters to guarantee stability.

The condition on the matrix Λ—that its eigenvalues have negative real part—has distinct bio-medical interpretation. Parameters E, J, and Q_1 are the rates of foam cell production by binding of macrophages to oxidized LDL. If these are large, then they are a source to the lesion. If each of these is small (conditions 4.1.1 and 4.1.6), then to leading order Λ is block diagonal. The parameters Q_2 and R_1 are the oxidation rates of LDL. If $Q_2<<1$ and $R_1<<1$–so that $C_z,C_s>0$, then the eigenvalues of the lower 3×3 block has negative eigenvalues $-P_1$, $-(Q_3+Q_4)$, and $-(R_2+R_3)$. A healthy system would be dominated by the antioxidant reactions which correspond to large values of P_1,Q_3,Q_4,R_2, and R_3. If in addition $L<<1$ (condition 4.1.4), then the production of chemoattractant due to the presence of the lesion is small, and the eigenvalues of the upper 3×3 block are to leading order

$$-M_1,\quad -\frac{1}{2}(H_1+A_1)\pm\sqrt{(H_1+A_1)^2-4(A_1 H_1-DG_1)}.$$

Large M_1 indicates a fast degradation of chemoattractant and sufficient uptake of chemokines by macrophages to minimize immune cell migration (reduce inflammation.) The parameters D and G_1 are large (condition 4.1.5) when the uncorrupted, healthy immune function dominates through normal phagocytosis of lesion debris. Similarly, large values for A_1 (due to dependence on A and C) and large H_1 correspond to degradation of the lesion and clearing by macrophages. The sufficient condition for stability is the inequality

$$\sqrt{(H_1 - A_1)^2 + 4DG_1} < H_1 + A_1.$$

Several of the requirements for stability rest on the interplay between chemotactic effects and diffusion/motility. This is typical of systems characterized by chemotaxis. Conditions 4.1.2 and 4.1.3 as well as the positivity of each parameter in the array (4.15) provide a minimal requirement of the diffusivity of the intimal layer and the motility of macrophages—motility unrelated to chemotaxis—to guarantee that a perturbation off of the healthy equilibrium state decays.

4.2 Stability with transport of macrophages and LDL across the endothelium

We again consider the simplified system (4.1)–(4.6) and perturb off of a healthy equilibrium solutions $(\mathcal{I}_e, \ldots, \mathcal{R}_e)$. However, we consider the boundary conditions (3.9), (3.10), (3.11), and (3.12) with $\alpha_C > 0$, $\alpha_L \neq 0$, and the form of α_I appearing in (3.11) as

$$\alpha_I(\mathcal{C}) = \alpha_I^0(\mathcal{C} - \mathcal{C}_*) \tag{4.16}$$

where $\mathcal{C}_*$ is a base line serum level of chemoattractant and α_I^0 is a positive constant. If the level of chemotaxis inducing agents at the endothelial interface is greater than an average level in the blood stream, then macrophages (or monocytes which differentiate) will enter into the subendothelial intima.

The perturbation variables, $u, \ldots, s$ are defined in the same manner as in 4.1, and the linearized system (4.7)–(4.12) is again studied. However, the boundary conditions on Γ_I for the variables u, w, and z (corresponding to immune cells, chemoattractant, and native LDL, respectively) in the present analysis are nonhomogeneous and must be derived from (3.9), (3.10), and (3.11). It should be noted that the existence of a spatially uniform equilibrium requires

$$\mathcal{C}_e = \mathcal{C}_* \quad \text{and} \quad \mathcal{L}_e = \mathcal{L}_B$$

with $\mathcal{C}_*$ and $\mathcal{L}_B$ the serum levels of chemoattractant and native LDL introduced in section 3.2. From (3.11)

$$\mu_I \frac{\partial(\mathcal{I}_e + u)}{\partial \mathbf{n}} = \alpha_I^0(\mathcal{C}_e + w - \mathcal{C}_*) \quad \text{so that} \quad \mu_I \frac{\partial u}{\partial \mathbf{n}} = \alpha_I^0 w. \tag{4.17}$$

Similarly

$$\mu_C \frac{\partial w}{\partial \mathbf{n}} = -\alpha_C w, \quad \text{and} \quad \mu_L \frac{dz}{d\mathbf{n}} = -\alpha_L z \quad \text{on } \Gamma_I. \tag{4.18}$$

The additional boundary conditions on both Γ_I and on Γ_O remain as in section 4.1.

The approach applied previously must be modified here to account for the effect of the boundary terms on the total energy of each perturbation variable. In addition to the Poincaré inequality, we require the well known Sobolev trace and generalized Friedrich's inequalities

$$\text{(Sobolev Trace)} \quad \int_{\partial\Omega} u^2 \, ds \leq C_1 \left(\int_\Omega u^2 + |\nabla u|^2 \right) dx, \quad \text{and}$$

(Generalized Friedrich) $C_2 \int_\Omega u^2 \, dx \leq \int_\Omega |\nabla u|^2 \, dx + C_3 \int_{\partial\Omega} u^2 \, ds.$

We note that these inequalities also depend on the geometry of the domain through the constants C_1, C_2, and C_3. The consideration of best estimates for these constants has received much attention (Acosta & Durán, 2003; Mazya, 1985). For the tubular domain considered herein, the present authors provide estimates of the constants appearing in each of these inequalities (including the Poincaré inequality) in (Ibragimov et al., 2010b).

The procedure is similar to that used in 4.1, and we obtain a set of inequalities relating the parameters of the system that provide sufficient conditions under which the perturbations will decay. Again, much of the computational details are omitted (the interested reader is referred to (Ibragimov et al., 2010a) and to (Ibragimov et al., 2008; 2010b) for similar results). Instead, we highlight a number of inequalities in light of the bio-medical significance and state the primary result.

To facilitate the analysis, we assume that the decrease of oxidized LDL due to attempted phagocytosis by macrophages is negligible compared the increase and decreases resulting from the chemical reactions with free-radical and antioxidant species. (This is to say that uptake by macrophages is a minor effect on the oxidized LDL concentration, not that foam cell formation is negligible especially as it relates to debris growth or decay.) This is equivalent to the previous case where Q_1 is small and corresponds to $f = 0$ so that $c = \hat{c}$, $Q_1 = Q_4 = 0$. Here, we no longer consider the transition matrix because we cannot impose any physically reasonable constraints to guarantee that the integrals $\left(\int_\Omega y\right)^2$ and $\left(\int_\Omega s\right)^2$ can be ignored throughout the construction. (The terms $\frac{1}{|\Omega|} \int_\Omega y$ and $\frac{1}{|\Omega|} \int_\Omega s$ are the average values of the total perturbations of oxidized LDL and free radicals, respectively, over the entire domain.) Instead, these are treated in the same manner as each of the perturbation variables.

The competing effects of diffusion (cellular motility) and chemotaxis are prominent in the result in section 4.1, and the same is true when considering boundary transport. In the present case, however, the sufficient conditions require the diffusion to overcome both chemotaxis within the intima as well as that across the endothelial layer. In particular, stability will rest on the conditions

[Condition 4.2.1] $\mu_I - C_1 \left(\alpha_I^0 + \frac{\chi \alpha_C}{\mu_C} \right) - \frac{\chi}{2} \equiv \bar{\mu}_I \geq 0$

and

[Condition 4.2.2] $\mu_C - \frac{\chi}{2} \equiv \bar{\mu}_C > 0.$

The latter condition arose in the previous result, however the former relates the impact of chemotaxis at the boundary through the parameters α_I^0 and α_C on the net motility of macrophages within the intima. A direct comparison with $C_{\nabla u}$ appearing in (4.15) reveals the additional requirement on this motility to overcome chemotactic effects when boundary transport is accounted for.

The diffusion and degradation of chemoattractant are also required to significantly increased in this case. Set $C(\bar{\alpha}, \bar{\mu}_C) = \min(\frac{\bar{\alpha}}{C_3}, \bar{\mu}_C)$ where

$$\bar{\alpha} = \alpha_C \left[1 - \frac{1}{2} \left(\frac{\alpha_I^0}{\alpha_C} + \frac{\chi}{\mu_C} \right) \right].$$

(C_3 is the constant from the Friedrich inequality.) The function $C(\bar{\alpha}, \bar{\mu}_C)$ is nondecreasing in $\bar{\alpha}$ and $\bar{\mu}_C$ independently, and will increase if both of these increase. The condition $C_w > 0$ in theorem 1 will be replaced by

$$M_1 + C(\bar{\alpha}, \bar{\mu}_C)C_2 - \frac{L}{2} > 0.$$

Recall that M_1 is the rate at which the chemoattractant is reduced within the intima due to natural degradation and through uptake by macrophages during chemotaxis. The added source of chemoattractant from the endothelial boundary is reflected in the new requirement on the size of this parameter.

Of particular interest are the two cases of LDL transport—forward and reverse—that can be admitted by allowing α_L to be either positive or negative. When $\alpha_L < 0$, LDL enters into the intima through the endothelial layer. Stability in this case will require

[Condition 4.2.3(-)] $\mu_L > |\alpha_L|$ and $P_1 - |\alpha_L|C_1 - \dfrac{P_2 + P_3 + R_1 + Q_2}{2} - \dfrac{(R_1 + Q_2)|\Omega|}{2} > 0.$

The second in condition 4.2.3(-) gives a specific requirement on the removal rate of LDL (P_1), especially due to chemical degradation, relative to influx across the endothelial layer (α_L), the oxidation kinetics within the intima ($\frac{P_2+P_3+R_1+Q_2}{2}$), and the size of the intima ($|\Omega|$). This particular inequality indicates that intimal thickening is destabilizing mathematically. The role of diffuse intimal thickening (DIT) as a precursor to, and in the early stages of, atherosclerosis has been the subject of a number of studies (Nakashima et al., 2008). Those arteries that are prone to atherosclerotic lesions such as the abdominal aorta, carotid, and coronary arteries are observed to express DIT whereas arteries known to be resistant to atherosclerosis do not (Nakashima et al., 2002). Accumulation of oxidized LDL relative to native LDL in the deep region of DIT in human coronary arteries has been observed (Fukuchi et al., 2002).

The stability requirement on the degradation of LDL in the case of reverse transport is significantly weaker provided the rate of diffusion of LDL and the rate at which LDL leaves the intima through the endothelial boundary are sufficiently high. Let

$$\phi_0 = \frac{P_2 + P_3 + R_1 + Q_2 + (R_1 + Q_2)|\Omega|}{2}.$$

Then ϕ_0 is a measure of the total oxidation rate of LDL and depends on the thickness of the intima. If LDL is transported from the intima back to the blood stream, then stability will require

[Condition 4.2.3(+)] $\mu_L > \phi_0/C_2,$ $\alpha_L > \phi_0 C_3/C_2,$ and $P_1 > 0,$ if $\alpha_L > 0.$

If conditions 4.2.1, 4.2.2, and the appropriate version of 4.2.3 (- or +) hold, and we follow the techniques used in section 4.1, we obtain our primary inequality

$$\frac{1}{2}\frac{d}{dt}\int_\Omega \left[u^2 + v^2 + w^2 + z^2 + y^2 + s^2\right] + \frac{1}{2}\frac{d}{dt}\left[\left(\int_\Omega y\right)^2 + \left(\int_\Omega s\right)^2\right] \le$$

$$-\left[C_u \int_\Omega u^2 + C_v \int_\Omega v^2 + C_w \int_\Omega w^2 + C_z \int_\Omega z^2 + C_y \int_\Omega y^2 + C_s \int_\Omega s^2\right.$$

$$+ (D + G_1)\int_\Omega uv + E\int_\Omega uy + K\int_\Omega uw + C_{\int y}\left(\int_\Omega y\right)^2 + C_{\int s}\left(\int_\Omega s\right)^2\bigg]. \qquad (4.19)$$

The coefficients appearing on the right hand side are defined by

$$
\begin{aligned}
C_u &= A_1 - \tfrac{C_1}{2}\left(\alpha_I^0 + \tfrac{\chi\alpha_C}{\mu_C}\right), & C_s &= \tfrac{\mu_R}{C_p} + R_2 + R_3 - \tfrac{P_3 + R_1 + Q_5}{2}, \\
C_v &= H_1 - \tfrac{I+L}{2}, & C_{fy} &= Q_3 - \tfrac{Q_2 + Q_5}{2}, \\
C_w &= M_1 + C(\bar\alpha, \bar\mu_C)C - \tfrac{L}{2}, & C_{fs} &= R_2 + R_3 - \tfrac{R_1 + Q_5}{2}, \\
C_y &= \tfrac{\mu_{Lox}}{C_p} + Q_3 - \tfrac{I + P_2 + Q_2 + Q_5}{2},
\end{aligned}
\tag{4.20}
$$

and

$$
C_z = \begin{cases}
P_1, & \alpha_L > 0 \\
P_1 - |\alpha_L|C_1 - \tfrac{P_2 + P_3 + R_1 + Q_2}{2} - \tfrac{(R_1 + Q_2)|\Omega|}{2}, & \alpha_L < 0.
\end{cases}
$$

Provided

$$[\text{Condition 4.2.4}] \quad \min\{C_u, C_v, C_w, C_z, C_y, C_s, C_{fy}, C_{fs}\} > 0,$$

we define the parameters

$$
\beta_u = \sqrt{\tfrac{1}{3}C_u}, \quad \beta_v = \sqrt{C_v}, \quad \beta_w = \sqrt{C_w}, \quad \text{and} \quad \beta_y = \sqrt{C_y}.
$$

The primary result of the current anaylsis is

Theorem 4.2. *The equilibrium solution* $(\mathcal{I}_e, \mathcal{D}_e, \mathcal{C}_e, \mathcal{L}_e, \mathcal{L}_{oxe}, \mathcal{R}_e)$ *of (4.1)–(4.6) subject to the nonhomogeneous Neumann boundary conditions (3.9), (3.10), (3.11) and (4.16) is asymptotically stable provided conditions 4.2.1–4.2.4 hold and*

$$\beta_u \beta_v \geq D + G_1, \quad \beta_u \beta_w \geq K, \quad \text{and} \quad \beta_u \beta_y \geq E.$$

The proof involves the pair of functionals

$$
\mathcal{F}_1(\mathbf{V}) = \left(\sum_{i=1}^{6} \int_\Omega V_i^2\right) + V_7^2 + V_8^2,
$$

and

$$
\mathcal{F}_2(\mathbf{V}) = \int_\Omega \tfrac{1}{2}(\beta_u u + \beta_v v)^2 + \tfrac{1}{2}(\beta_u u + \beta_w w)^2 + \tfrac{1}{2}(\beta_u u + \beta_y y)^2 +
$$

$$
+ M\left[\int_\Omega (z^2 + s^2) + \left(\int_\Omega y\right)^2 + \left(\int_\Omega s\right)^2\right]
$$

where $\mathbf{V} = (u, v, w, z, y, s, \int_\Omega y, \int_\Omega s)$ and $M = \min\{C_z, C_s, C_{fy}, C_{fs}\}$. The hypotheses of theorem 4.2 ensure

$$\frac{d}{dt}\mathcal{F}_1(\mathbf{V}) \leq -\mathcal{F}_2(\mathbf{V})$$

establishing asymptotic stability for this case.

4.3 Instability of the equilibrium solution

The theorems obtained in sections 4.1 and 4.2 establish sufficient conditions under which the uniform healthy state is guaranteed to be stable to small perturbations. It is not readily clear whether the inequalities derived are tight—in the sense that they are *nearly* necessary conditions. One can ask the degree to which these conditions must be violated to result in the existence of a perturbation that will blow up.

The existence of perturbations that blow up, in particular spatially nonhomogeneous perturbations, is typically addressed through construction of an explicit example. The classical approach is adopt the ansatz for the perturbation variables

$$u(\mathbf{x}, t) = e^{\sigma t} \bar{u}(\mathbf{x}), \quad v(\mathbf{x}, t) = e^{\sigma t} \bar{v}(\mathbf{x}), \quad \dots, \quad s(\mathbf{x}, t) = e^{\sigma t} \bar{s}(\mathbf{x}). \tag{4.21}$$

Expressing the perturbation as $\mathbf{U}$ as in definition 4.1, this gives $\mathbf{U}(\mathbf{x}, t) = e^{\sigma t} \bar{\mathbf{U}}(\mathbf{x})$, and the system (4.7)–(4.12) can be written in the vector/matrix formulation as

$$\sigma \bar{\mathbf{U}} = \nabla \cdot (\mathbf{M}_e \nabla \bar{\mathbf{U}}) + \Lambda \bar{\mathbf{U}}. \tag{4.22}$$

The diffusion-chemotaxis coefficient matrix $\mathbf{M}_e$ has the diffusion coefficients on the main diagonal, $\chi(\mathcal{I}_e, \mathcal{C}_e)$ in the first row and third column, and zeroes everywhere else. When considering the case without boundary transport, using the fact that $\mathbf{M}_e$ and Λ are constant matrices, the ansatz can be further refined to seek solutions of the form

$$\bar{\mathbf{U}} = \phi_\lambda(\mathbf{x}) \vec{\xi}.$$

Here $\vec{\xi}$ is a constant vector and ϕ_λ an eigenfunction of the Laplacian on Ω,

$$-\nabla^2 \phi_\lambda = \lambda \phi_\lambda,$$

subject to the completely homogeneous Neumann boundary conditions (4.13). The system (4.7)–(4.12) reduces to the algebraic equation in σ, λ, and $\vec{\xi}$

$$\sigma \vec{\xi} = (\Lambda - \lambda \mathbf{M}_e) \vec{\xi}. \tag{4.23}$$

Solutions to (4.23) for which the real part of σ is positive will grow; this is the classic Turing instability problem (Turing, 1952). For the Turing stability problem, one considers the case for which Λ has only negative eigenvalues and $\mathbf{M}_e^s$, the symmetric part of $\mathbf{M}_e$, has only positive eigenvalues. (This latter condition will hold if and only if $\chi(\mathcal{I}_e, \mathcal{C}_e) < 2\sqrt{\mu_I \mu_C}$, and this inequality follows from the conditions $C_{\nabla u} > 0$ and $C_{\nabla w} > 0$ appearing in theorem 4.1.) For any domain Ω, the first eigenpair is $\lambda_0 = 0$ and $\phi_0 = constant$, and it is well known that there is an enumerable set of positive eigenvalues $0 < \lambda_1 < \lambda_2 < \cdots$ and corresponding eigenfunctions $\{\phi_{\lambda_n}\}$ that form an orthonormal basis for $L^2(\Omega)$. In the case that Λ has only negative eigenvalues, an instability must come from one of the larger eigenvalues. Unfortunately, finding these eigenvalues explicitly for a general domain is not possible. For an annulus ($\mathbb{R}^2$), or an annular cylinder ($\mathbb{R}^3$), they can be found by separation of variables. The corresponding eigenmodes in these cases are nonaxisymmetric suggesting that lesion initiation should also be nonaxisymmetric—this is consistent with clinical observations.

For the present case with no transport of any species across the endothelial layer, we can study the effect of the antioxidant level on the stability of the healthy state. If $M\phi_0$ in equation (4.1) is replaced with $M\phi_0 C$ (to make the source explicitly dependent on the chemoattractant), or if $M\phi_0 = 0$, then the equilibrium solution is $(\mathcal{I}_e, \mathcal{D}_e, \mathcal{C}_e, \mathcal{L}_e, \mathcal{L}_{oxe}, \mathcal{R}_e) = (0, 0, 0, \mathcal{L}_e, \mathcal{L}_{oxe}, \mathcal{R}_e)$.

We can, after some lengthy calculations, show that in the limiting cases as $A_{ox} \to 0^+$ and $A_{ox} \to \infty$ (Ibragimov et al., 2010b)

$$\mathcal{L}_{oxe} \propto A_{ox}^{-1}, \quad \text{and} \quad \mathcal{R}_e \propto p_R, \quad \text{as} \quad A_{ox} \to 0^+$$

and

$$\mathcal{L}_{oxe} \propto A_{ox}^{-2}, \quad \text{and} \quad \mathcal{R}_e \propto A_{ox}^{-1}, \quad \text{as} \quad A_{ox} \to \infty.$$

The latter result demonstrates that the antioxidants strongly control free radical production and LDL oxidation. When studying the spectrum of $\Lambda - \lambda \mathbf{M}_e$, this asymptotic result shows that for A_{ox} sufficiently large, the lower 3×3 block corresponding to the lipid chemistry produces no eigenvalues with positive real part. The question of most interest is what conditions are required for stability (or produce an instability) for the full system in the case that the lipid chemistry alone is stable. If $(\mathcal{L}_e, \mathcal{L}_{oxe}, \mathcal{R}_e)$ is a stable equilibrium for the lipid equations in isolation, what effect does the antioxidant level have on the stability of the equilibrium $(0, 0, 0, \mathcal{L}_e, \mathcal{L}_{oxe}, \mathcal{R}_e)$? In the limit as the antioxidant level vanishes, the equilibrium will be unstable whenever

$$(\lambda \mu_D + d_2)(\lambda \mu_C + d_3) < (\lambda \chi(0,0) - M\phi_0) \left(\frac{\hat{c}p}{c} \right). \tag{4.24}$$

The critical and competing roles of diffusion and chemotaxis are prominent in this criterion providing an unstable equilibrium. For any positive eigenvalue λ and diffusive capacity of the chemoattractant μ_C, if the chemotactic sensitivity $\chi(0,0)$ is large enough, the perturbation will grow away from the healthy equilibrium to some other state.

An analysis like the above can be employed with any variation of the system (3.1)–(3.8) provided the boundary conditions considered are completely homogeneous of Neumann type. For example, in (Ibragimov et al., 2008) the present authors consider a system characterized by two distinct macrophage phenotypes each subject to diffusion, chemotaxis, the potential to change phenotypes, but for which only one subspecies was subject to foam cell formation. We showed that the stability result provided therein—that analogous to theorem 4.1 here—was strongly dependent on the dominance of diffusion over chemotaxis. As is seen here, for any set of other parameter values, the chemotactic sensitivity coefficient can always be taken sufficiently large to produce an unstable equilibrium.

The question of unstable equilibria for the case with boundary transport can likewise be considered. Not surprisingly this presents a far more complicated situation mathematically. Even if we only consider constant equilibria, the special approach based on the ansatz (4.21) and the spectral analysis above does not yield any instability examples. Moreover, the coupled boundary conditions provide a Laplacian that is not self-adjoint and does not allow us the option to expand all of the perturbation variables using any single family of eigenfunctions. Nevertheless, a careful construction within the appropriate mathematical framework will provide conditions for which an unstable equilibrium exists. The effect of antioxidant concentration on stability can be analyzed. The reader is encouraged to see (Ibragimov et al., 2010b) for a construction in this case.

5. Conclusion

The purpose of this work is twofold. We have formulated a mathematical model of the inflammatory process that characterizes atherogenesis. This model given in equations (3.1)–(3.8) is presented in general terms to provide a framework for the ongoing modeling process. With this in mind, adaptations are easily included as our understanding of this complex medical process increases. We believe that mathematical modeling provides a useful tool to meet the goals of medical research on atherogenesis—identifying vulnerability to disease, development of treatments, and promotion of preventative interventions. Computer simulation (*in silico* analysis) requires a model consistent with and able to capture the characteristics of disease as observed *in vivo*.

Here, we have also studied the model by performing stability analyses under two different assumptions regarding the supply of inflammatory components—macrophages, chemotactic chemokines, and LDL. Taking the vasa vasorum as the sole source of these species, we arrive at a distinct set of inequality conditions on the system parameters that will guarantee that perturbations off of the healthy equilibrium state will decay. Bio-medically, the perturbations are interpreted as the start of inflammation, and the starting equilibrium as a disease-free state. A stable equilibrium is then seen as representing a cellular configuration that is robust—where a lesion is unlikely to develop in the short term. An unstable one suggests that (bio-chemically) the location is vulnerable to atherogenesis and the potential for development of a fibrofatty lesion or latter fibrous plaque. In addition to the positive stability criteria obtained using the energy estimate, we offer a negative result in the form of construction of an instability example. This latter condition highlights the inflammation mitigating effects of antioxidant presence and the significant interplay between chemotaxis and diffusion when the antioxidant level becomes negligible.

We also raise this same stability question under the assumption that the supply of inflammatory components is from influx from the blood flow via the endothelial interface. We again produce several inequalities that when satisfied by the system parameters ensure that the equilibrium solution is linearly asymptotically stable to small perturbations. Of particular interest in this latter case is the stabilizing effect of reverse transport of native LDL from the intima back to the blood stream. That reverse transport of LDL is stabilizing is not surprising given the corruptive nature of oxidized LDL on macrophage function. Our finding further supports the development of treatment modalities aimed at not only reducing serum LDL levels but at facilitating reverse transport of cholesterol (Superko, 2006). Although the conditions are numerous, clinical values of the various parameters can be easily compared in light of the various inequalities derived and presented in theorems 4.1 and 4.2.

The availability of clinical values for several parameters is lacking. Moreover, the parameters appearing in table 1 need not be constant, and determination of appropriate functional forms is an important and difficult task. This will require a process of "fine tuning" through collaboration with clinicians and experimental scientists.

6. References

Acosta G. & Durán, R. G. (2003). An optimal Poincaré inequality in L^1 for convex domains, *Proc. Am. Math. Soc.* 132(1): 195–202.

Baek, S., Gleason, R. L., Rajagopal, K. R., & Humphrey, J. D. (2007). Theory of small on large: Potential utility in computations of fluidâĂŞsolid interactions in arteries *Comput. Methods Appl. Mech. Engrg.* 196(31-32): 3070–3078

Boullier, A., Bird, D. A., Chang, M., Dennis, E. A., Friedman, P., Gillotte-Taylor, K., Hörkkö, S., Palinski, W., Quehenberger, O., Shaw, P., Steinberg, D., Terpstra, V., & Witztum, J. L. (2001). Scavenger receptors, oxidized LDL, and atherosclerosis, *Ann. N. Y. Acad. Sci.* 947: 214–223

Cobbold, C. A., Sherratt, J. A., & Maxwell, S. J. R. (2002). Lipoprotein oxidation and its significance for atherosclerosis: a mathematical approach, *Bull. Math. Biol.* 64: 65–95.

M. A. Creager, M. A. & Braunwald, E. eds. (2003). *Atlas of Vascular Disease,* Current Medicine, Inc. 2nd edition

Cui, D., Thorp, E., Li, Y., Wang, N., Yvan-Charvet, L., Tall, A. R., & Tabas, I. (2007). Pivital advance: Macrophages become resistant to cholesterol-induced death after phagocytosis of apoptotic cells, *J. Leuk.Bio.* 82: 1040–1050

Davignon, J. & Ganz, P. (2004). Role of endothelial dysfunction in atherosclerosis, *Circulation* 109(3 supplement 1): 27–32

Esterbauer, H., Gebicki, J., Puhl, H. & Jurgens, G. (1992). Review Article: The role of lipid peroxidation and antioxidants in oxidative modification of LDL, *Free Radic. Biol. Med.* 13: 341–390

Fan, J., & Watanabe, T. (2003). Inflammatory reactions in the pathogenesis of atherosclerosis, *JAT* 10(2): 63–71.

Fukuchi, M., Watanabe, J., Kumagai, K., Baba, S., Shinozaki, T., Miura, M., Kagaya, Y. & Shirato, K. (2002). Normal and oxidized low density lipoproteins accumulate deep in physiologically thickened intima of human coronary arteries, *Lab Invest* 82(10): 1437–1447

Goldstein, J. L., Ho, Y. K., Basu, S. K. & Brown, M. S. (1977). Binding site on macrophages that mediates uptake and degradation of acetylated low density lipoproteins, producing massive cholesterol deposition, *Proc. Natl. Acad. Sci. USA* 76: 333–337

Hajjar, D. P. & Haberland, M. E. (1997). Lipoprotein trafficking in vascular cells; Molecular trojan horses and cellular saboteurs, *J. Bio. Chem.* 272: 22975–22978.

Holzapfel, G. A., Gasser, T. C. & R. W. Ogden, R. W. (2000). A new constitutive framework for arterial wall mechanics and a comparative study of material models, *J. Elast.* 61: 1–48

Humphery, J. D. & Rajagopal, K. R. (2002). A constrained mixture model for growth and remodeling of soft tissues, *Math. Models Methods Appl. Sci.* 12: 407–430.

Ibragimov, A. I., McNeal, C. J., Ritter, L. R. & Walton, J. R. (2005). A mathematical model of atherogenesis as an inflammatory response, *Math. Med. and Biol.* 22: 305–333

Ibragimov, A. I., McNeal, C. J., Ritter, L. R. & Walton, J. R. (2008). Stability analysis of a model of atherogenesis: An energy estimate approach, *J. of Comp. and Math. Meth. in Med.* 9(2): 121–142

Ibragimov, A. I., McNeal, C. J., Ritter, L. R. & Walton, J. R. (2010). Stability analysis of a model of atherogenesis: An energy estimate approach ii, *J. of Comp. and Math. Meth. in Med.* 11(1): 67–88

Ibragimov, A. I., Ritter, L. R. & Walton, J. R. (2010). Stability analysis of a reaction-diffusion system modeling atherogenesis, *SIAM J. Appl. Math.* 70(7): 2150–2185

Kadl, A., Meher, A. K., Sharma, P. R., Lee, M. Y., Doran, A. C., Johnstone, S. R., Elliott, M. R., Gruber, F., Han, J., Chen, W., Kensler, T., Ravichandran, K. S., Isakson, B. E., Wamhoff, B. R. & Leitinger, N. (2010). Identification of a novel macrophage phenotype that develops in response to atherogenic phospholipids via Nrf2, *Circ. Res.* 107(6): 737–746

Keller, E. F. & Segel, L. A. (1971). Model for chemotaxis, *J. Theor. Biol.* 30: 235–248

Martín-Fuentes, P., Civeire, F., Recalde, D., García-Otín, A. L., Jarauta, E., Marzo, I. & Cenarro, A. (2007). Individual Variation of Scavenger Receptor Expression in

Human Macrophages with Oxidized Low-Density Lipoprotein Is Associated with a Differential Inflammatory Response *J. Immunol.* 179: 3242–3248

Mazya, V. G. (1985). *Sobolev Spaces*, Springer-Verlag, Berlin (Russian version: Leningrad Univ., Leningrad)

Mosser, D. M., & Edwards, J. P. (2008). Exploring the full spectrum of macrophage activation, *Nature Rev. Immunol.* 8: 958–969

Murray, J. D. (2002). *Mathematical Biology II: Spatial models and biomedical applications* 3rd ed., Springer-Verlag, New York, Berlin

Nakashima, Y., Chen, X. Y., Kinukawa, N., & Sueishi, K. (2002). Distribution of diffuse intimal thickening in human arteries: preferential expression in atherosclerosis-prone arteries from an early age, *Virchows Arch* 441: 279–288

Nakashima, Y., Wight, T. N., & Sueishi, K. (2008). Early atherosclerosis in humans: role of diffuse intimal thickening and extracellular matrix proteoglycans, *Cardiovasc Res.* 79(1): 14–23

Neumann, S. J., Berceli, S. A., Sevick, E. M., Lincoff, A. M., Warty, V. S., Brant, A. M., Herman, I. M. & Borovetz, H. S. (1990). Experimental determination and mathematical model of the transient incorporation of cholesterol in the arterial wall, *Bull. Math. Biol.* 52: 711–732.

Niki, E., Saito, T., Kawakami, A. & Kamiya, Y. (1984). Inhibition of oxidation of methyl linoleate in solution by vitamin E, *J. Biol. Chem.* 259: 4177–4182

Parthasarathy, S., Steinberg, D., & Witztum, J. L. (1992). The role of oxidized low-density lipoproteins in the pathogenesis of atherosclerosis, *Annu. Rev. Med.* 43: 219–225

Podrez, E. A., Poliakov, E., Shen, Z., Zhang, R., Deng, Y., Sun, M., Finton, P. J., Shan, L., Gugiu, B., Fox, P. L., Hoff, H. F., Salomon, R. G. & Hazen, S. L. (2002). Identification of a novel family of oxidized phospholipids that serve as ligands for the macrophage scavenger receptor CD36, *J. Biol. Chem.* 277: 38503–38516

Quarteroni, A. (2001). Modeling the cardiovascular system: a mathematical challenge, *in* Engquist, B. & Schmid, W. (eds.) *Mathematics Unlimited- 2001 And Beyond: 2001 And Beyond*, Springer-Verlag, Berlin, New York, pp. 961–972

Ross, Russell (1995). Cell biology of atherosclerosis, *Annu. Rev. Physiol.* 57: 791–804.

Ross, Russell (1999). Atherosclerosis–An inflammatory disease, *N. Engl. J. Med.* 340(2): 115–126

Saidel, G. M., Morris, E. D. & Chisolm, G. M. (1987). Transport of macromolecules in arterial wall in vivo: a mathematical model and analytic solutions, *Bull. Math. Biol.* 49: 153–169.

Steinberg, D. (1997). Low density lipoprotein oxidation and its pathobiological significance, *J. Biol. Chem.* 272: 20963–20966

Steinberg, D. (2002). Atherogenesis in perspective: hypercholesterolemia and inflammation as partners in crime, *Nat. Med.* 8: 1211–1217

Stocker, R. (1999). The ambivalence of vitamin E in atherogenesis, *Trends Biochem. Sci.* 24: 219–223

Stout, R. D., Jiang, C., Matta, B., Tietzel, I., Watkins, S. K. & Suttle, J. (2005). Macrophages sequentially change their functional phenotype in response to changes in microenvironmental influences, *J. Immunol.* 175(1): 342–349

Superko, H. R. (2006). The Failure of LDL Cholesterol Reduction and the Importance of Reverse Cholesterol Transport. The Role of Nicotinic Acid, *Br. J. Cardiol.* 13(2): 131–136

Tabas, I. (2004). Apoptosis and plaque destabilization in atherosclerosis: the role of macrophage apoptosis induced by cholesterol, *Cell Death and Differentiation* 11: S12–S16

Tall, A. R. (1998). An overview of reverse cholesterol transport, *Euro. Heart J.* 19(A): A31–A35

Taylor, C. A. & Humphrey, J. D. (2009). Open problems in computational vascular biomechanics: Hemodynamics and arterial wall mechanics, *Comput. Methods Appl. Mech. Engrg.* 198(45-46): 3514–3523

Turing, A. (1952). The chemical basis of morphogenesis, *Phil. Trans. Royal Soc. Lond.* B237: 37–72

Veneziani, A. (1998). Mathematical and numerical modeling of blood flow problems, Ph.D. Thesis, Politecnico di Milano, Italy

Watanabe, A., Noguchi, N., Takahashi, M. & Niki, E. (1999). Rate constants for hydrogen atom abstraction by α-tocopherol radical from lipid, hydroperoxide and ascorbic acid, *Chem. Lett.* 7: 613–614

Wilson, P. W. F. (ed.) (2000). *Atlas of Atherosclerosis: Risk Factors and Treatments*, Current Medicine, Inc. 2 edition

Young, I. S., & McEneny J. (2001). Lipoprotein oxidation and atherosclerosis, *Biochem. Soc. Trans.* 29: 358–362

Zhang, Y. & Wahl, L. M. (2006). Synergistic enhancement of cytokine-induced human monocyte matrix metalloproteinase-1 by C-reactive protein and oxidized LDL through differential regulation of monocyte chemotactic protein-1 and prostaglandin E2, *J. Leukoc. Bio.* 79: 105–113

2

Spontaneous Atherosclerosis in Pigeons: A Good Model of Human Disease

J. L. Anderson, S. C. Smith and R. L. Taylor, Jr.

University of New Hampshire, Durham
U.S.A.

1. Introduction

Avian models of human atherosclerosis such as the chicken, turkey, quail, and pigeon are not currently in widespread use, but have a longer and richer history than most mammalian models of cardiovascular disease. In 1874, the first angioplasty surgery of the aortic wall was performed in birds (Roberts & Strauss, 1965). Spontaneous (non-induced) atherosclerosis in the chicken was first described in 1914 (Roberts & Strauss, 1965), and it has been repeatedly observed that avian lesions bear close resemblance to their human counterparts (Clarkson et al., 1959; Herndon et al., 1962; Cornhill et al., 1980b; Qin & Nishimura, 1998). The pigeon (*Columba livia*) is especially suited for genetic studies of atherosclerosis because susceptible and resistant strains exist in the natural population (Herndon et al., 1962; St. Clair, 1983) eliminating the need to construct an artificial phenotype through genetic or dietary manipulation. In fact, it has been suggested that the White Carneau (WC) pigeon may be one of the most appropriate models of early human lesions (Cornhill et al., 1980b; St. Clair, 1998; Moghadasian et al., 2001). This review is comprised of background information on human atherosclerosis, a description of other animal models and details of the pigeon model.

Atherosclerosis is the most common form of heart disease, a general term encompassing a variety of pathologies affecting the heart and circulatory system. More specifically, atherosclerosis is a disease of the blood vessel itself, and is most likely to develop at branch points and other regions of low shear stress along the arterial tree, such as the celiac bifurcation of the aorta, and in coronary and carotid arteries (Bassiouny et al., 1994; Kjaernes et al., 1981). The disease is a chronic and multifactorial result of both environmental and genetic factors, as well as their interactions (Breslow, 2000; Moghadasian et al., 2001). It remains the number one cause of morbidity and mortality in the United States and other developed countries (Gurr, 1992; Wagner, 1978).

Arterial lesions begin to develop during childhood as lipid-filled foam cells making up "fatty streaks" (Napoli et al., 2002; Stary, 1989), and slowly progress into complex plaques consisting of multiple cell types, intra- and extracellular cholesterol esters, calcium deposits, proteoglycans, and extensive connective tissue. The final and terminating atherosclerotic event is blood vessel occlusion, often caused by plaque rupture, which can lead to a heart attack, stroke, or embolism, depending on the location of the affected artery. However, not all fatty streaks progress to advanced lesions (Getz, 2000), and their progression/regression rate, although well correlated with classical risk factors, is unique to each individual.

Clinical symptoms do not usually appear until later in life (Munro & Cotran, 1988; Stary, 1989). Therefore, research and intervention strategies have focused on delaying the progression of plaque formation rather than preventing the appearance of foam cells or fatty streaks. There is a strong familial component to all forms of heart disease, and many genetic disorders have been identified that contribute to lesion progression and the probability of plaque rupture in the general population. However, little is known about the specific genes that determine predisposition to the disease, nor how these genes interact with each other and the environment to initiate atherosclerotic foam cell formation in any one individual.

2. Human atherogenesis

2.1 The observed beginning: Foam cells and lesion development

In human lesions, early foam cells originate primarily from vascular smooth muscle cells (VSMC) [Wissler et al., 1996]. They are the first cell type to appear in susceptible regions of the aorta (Balis et al., 1964; Ross & Glomset, 1973), and the most abundant cell type in developing fatty streaks (Gabbiani et al., 1984; Katsuda & Okada, 1994; Mosse et al., 1985, 1986; Wissler et al., 1996;). Early electron microscopy studies noted that VSMC were often filled with lipid when there was no lipid in either existing macrophages or in the extracellular space, but the reverse was never observed.

Since those observations, multiple investigators have reported that abnormal VSMC accumulation in susceptible aortic regions precedes the actual lipid accumulation (Mosse et al., 1985; Ross & Glomset, 1973). Atherosclerotic foam cells can be derived from both VSMC and macrophages (Adelman & St. Clair, 1988; Wissler et al., 1996), depending on their physical location (Strong et al., 1999) and the cause of initiation. For example, plaques that develop along the descending thoracic aorta have more macrophages than VSMC, whereas plaques along the abdominal aorta and coronary arteries are comprised mostly of VSMC, with very few macrophages. Human thoracic plaques are very rare, and those that do progress are usually secondary to other chronic conditions such as hypertension and hyperlipidemia (Wissler et al., 1996).

Although VSMC are the first cell type to accumulate lipid and initiate the fatty streak (Doran et al., 2008), much emphasis is placed on macrophage foam cells rather than myogenic foam cells. Macrophage-derived foam cells are quick to develop into lesions and are easy to induce with a high-fat and/or high-cholesterol diet (Knowles & Maeda, 2000; Xu, 2004; Zhang et al., 1992), in common animal models of human atherosclerosis, especially transgenic mice. Unlike VSMC, which can alternate between contractile and synthetic phenotypes, macrophage cells do not change during the disease progression, and so are easier to identify in the laboratory under controlled conditions.

Greater emphasis on macrophage-derived foam cells is problematic because the pathogenic lipid accumulation mechanism appears to be dissimilar for the two cell types. Also, rather than being a primary initiative event in humans, the arrival of macrophages appears to be a secondary response, as they are far more common in advanced plaques than in early lesions (Balis et al., 1964; Nakashima et al., 2007; Stary, 1989; Wissler et al., 1996; Zhang et al., 1992;).

2.2 Atherogenesis risk factors

Major physiological conditions such as high blood cholesterol, high blood pressure, diabetes, a skewed lipoprotein profile, heredity, advanced age, and maleness can increase an individual's chance of developing atherosclerosis. Collectively, these risk factors, along with lifestyle patterns such as physical inactivity, smoking, obesity, and stress have been statistically correlated with specific stages of lesion development, plaque stability, and overall disease outcome in the general population. Although genotype clearly influences many quantitative traits such as LDL/HDL levels, blood pressure, and adiposity (Gibbons et al., 2004), progress has been made on minimizing the effects of the controllable risk factors in order to disrupt, delay, reverse, or otherwise deter plaque rupture and aortic occlusion in high risk individuals.

Despite moderate success, especially in the realm of cholesterol-lowering drugs, unknown genetic factors continue to influence both the age of onset as well as the frequency/severity of clinical symptoms (Funke & Assmann, 1999). Unfortunately, by the time most people manifest clinical symptoms, it is too late to implement preventative measures because the disease is well into the progressive stage. Early identification of susceptible individuals allows timely therapeutic treatment. Less than 50% of the mortality risk from coronary heart disease can be explained by currently recognized risk factors (Ridker, 2000), even with early diagnosis.

In order to understand events in the at-risk population that remain unidentified under current screening methods, the specific contributions of heredity, diet, and lifestyle influences on atherogenesis and progression must be determined. Towards this end, research emphasis has recently shifted towards identifying cardiovascular disease markers that may be detectable prior to the manifestation of clinical symptoms. Markers are simply variations in alleles that are known to associate with a specific disease phenotype. Markers do not necessarily cause the disease, but can be used to improve diagnosis and risk assessment (Gibbons et al., 2004). Inflammatory markers such as C-reactive protein (CRP) factors [Tsimikas et al., 2006; Ridker, 2000] plus markers of oxidative damage such as myeloperoxidase (Shao et al., 2006) and paraoxanase (Visvikis-Siest & Marteau, 2006) have already increased clinicians' predictive power. As more markers of atherosclerosis are correlated with disease progression and outcome, the genetic variation contributing to predisposition and initial manifestation will become clear.

Until the genetic basis for susceptibility to atherosclerosis is understood, correlation of various risk factors with specific metabolic or pathological features will be difficult to assess, and efforts for prevention will remain equivocal. Understanding the inheritance mechanisms for atherosclerosis is an important step towards reducing the morbidity and mortality from the disease by customizing intervention strategies for individuals based upon unique genotypes and environmental risk exposures.

3. Genetic defects in human atherogenesis

The relative risk for atherosclerosis is clearly higher in individuals with a familial history compared with those having a susceptible lipid profile (Funk & Assmann, 1999; Ordovas & Shen, 2002; Palinski & Napoli, 2002). Many studies have explored the relationship, or concordance, between heredity and atherosclerosis. Heritability for early-onset coronary heart disease has been estimated at 0.63 (Galton & Ferns, 1989). The relationship becomes even clearer after analyzing concordance in twin studies. Twins fertilized from one egg (monozygotic) have a concordance rate of 0.83, whereas twins that arose from two separate fertilizations (dizygotic) demonstrate a concordance rate of 0.22 (Galton & Ferns, 1989).

These concordance values suggest an intimate relationship between the genotype of an individual and the incidence of heart disease. The fact that the concordance rate in monozygotic twins is less than 1.0 (indicating 100% correlation) most likely reflects the attenuating environmental effects on atherosclerosis initiation and progression. This gap in causality underscores the importance of understanding the genetic profile of a client before attempting intervention, because even among those sharing the same set of alleles, the atherosclerosis phenotype will vary depending on individual exposures.

Genetic research on human atherosclerosis has focused primarily on the role of cholesterol metabolism. It is estimated that several hundred genes (Ordovas & Shen, 2002) are involved in the absorption, conversion, transport, deposition, excretion, and biosynthesis, of cholesterol and other lipid substrates in the body (Knowles & Maeda, 2000; Stein et al., 2002). Very few of these genes have been characterized. A defect in any of these pathways may contribute to atherosclerotic susceptibility, because the net result can be a significant increase in plasma lipoprotein concentration, especially LDL, and/or the inappropriate deposition of cholesterol in peripheral tissues such as skin, tendons, and arteries (Garcia et al., 2001).

Blood lipid homeostasis and cellular cholesterol metabolism are highly regulated (Attie, 2001). Genetic defects have been found to impact overall cholesterol metabolism at many steps. In humans, most plasma cholesterol is in the form of LDL, having a half-life of about 2.5 days (Goldstein & Brown, 2001). Some of the cholesterol component of LDL is transferred to HDL via the action of cholesterol ester transfer protein (CETP). However, as much as 70% of LDL is removed from the blood by LDL receptors (LDLR) in the liver (Garcia et al., 2001). A variety of single gene defects have been identified that increase the incidence of atherosclerosis by influencing the LDLR activity (Funke & Assmann, 1999).

Probably the most studied of these LDLR defects is familial hypercholesterolemia (FH), an autosomal dominant Mendelian disorder (Brown et al., 1981; Funke & Assmann, 1999; Goldstein & Brown, 2001). This mutation renders the hepatic receptors nonfunctional, so that they are unable to clear circulating LDL from the blood. A second type of hypercholesterolemia, autosomal recessive hypercholesterolemia (ARH), also impacts the LDLR (Garcia et al., 2001; Goldstein & Brown, 2001). ARH is similar to FH, in that both of these hereditary defects result in chronically elevated blood cholesterol. This imbalance has the potential to change the physiology of the arterial wall, making it exceptionally vulnerable to atherogenesis. However, unlike FH, the LDLR in ARH, are believed to be functional, but their altered location in the liver makes them inaccessible to circulating LDL.

Brown and Goldstein also identified a single gene defect known as familial ligand defective apoB-100, the primary human LDL (Fielding et al., 2000) apoprotein. This inherited defect lies in the composition and binding capacity of the apoB-100 to the LDLR, decreasing the ability of the LDL to be picked up by the LDLR (Goldstein & Brown, 2001; Gurr, 1992). In the healthy human aorta, LDL particles are thought to be incorporated into SMC by receptor mediator endocytosis. Chemically modified or oxidized LDL enters via scavenger receptors. Once inside the cell, the LDL cholesterol esters (CE) are transported to the lysosomes where they are hydrolyzed by lysosomal acid lipase (LAL), also known as acid cholesterol ester hydrolase (ACEH). This enzyme breaks each CE into its free fatty acid (usually linoleate), and free cholesterol. There are several known LAL gene mutations that result in the abnormal accumulation of cholesterol esters in the lysosome.

Two of the more common lysosomal storage disease phenotypes of a LAL mutation are Wolman's Disease (Kuriyama et al., 1990; Lohse et al., 1999) and cholesterol ester storage disease (CESD). Both are inherited as an autosomal recessive trait, although Wolman's disease is usually fatal within the first year of life, and so not directly related to atherogenesis in the general population. However, individuals with CESD do demonstrate premature atherosclerosis, in addition to accumulating CE and triglycerides (TG) in the liver, adrenal glands and intestines (Pagani et al., 1996). Niemann-Pick Type C is a third form of lysosomal storage disease that directly impacts cholesterol metabolism at the cellular level (Blanchette-Mackie et al., 1988). In this condition, the CE is successfully hydrolyzed by ACEH, but the released cholesterol component is unable to leave the lysosome to travel to the endoplasmic reticulum, causing the accumulation of free cholesterol in the lysosome.

Lysosomes are also responsible for the degradation of glycosaminoglycan (GAG) chains after the core proteoglycan has been broken down by extracellular proteases such as matrix metallopeptidases (MMP) and disintigrins (ADAMs) [Arndt et al, 2002; Seals & Courtneidge, 2003). There is an extensive repertoire of catalytic lysosomal enzymes, and their functions have been revealed mostly by observing the consequences of their absence (Santamarina-Fojo et al., 2001). Defective enzymes lead to a wide variety of diseased phenotypes known as mucopolysaccharidoses (MP) ranging from the mild Schie Disease to the severe Hurler Disease, which results in childhood mortality. In these two examples, GAGs are not properly degraded, and so will accumulate in the lysosomes and in the extracellular space. GAGs in the ECM will attract LDL that has entered the intima by binding to apoB-100 as previously described, where the cholesterol is most likely endocytosed by macrophages and SMC within the developing plaque.

Once in the cytoplasm, cholesterol that is not needed for routine cellular functions is esterified by acyl CoA: cholesterol acyltransferase (ACAT) and stored in vacuoles. Intracellular CE remains trapped in the cytoplasm until hydrolyzed by neutral cholesterol ester hydrolase (NCEH). This enzyme releases the free cholesterol so it can be removed by HDL and transported to the liver. A pair of ATP binding cassette proteins has been identified that are believed to control this efflux of cellular cholesterol. One of these, ABCP-1 is defective in Tangier Disease (Faber et al., 2002), an inherited condition where cholesterol is unable to exit the cell via reverse cholesterol transport. There is a moderate risk of atherogenesis associated with Tangier Disease, which is increased in the presence of additional risk factors (Tall et al., 2001)

Research is directed towards a range of HDL-associated apoproteins. Genetic factors account for approximately 50% of the variance of HDL composition and plasma concentration in the general population (Tall et al., 2001). The primary apoprotein in HDL is apoA1, followed by apoA2, apoC, and apoE (Fielding, 2000). ApoE is an important ligand for receptor-mediated clearance of HDL from arterial cells (Moghadasian et al., 2001; Stein et al., 2002), whose role is of great interest to investigators of atherosclerotic resistance because most patients with familial dysbetalipoproteinemia (FD) are homozygous for the E2 isoform of apoE (Johns Hopkins University, 2011). Although this defect has been shown to be relevant in some animal models, especially apoE null mice (Smith et al., 2006; Zhang et al., 1992), only 1-4% of humans with the E2/E2 apoE phenotype actually develop FD (Johns Hopkins University, 2011). The pathological influence of apoE dysfunction is important in these genetically susceptible individuals, but may not be relevant to the more common forms of atherosclerosis in the overall population.

Any of the currently identified monogneic defects that directly or indirectly influence cholesterol metabolism and/or the inflammatory response will increase the likelihood of atherosclerotic events. However, individual genes do not work in a vacuum, and additional genetic and/or environmental factors are often required to determine the overall susceptibility or resistance to disease. Nuclear hormone receptors and other types of transcription factors are under investigation to determine how they exert their regulatory effects (Cohen & Zannis, 2001; Desvergne al., 2006). For example, although the binding capacity of apoB-100 is genetically determined (Goldstein & Brown, 2001), the specific number of hepatic LDLR being expressed at any given time is dependent on dietary and hormonal factors (Gurr, 1992). In a hypothetical situation, the apoB domain of LDL may be functional (non-mutated), but without the adequate expression of the LDLR to bind circulating LDL, the end result could still be high blood cholesterol.

Clinical studies have demonstrated that not all individuals afflicted with FH will develop early onset atherosclerosis. Of those manifesting the heterozygous form of the disease, where circulating LDL levels tend to range between 300-400 mg/dL, only 50% will actually develop cardiovascular disease (Stein et al, 2002). Even though there are both hyper- and hypo- responders to the effects of dietary cholesterol on serum levels, some individuals demonstrate relative resistance to atherogenesis, even in the face of hypercholesterolemia. Equal emphasis should be placed on the search for genes that contribute to individual susceptibility and those that confer resistance.

The ultimate sequence of atherosclerotic events is a result of the combined effects of many genes, regulatory factors, and environmental exposures (Hartman et al., 2001). This synergistic influence on phenotype may give the appearance of a polygenic or multifactorial effect (Funke & Assmann, 1999; Goldstein & Brown, 2001), even when a monogenic abnormality has been clearly implicated. These interactions have made it difficult to establish a universally accepted mechanism of atherogenesis (Peltonen & McKusick, 2001), because the sample sizes needed to test these gene-gene and gene-environment interactions are much larger than those needed for simpler genotype-phenotype associations (Ordovas & Shen, 2002).

Pathways that trigger atherosclerosis in the general population have yet to be elucidated (Visvikis-Siest & Marteau, 2006). Most genomic scale experiments have compared either full-blown plaques against non-affected aortic segments (Archacki et al., 2003; Forcheron et al., 2005; Hiltunen et al., 2002; Shanahan et al., 1997), or they have analyzed differences between ruptured and unruptured plaques (Adams et al., 2006; Faber et al., 2001; Papaspyridonos et al., 2006). In both types of comparisons, differentially expressed genes have been identified that illuminate plaque development and mortality risk. However, genes responsible for initiating foam cell formation could not be discriminated from those involved in later events. This gap is not an oversight by the investigators, but rather reflects the limited availability of human tissue samples at early stages of atherosclerosis for relevant comparative studies. One of the major limitations of elucidating the sequence of events that occur during atherogenesis is that an investigator can "observe and study a single site in the arterial vasculature" only once (Ross & Glomset, 1973). For this and other reasons, most atherogenic research requires animal and in-vitro models of the human disease.

4. Animal models of atherogenesis

4.1 Mammals

No animal model of human disease can fully encompass the unique complexity of molecular machinery and the wide range of expressed clinical phenotypes. However, many important metabolic pathways have been explained by the judicious use of animal models (Hartman et al., 2001). Therefore, the most appropriate choice of a disease model for genetic inquiry will ultimately depend on the specific hypothesis or research question being investigated.

There are some general guidelines to follow when choosing an animal model of human disease. The phenotype should resemble the human physiological condition as closely as possible in both the normal and diseased state (Moghadasian et al., 2001). There are additional practical issues to consider such as the size of the animal and housing requirements, generation times, and the specific cost of overall maintenance, including food, daily care, and experimental treatment (Moghadasian et al., 2001; Suckling, & Jackson, 1993). These concerns become especially important with the development of transgenic models, in that the associated investment costs are much higher than with traditional animal studies.

Several animal models are used currently to investigate various clinical manifestations and genetic mechanisms of human atherosclerosis. Mice (regular laboratory and transgenic), rabbits, and hamsters, are the most common models but miniature swine, primates, rats, dogs, and pigeons are also employed. These models have been used to elucidate the role of specific molecules in atherogenesis, lesion progression, thrombosis, and plaque rupture by direct hypothesis testing. Selected disease characteristics in animal models with their relationship to the human atherosclerosis are presented in **Table 1**.

Animal lipid metabolism studies become complicated because the majority of circulating cholesterol is in HDL (Suckling & Jackson, 1993) for most species except humans who utilize LDL (Garcia et al., 2001). For example, a decrease in plasma HDL has been associated with a reduced risk of atherosclerosis in mice (Breslow, 2000). It does make sense that relatively low levels of HDL decreased the clinical atherosclerosis incidence because HDL (Moghadasian et al., 2001) is 70% of mouse total cholesterol.

However, in humans, decreased HDL levels are associated with an increased risk of atherosclerosis. Despite this marked inconsistency, the successful extrapolation of animal studies to human atherosclerosis is exemplified by the fact that it was impossible to raise circulating LDL levels, and thus increase atherosclerosis risk in experimental models, without LDLR that were compromised, either genetically or in response to dietary overload (Brown et al., 1981; Goldstein & Brown, 2001). Subsequently, over 600 human LDLR gene mutations similar to FH that trigger varying degrees of hypercholesterolemia have been identified (Goldstein & Brown, 2001). In addition, hamsters, rabbits and primates have repeatedly shown reduced functional capacity of hepatic receptors in response to a high fat (Suckling & Jackson, 1993) diet. Individual LDLR activity varied in response to dietary fat and cholesterol because primates, like humans, dogs, and rabbits can be hypo- or hyper-responsive to diet (Goldstein & Brown, 2001; Moghadasian et al., 2001; Overturf et al., 1990; Stein et al., 2002), with some individuals demonstrating unique resistance.

In newborn humans and many animal species, hepatic LDLR have a maximum operative capacity when circulating LDL levels are approximately 0.25 mg/dL (Khosla & Sundram, 1996). Approximately 60% of plasma LDL in hamsters is removed by hepatic receptors. The clearance rate in hamsters is much faster than that of humans, with the hamster LDLR taking up 3.1 mg/hr whereas the companion human LDLR only removes 0.6 mg/hour

(Suckling & Jackson, 1993). However, the fact that hamsters and humans share a common LDL clearance mechanism makes the hamster a suitable model for this aspect of cholesterol metabolism.

Hamsters and humans also share CETP molecules (Suckling & Jackson, 1993) that transfer the cholesterol component of LDL to HDL, a key step in reverse cholesterol transport. These homologous features are in direct contrast to the mouse, which, despite being fed a high-fat high-cholesterol diet (Pitman et al., 1998) and its evolutionary relationship to hamsters, does not develop advanced atherosclerotic plaques resembling those in humans unless animals with sensitized genetic backgrounds (Xu, 2004) are used.

	Hamster	Mouse		Pig	Rabbit		Pigeon	Human
		Normal	Transgenic		Normal	WHHL/ MI		
Lipoprotein Profiles								
Predominant	LDL	HDL	HDL	LDL	HDL	HDL	HDL	LDL
CETP	+	-	-	-	+	+	+	+
LDLR	+	+	-	+	+	-	-	+
ApoE	+	+	-	+	+	+	-	+
ApoB100	+	+	+	+	+	+	+	+
ApoB-48	+	+	+	+	+	+	-	+
Lesions/Foam Cells								
Primary Location	Arch	Root	Root	Arch	Arch, Thoracic	Arch, Thoracic	Celiac branch	Coronary, Celiac branch
Primary Cell								
Macrophage	+	+	+	-	+	+	-	-
SMC	-	-	-	+	+	+	+	+
Characteristics								
Spontaneous	-	-	-	+	-	-	+	+
Diet-induced	+	+	+	+	+	+	+	+
Thrombosis	-	-	+	+	-	+	+	+
Myocardial infarction	-	-	+	-	-	+/-	+	+
Genome size (Gbp)	3.55	3.45	3.45	3.10	3.47	3.47	1.47	3.40
Wild-type diet								
Omnivore	+	+	+	+	-	-	+	+
Herbivore	-	-	-	-	+	+	-	-

Table 1. Comparison of selected characteristics of atherosclerosis between animal models and humans.

The mouse is technically advantageous because of its small size, short generation time, large litters, and the availability of many inbred strains (Breslow, 2000). However, laboratory mice fed on a chow diet do not develop spontaneous atherosclerotic lesions. Atherosclerosis must be experimentally induced by feeding a diet containing 15% fat, 1.25% cholesterol, and 0.5% cholic acid. These non-physiological conditions create serious limitations for comparison with human studies. The most important factor may be the presence of cholate in the diet. Cholate is enough, in and of itself, to induce a chronic inflammatory state in mice (Breslow, 2000; Shi et al., 2003) confounding the true atherogenic role of inflammation. This is further exacerbated by the fact that some mice are more sensitive to inflammatory cues (Rader & Pure, 2000) so that some genetic differences between susceptible and resistant mouse strains pertain to the diet used, rather than the atherogenic process as it is observed on Western diets (Breslow, 2000).

These and other genetic differences that exist between mouse strains can cause significant problems when interpreting and comparing the results of gene expression studies (Sigmund, 2000). For example, just because a specific inflammatory marker was identified in an atherosclerotic plaque and not in a healthy aorta does not mean that inflammation is causing the disease. Indeed, the molecule could be there to accelerate the cascade; but it could also be there in an attempt to reverse the pathology, or may even be responding to a cellular signal not specific to plaque progression (Knowles & Maeda, 2000) such as cholate. This is true even with transgenic mice because the foundation stock may be different. Also, because gene insertion is random, knock-in models do not by definition contain the gene of interest at the same locus. Therefore, simple transgenics may not be sufficient to prove the role of any given trait because of positional insertion effects on both absolute gene expression and copy number variation (Warden & Fisler, 1997). Delineating the specific function of a candidate gene is difficult, if not impossible, without being able to precisely correlate the phenotype to the initiating mechanism of foam cell formation. The heterogenic background of the mice combined with the variable responses to the atherogenic diet confound the interpretation.

Despite these often overlooked limitations of extrapolating mouse studies to the human disease, research using transgenic mice has enhanced the concept that atherosclerosis is not a simple lipid disorder. New atherogenic theories must be explored to explain the occurrence of atherosclerotic heart disease in individuals displaying no dyslipidemia. Most of the more than twenty unique quantitative trait loci (QTL) identified in mice (Smith et al., 2006) do not influence plasma lipid levels or blood pressure (Allayee et al., 2003; Colinayo et al., 2003). This finding has been especially interesting because these QTL were identified in hypothesis-driven experiments exploring cholesterol metabolism in LDLR and/or apoE knockout mice. Many of these studies have demonstrated the strong genetic influence in the arterial wall on the susceptible and resistant phenotypic differences between mouse strains (Lusis et al., 2004). For example the major mouse QTL, Ath29 on chromosome 9, in the BXH ApoE(-/-) cross fed a chow diet was associated with early lesion development but not with risk factors including circulating lipids (Wang et al., 2007).

Knockout models theoretically mirror homozygous recessive forms of inherited disease because of the loss of gene function (Knowles & Maeda, 2000). As in familial hypercholesterolemia (FH), LDLR null mice experience a 2X increase in plasma cholesterol levels, even on a regular diet, that is further exacerbated on the high-fat, high-cholesterol atherogenic diet (Knowles & Maeda, 2000). The same is true for apoE null mice, although the mutation's impact on plasma cholesterol is greater than in the LDLR negative mice, with 4-5 times the normal amount of circulating lipoproteins (Knowles & Maeda, 2000; Zhang et al., 1992;). However, preliminary studies revealed no relationship between these elevated lipid levels and lesion size in apoE null mice (Zhang et al., 1994). Only 2% of the homozygous apoE2 null mice developed aortic lesions at all, and the contribution of this mutation to the overall human disease burden has been questioned (Visvikis-Siest & Marteau, 2006). Subsequent studies have shown contradictory results, as the nature of the lesion appears to be dependent on the parental strain used in the experiment rather than the particular knockout gene (Allayee et al., 2003; Getz, 2000; Sigmund, 2000; Smith et al., 2006). The largest effect in these hyper-cholesterolemic models resulted from the macrophage colony stimulation factor (MCSF) impact on lesion progression (Knowles & Maeda, 2000). MCSF has been reported in advanced human atheromas, and this finding in mice lends experimental support to the role of the inflammatory response in atherosclerosis. However, the role of this molecule in atherogenesis per se is difficult to elucidate in the mouse, because of its chronically inflamed state.

Although not yet yielding consistent results applicable to human therapeutics (Yutzey & Robbins, 2007), transgenic mouse research has reinforced the importance of genetic background in determining atherosclerotic susceptibility or resistance in an individual. These studies have also suggested that the mechanism of foam cell formation varied among individuals under discrete experimental and/or environmental stimuli. The importance of the specific initiating mechanisms on the developing phenotype has been further demonstrated in rabbit models of atherosclerosis.

Rabbits, like hamsters, have CETP and do develop atherosclerotic foam cells when induced by an unnatural diet (Suckling & Jackson, 1993). Unlike the other animal models described in Table 1, rabbits are vegetarian, and so cholesterol is not a normal component of their wild-type diet. The Watanabe Heritable Hyperlipidemic (WHHL) rabbit was developed through selective breeding, and does not have LDLR (Watanabe et al., 1985;). WHHL rabbits get lesions along the aortic arch within six months, but do not experience thrombosis or myocardial infarction. However, these advanced atherosclerotic phenomena are observed in a sub-strain, the WHHLMI rabbit. This rabbit does get a heart attack similar to one of the human atherosclerotic (Shiomi et al., 2003) endpoints.

One of the important contributions of the rabbit model to understanding human disease was the observation that rabbit foam cells can be derived from smooth muscle cells (SMC) or macrophages, depending on the specific dietary perturbation (Weigensberg et al, 1985). This is in direct contrast to the mouse, where the predominant cell type in early lesions is always the macrophage, regardless of diet and genetic strain (Lusis, 2000). Rabbit myogenic foam cells are biochemically and morphologically distinct from macrophage derived foam cells, and both types of early lesions are structurally different from those produced by catheter injury (Weigensberg et al, 1985). Recognizing that different types of foam cells develop in response to different initiating mechanisms should help unravel the controversy of foam cell origin. In all probability, the predominant cell type in early atherogenesis is dependent on the pathological stimulus, and the specific model under study.

A second revelation from rabbit research has been that both macrophages and SMC express receptors for the MCSF protein (Inaba et al., 1992). The proto oncogene c-fms3 induces SMC migration and proliferation, as well as macrophage recruitment to the atherosclerosis-prone regions of the aorta (Mozes et al., 1998). This is important for atherogenesis investigations because the ratio of SMC to macrophages, both found in human lesions, changes as the disease progresses. The fact that both cell types share an activation mechanism means that the presence of MCSF in an experimental sample does not by definition mean that only macrophages will be recruited. This simple fact is not evident from the plethora of mouse studies, and is further evidence that multiple models are needed to grasp the complexity of human atherosclerosis, especially at the initiation stage.

Swine are unique among the other mammals depicted in Table 1 because, although they are LDL carriers like the hamster (Julien et al., 1981), and most lesions develop in the aortic arch, they also develop spontaneous lesions in the abdominal aorta. The initial foam cells are derived from intimal SMC (Scott et al., 1985), and appear similar to those found in early stages of the human disease. Unfortunately, these lesions do not progress to advanced atheromas without being induced by a 4% (w/w) cholesterol diet (Moghadasian et al., 2001). Even after 90 days on a hyperlipidemic diet, less than 5% of the cells are monocytes (Scott et al., 1985). Swine could adequately model the gradual transition from a myogenic fatty streak to an advanced lesion with activated macrophage cells, reflecting the inflammatory response in humans over time.

4.2 Pigeons

The WC pigeon is unique among non-primate models in that it develops naturally occurring (spontaneous) atherosclerosis at both the celiac bifurcation of the aorta and in the coronary arteries (Clarkson et al., 1959; Prichard et al., 1964). Foam cells develop into fatty streaks which progress into mature plaques in the absence of elevated plasma cholesterol and other traditional risk factors (Wagner, 1978; Wagner et al., 1979). These non-induced atherosclerotic lesions are morphologically and ultrastructurally similar to those seen in humans and occur at parallel anatomical sites along the arterial tree (Cornhill et al., 1980a, 1980b; Hadjiisky, et al., 1991; Kjaernes et al., 1981). Multiple studies have clearly demonstrated that susceptibility in the WC resides at the level of the arterial wall (St. Clair et al., 1986; Wagner et al., 1973, 1979;). Lesion site specificity, severity, and disease progression as a function of age are also highly predictable (Cooke & Smith, 1968; Santerre et al., 1972).

Show Racer pigeons (SR) are resistant to atherosclerosis, while consuming the same cholesterol-free diet. This susceptibility difference occurs despite similar plasma cholesterol and lipoprotein concentrations in both WC and SR (Barakat & St. Clair, 1985). WC pigeons are one of the few animal models to develop severe atherosclerosis while consuming a cholesterol free diet, and comparing results with the resistant SR enables pathological changes associated with the disease to be distinguished from changes due to the natural pigeon aging process. Virtually all WC and SR differences occur at the arterial tissue level as there are few system level differences (Fronek & Alexander, 1981).

Both pigeon breeds are hypercholesterolemic compared to humans, and, like mice and rabbits, they are primarily HDL carriers. However, pigeons are unique in that for the first three days of life, cholesterol is circulated in the form of LDL, after which time the lipoprotein profile switches to HDL (unpublished data) for the remainder of the pigeon's life. Neither breed has apoE (Randolph et al., 1984) or LDLR (Randolph & St. Clair, 1984; St. Clair et al., 1986), so the effect of these variables in other models of the human disease is not a factor in the pigeon pathology. Combined unpublished data gathered from several hundred birds aged 6 months to 3 years over a twenty-year period shows that the average plasma cholesterol concentration in pigeons ranges from 201 mg/dL in the SR to 242 mg/dL in the WC (+/- 16 mg/dL in both groups). Although these values are borderline significant, they do not change during disease progression, nor does it appear that blood cholesterol induces WC foam cell development. This fact is further supported in wild mourning doves, a close relative of the pigeon, that have 258 mg/dL average plasma cholesterol but do not get atherosclerosis (Schulz et al., 2000). Sterol balance studies have revealed that the WC excretes less neutral sterols than the SR breed (Siekert et al., 1975; Subbiah & Connelly, 1976), but this difference had much greater impact in diet-induced atherosclerosis than in the susceptible phenotype of the WC to the naturally occurring form of the disease (Hulcher & Margolis, 1982).

The most widely studied spontaneous atherosclerotic lesion in susceptible pigeons occurs at the celiac bifurcation of the aorta, and by three years of age reaches a size to be easily visible on gross examination (Nicolosi et al., 1972; Santerre et al., 1972). Early pathological and metabolic changes are apparent microscopically in this site by six months of age (Cooke & Smith, 1968). In contrast, diet-induced lesions in the WC aorta occur at various and unpredictable sites along the descending (Gosselin, 1979; Jerome & Lewis, 1985; Wagner, 1978) and abdominal aortas, and are pathologically very different from non-induced lesions. Foam cells in spontaneous lesions consist primarily of modified SMC (Cooke & Smith, 1968; St. Clair, 1983) while cholesterol-induced foam cells are mostly composed of macrophages (Denholm & Lewis, 1987; Gosselin, 1979; Jerome & Lewis, 1984; St. Clair, 1983).

As with mice, diet-induced lesions develop more rapidly in the pigeon than their spontaneous counterparts (Jerome & Lewis, 1984; Xu, 2004), but different atherogenic mechanisms appear to be involved (Santerre et al., 1972; St. Clair, 1983). One of the primary diet induction effects is to shift the physiological lipoprotein profile from HDL to LDL (Jones et al., 1991; Langelier et al., 1976). In fact, 1% diet supplementation with cholesterol causes such a rapid onset of atherosclerotic foam cells in both breeds that it becomes unfeasible to detect the influence of intrinsic factors (Lofland, 1966) contributing to either WC susceptibility or SR resistance. Therefore, the spontaneous lesion model is best suited for genetic studies to identify candidate genes for susceptibility or resistance as the introduction of an artificial diet confounds the interpretation of the earliest events occurring in atherogenesis.

Since 1959, many studies have been performed to systematically characterize the initiating factor in lesion development in the susceptible WC pigeon. However, the mechanism(s) leading to WC foam cell development is not known, and few studies have been conducted in the spontaneous model to identify the gene(s) or gene product(s) that are specific to initiation. Clarkson and associates (1959) observed that age and heredity were the biggest factors in atherosclerotic susceptibility. Diet, exercise, and gender were not primary factors in the WC pathology.

Further studies of age and heredity effects demonstrated that genetics play a larger role in lesion development than the normal aging process (Goodman & Herndon; 1963). The authors hypothesized that inheritance was a polygenic trait. Wagner and co-workers (1973) compared susceptibility to lesion development between the WC and SR celiac bifurcation of the aorta. The authors found a greater number of advanced lesions in the WC than in the SR, and concluded that the genetic control conferring susceptibility or resistance in the pigeon appeared to be at the level of the artery. Supplementary experiments by that group showed that blood cholesterol, triacylglycerol, and glucose levels were not different between the two breeds (Wagner, 1978), and that elevated blood pressure is actually a consequence of pigeon atherosclerosis, rather than being an initiating factor (Wagner et al., 1979). The latter study provided initial indications that although diet is not the primary factor contributing to atherosclerotic susceptibility in the pigeon, it can impact the severity of a lesion once formed; thus indicating a role in progression.

A range of metabolic differences between the arterial wall of WC and SR pigeons have been identified. In vivo, differences in the WC susceptible foci include increased glycosaminoglycans, especially chondroitin-6-sulfate (Curwen & Smith, 1977), greater lipid content, predominantly in the form of cholesterol esters (Hajjar et al., 1980b; Nicolosi et al., 1972), lower oxidative metabolism(Hajjar et al., 1980a; Santerre et al., 1974), relative hypoxia (Hajjar et al., 1988), decreased acid cholesterol hydrolase (Sweetland et al., 1999), and neutral cholesterol ester hydrolase (Fastnacht, 1993) activities, increased glycolysis (Zemplenyi & Rosenstein, 1975), decreased tricarboxylic acid cycle activity (Zemplenyi & Rosenstein, 1975), and the increased synthesis of prostaglandin E2, which also decreased cholesterol ester hydrolase activity (Subbiah et al., 1980). Although these studies did not distinguish the primary or underlying problem from secondary effects, increases in non-esterified fatty acids (NEFA) and in chondroitin-6-sulfate (C6S) seem to precede many of the other observed differences. The role of excess NEFA and C6S in pigeon atherogenesis is not yet clear, although the presence of C6S in the susceptible pigeon by six weeks of age does support the response to retention theory. Both human and pigeon smooth muscle cells synthesize C6S as part of the ECM (Edwards et al., 1995; Wight, 1985), where it has been observed to complex with plasma LDL entering the vascular wall (Nakashima et al., 2007; Tovar et al., 1998; Wagner et al., 1989; Wight, 1980).

Human atherosclerosis is considered to be a multifactorial disease, with many genes and environmental factors contributing to the specific phenotype and ultimate endpoint. In pigeons, where individual lifestyle choices are not a factor, the numbers and types of genes contributing to baseline susceptibility and resistance may be easier to elucidate. Preliminary crossbreeding studies indicated a polygenic mechanism of inheritance (Goodman & Herndon, 1963) with resistance being the dominant trait. However, the authors noted that each breed responded differently to dietary manipulation (Herndon et al., 1962), so it is possible that the genetic differences observed may have reflected the confounding influence of diet, rather than the spontaneous expression profile.

Pigeons are not as well suited for traditional inheritance studies as mammalian species because the birds mate for life, and do not reach sexual maturity until seven months of age (Brannigan, 1973). Although excess cholesterol esters can be detected biochemically at 12 weeks, three years are required in order to definitively characterize the complete atherosclerotic phenotype. However, the pigeon genome is approximately half the size of its counterpart mammalian models, and comparative genomic studies are facilitated by the published chicken (Gallus gallus) genome, which is similar in size (Hillier et al., 2004) to the pigeon.

A 15-year cross breeding study at the University of New Hampshire examined grossly visible lesions (or lack thereof) at three years of age in the celiac foci of susceptible WC, resistant SR, and in F1, F2, and backcross progeny. The results supported autosomal recessive inheritance of susceptibility to spontaneous atherosclerosis in the pigeon (Smith et al., 2001). This finding contrasted earlier results (Herndon et al., 1962) that indicated a polygenic mechanism based only on the F1 progeny, but the latter researchers carried the experiments through the backcross generations and did not use a cholesterol-supplemented diet (Smith et al., 2001). In addition, and probably of greater importance to the experimental results, all pigeons consumed the same cholesterol-free diet. Parallel investigation of the smooth muscle cells cultured from several tissues of the WC, SR, and F1 pigeons demonstrated that lipid accumulation observed at the celiac bifurcation is a constitutive property of WC (Smith et al., 2001).

The finding that spontaneous atherosclerosis in the susceptible WC appears to be the result of a single gene, and not the net result of many interacting genes, as is thought to be the case in humans, makes the pigeon model a simplest case system. Identification of the gene responsible for predisposition, and an understanding of how this gene influences the described metabolic and morphological changes could reveal an initiating mechanistic pathway that remains undetected in more confounded models of atherogenesis.

Experiments have demonstrated that the SMC monolayers grown in vitro accumulate lipid and synthesize proteoglycans in the same manner as aortic cells in vivo (Cooke & Smith, 1968; Smith et al., 1965; Wight, 1980; Wight et al., 1977) but at an accelerated rate. A comparison of the maturation and degeneration of pigeon aortic cells in vivo and in vitro is presented in **Table 2**. In culture, foam cell development is evident in WC SMC by 8-10 days, where several weeks are needed in order to observe the same phenomena in vivo. Other differences in the WC SMC include more esterified cholesterol present in lipid vacuoles, less arachidonate, and decreased mitochondrial metabolism. Although it has been demonstrated that the act of culturing aortic cells can change the SMC phenotype from contractile to synthetic (Worth et al., 2001), this has not been observed in primary cultures, where the lack of sub-culture minimizes potential genetic alterations. WC aortic cells obtained in vitro demonstrate a similar degenerative progression as those cells observed in the celiac bifurcation (Cooke & Smith, 1968; Wight et al., 1977), offering further evidence that the gene expression profile is comparable between the two model systems.

In vitro, there is no signal communication between SMC and endothelial cells, monocytes, hormones, neurotransmitters, other humoral factors, and whole body feedback systems (Shanahan & Weissberg, 1998; Thyberg et al., 1990). The only source of interaction is between the SMC and the media components, resulting in cell growth and ECM synthesis. This makes it possible to observe the intrinsic characteristics of WC and SR aortic cell development in a controlled, time-compressed setting, while limiting the number of genes under investigation to those specific to aortic SMC. Interestingly, although only the SMC of the WC celiac and coronary bifurcations are susceptible to atherogenesis in vivo, SMC taken from other WC tissue such as the gizzard or small intestine exhibit features in vitro similar to atherogenesis in aortic cells. This is not the case in the SR, where neither SMC from the celiac foci, nor SMC from any other tissue undergo phenotype modification when cultured under identical conditions.

The aforementioned experiments provide additional evidence that the genetic defect predisposing the WC to atherosclerosis is conditionally expressed in SMC. Factors that stimulate the expression of atherogenic genes at the celiac bifurcation in vivo appear to be present in vitro, as the cultured WC cells undergo degeneration parallel to their counterparts in aortic tissue (Cooke & Smith, 1968; Wight et al., 1977). Genetic factors denoting resistance in the SR remain expressed in both experimental environments.

Approximate Age *(in vivo)* variable starting at 6 weeks	Salient Morphological Features		Approximate Age *(in vitro)*
1-10 days	Myoblasts ⬇		1-2 days
10-18 days	Myofilaments increase Organelles increase Myofilaments align ⬇ Formation of myofibrils Dilation of ER ⬇ ⬇		2-4 days
	Show Racer	White Carneau	
1 day–6 months	Myofibrils enlarge ⬇	Extension & dilation of ER Modified smooth muscle cell ⬇	4-6 days
2 weeks–2 years	Myofibrils increase Organelles decrease ⬇	Pinched off cisternae of ER Loss of ribosomes Mitochondrial abnormalities Lipid inclusions, vacuoles Cell rounding ⬇	6-8 days
	Mature smooth muscle cell	Foam cell	8-10 days

Table 2. Maturation and degeneration of pigeon aortic cells.

Anderson (2008) analyzed differential gene expression in vitro at day seven of cellular growth. Ninety-one genes were uniquely expressed in the susceptible WC cells compared to 101 genes exclusive to the resistant SR. There was a marked difference in energy metabolism between the two breeds. The SR VSMC expressed genes related to oxidative phosphorylation such as cytochrome B, cyctochrome C oxidase subunit I, NADH dehydrogenase subunit 4, ubiquinone, and ATP synthase subunit 4B. This was in direct contrast to the glycolytic genes expressed by the WC which included enolase, glucose phosphate isomerase, and lactate dehydrogenase subunit B.

In addition, genes expressed by the SR were indicative of a contractile VSMC phenotype whereas susceptible WC pigeons expressed genes that reflected a synthetic phenotype. Spondin, decorin, vimentin and beta actin were upregulated in the WC. Myosin heavy chain, myosin light chain kinase, tropomyosin, and alpha actin were expressed in the SR. The resistant SR appeared to develop and maintain an extracellular matrix with structural integrity, whereas the susceptible WC was already expressing proteases and immune signals.

Although many genes were different between the two breeds, the compressed time frame made it difficult to determine what happens first: changes in energy metabolism or changes in cellular phenoptye. Future in vivo studies are necessary to elucidate the chronological sequence of events and determine the single gene responsible for atherogenesis in the WC pigeon.

Analysis of SMC soluble proteins from WC and SR pigeons revealed differential expression between the two breeds. Eight discrete zones of molecular weight versus pI were identified, five which included only proteins unique to susceptible cells and three which included proteins unique to resistant cells. Eighty-eight differentially-expressed proteins were found in susceptible cells with 41 located in unique zones. Resistant cells had 29 of 82 differentially-expressed proteins in unique zones. Some annotated proteins, including smooth muscle myosin phosphatase, myosin heavy chain, fatty acid binding protein, ribophorin, heat shock protein, TNF alpha-inducing factor, and lumican, corresponded to genes identified previously or to current hypotheses to explain atherogenesis (Smith et al., 2008).

Additional research to identify the causative gene for spontaneous atherosclerosis will be facilitated by pigeon genome sequencing. Comparative studies between the resistant versus susceptible breeds may reveal sequence variation contributing to the disease. The pigeon remains an important model to study the genetic role at the site of lesion development that is associated with human atherosclerosis.

5. Acknowledgements

This is Scientific Contribution Number 2455 from the New Hampshire Agricultural Experiment Station.

6. References

Adams, L.D., Geary, R.L., Li, J., Rossini, A., & Schwartz, S.M. (2006). Expression profiling identifies smooth muscle cell diversity within human intima and plaque fibrous cap: loss of RGS5 distinguishes the cap. *Arteriosclerosis Thrombosis and Vascular Biology*, Vol. 26, 319-325

Adelman, S., & St. Clair, R. (1988). Lipoprotein metabolism by macrophages from atherosclerosis-susceptible White Carneau and resistant Show Racer pigeons. *Journal of Lipid Research*, Vol. 29, 643-656

Allayee, H., Ghazalpour, A., & Lusis, A.J. (2003). Using mice to dissect genetic factors in atherosclerosis. *Arteriosclerosis Thrombosis and Vascular Biology*, Vol. 23, 1501-1509

Anderson, J. L. (2008). Differentially expressed genes in aortic cells from atherosclerosis-resistant and atherosclerosis-susceptible pigeons. *Ph. D. Dissertation*, University of New Hampshire, Durham

Archacki, S.R., Angheloiu, G., Tian, X.L., Tan, F.L., DiPaola, N., Shen, G.Q., Moravec, C., Ellis, S., Topol, E.J., & Wang, Q. (2003). Identification of new genes differentially expressed in coronary artery disease by expression profiling. *Physiological Genomics*, Vol. 15, 65-74

Arndt, M., Lendeckel, U., Röcken, C., Nepple, K., Wolke, C., Spiess, A., Huth, C., Ansorge, S., Klein, H.U. & Goette, A. (2002). Altered Expression of ADAMs (a disintegrin and metalloproteinase) in fibrillating human atria. *Circulation*, Vol. 105, 720-725

Attie, A.D. (2001). *Atherosclerosis modified*. Circulation Research, Vol. 89, 102-104

Balis, J.U., Haust, M.D., & More, R.H. (1964). Electron-microscopic studies in human atherosclerosis: cellular elements on aortic fatty streaks. *Experimental and Molecular Pathology*, Vol. 3, 511-525

Barakat, H., & St. Clair, R. (1985). Characterization of plasma lipoproteins of grain- and cholesterol-fed White Carneau and Show Racer pigeons. *Journal of Lipid Research*, Vol. 26, 1252-1268

Bassiouny, H., Zarins, C., Kadowaki, M., & Glagov, S. (1994). Hemodynamic stress and experimental aortoiliac atherosclerosis. *Journal of Vascular Surgery*, Vol. 19, 426-434

Blanchette-Mackie, E.J., Dwyer, N.K., Amende, L.M., Kruth, H.S., Butler, J.D., Sokol, J., Comly, M.E., Vanier, M.T., August, J.T., Brady, R.O., & Pentchev, P.G. (1988). Type-C Niemann-Pick disease: low density lipoprotein uptake is associated with premature cholesterol accumulation in the golgi complex and excessive cholesterol storage in lysosomes. *Proccedings of the National Academy of Sciences USA*, Vol. 85, 8022-8026

Brannigan, D. (1973). Reproductive behavior and squab development in atherosclerosis-susceptible White Carneau and atherosclerosis-resistant show racer pigeons. *Ph. D. Dissertation*, University of New Hampshire, Durham

Breslow, J.L. (2000). Genetic differences in endothelial cells may determine atherosclerosis susceptibility. *Circulation*, Vol. 102, 5-6

Brown, M., Kovanen, P., & Goldstein, J. (1981). Regulation of plasma cholesterol by lipoprotein receptors. Science, Vol. 212, 628-635

Clarkson, T.B., Prichard, R.W., Netsky, M.G., & Lofland, H.B. (1959). Atherosclerosis in pigeons: its spontaneous occurrence and resemblance to human atherosclerosis. *American Medical Association Archives of Pathology*, Vol. 68, 143-147

Cohen, J.C., & Zannis, V.I. (2001). Genes affecting atherosclerosis. *Current Opinion in Lipidology*, Vol. 12, 93-95

Colinayo, V., Qiao, J.H., Wang, X., Krass, K.L., Schadt, E., Lusis, A.J., & Drake, T.A. (2003). Genetic loci for diet-induced atherosclerotic lesions and plasma lipids in mice. *Mammalian Genome*, Vol. 14, 464-471

Cooke, P., & Smith, S. C. (1968). Smooth muscle cells: source of foam cells in atherosclerotic White Carneau pigeons. *Experimental and Molecular of Pathology*, Vol. 8, 171-189

Cornhill, J., Akins, D., Hutson, M., & Chandler, A. (1980a). Localization of atherosclerotic lesions in the human basilar artery. *Atherosclerosis*, Vol. 35, 77-86

Cornhill, J., Levesque, M., & Nerem, R. (1980b). Quantitative study of the localization of sudanophilic coeliac lesions in the White Carneau pigeon. *Atherosclerosis*, Vol. 35, 103-10

Curwen, K., & Smith, S. (1977). Aortic glycosaminoglycans in atherosclerosis-susceptible and -resistant pigeons. *Experimental and Molecular Pathology*, Vol. 27, 121-133

Denholm, E., & Lewis, J. (1987). Monocyte chemoattractants in pigeon aortic atherosclerosis. *American Journal of Pathology*, Vol. 126, 464-475

Desvergne, B., Michalik, L., & Wahli, W. (2006). Transcriptional regulation of metabolism. *Physiological Reviews*, Vol. 86, 465-514

Edwards, I. J., Xu, H., Obunike, J. C., Goldberg, I. J., & Wagner, W. D. (1995). Differentiated macrophages synthesize a heparan sulfate proteoglycan and an oversulfated chondroitin sulfate proteoglycan that bind lipoprotein lipase. *Arteriosclerosis Thrombosis and Vascular Biology*, Vol. 15, 400-409

Faber, B., Heeneman, S., Daemen, M., & Cleutjens, K. (2002). Genes potentially involved in plaque rupture. *Current Opinion in Lipidology*, Vol. 13, 545-552

Faber, B.C., Cleutjens, K., Niessen, R.L., Aarts, P., Boon, W., Greenberg, A.S., Kitslaar, P., Tordoir, J. & Daemen, M. (2001). Identification of genes potentially involved in rupture of human atherosclerotic plaques. *Circulation Research*, Vol. 89, 547-554

Fastnacht, C. (1993). Egasyn-esterase activity in atherosclerosis-susceptible White Carneau and atherosclerosis-resistant Show Racer pigeon aortas. *M.S. Thesis*, University of New Hampshire, Durham

Fielding, C. (2000). Lipoprotein synthesis, transport, and metabolism, In: *Genetic Biochemical and Physiological Aspects of Human Nutrition*, M. Stipanuk, (Ed). pp 351-364, W.B. Saunders, ISBN 072164452X, Philadelphia

Forcheron, F., Legedz, L., Chinetti, G., Feugier, P., Letexier, D., Bricca, G., & Beylot, M. (2005). Genes of cholesterol metabolism in human atheroma: overexpression of perilipin and genes promoting cholesterol storage and repression of ABCA1 expression. *Arteriosclerosis Thrombosis and Vascular Biology*, Vol. 25, 1711-1717

Fronek, K. & Alexander, N. (1981). Genetic difference in the sympathetic nervous activity and susceptibility to atherosclerosis in pigeon. *Atherosclerosis*, Vol. 39, 25-33

Funke, H. & Assmann, G. (1999). Strategies for the assessment of genetic coronary artery disease risk. *Current Opinion in Lipidology*, Vol. 10, 286-291

Galton, D.J., & Ferns, G.A. (1989). Candidate genes for atherosclerosis, In: *Genetic Factors in Atherosclerosis: Approaches and Model Systems*, R.S. Sparkes & A.J. Lusis, (Eds). pp 95-109, Karger, ISBN 3805548907, Basel

Garcia, C.K., Wilund, K., Arca, M., Zuliani, G., Fellin, R., Maioli, M., Calandra, S., Bertolini, S., Cossu, F., Grishin, N., Barnes, R., Cohen, J.C., & Hobbs, H.H. (2001). Autosomal recessive hypercholesterolemia caused by mutations in a putative LDL receptor adaptor protein. *Science*, Vol. 292, 1394-1398

Getz, G.S. (2000). When is atherosclerosis not atherosclerosis? *Arteriosclerosis Thrombosis and Vascular Biology*, Vol. 20, 1694

Gibbons, G.H., Liew, C.C., Goodarzi, M.O., Rotter, J.I., Hsueh, W.A., Siragy, H.M., Pratt, R., & Dzau, V.J. (2004). Genetic markers: progress and potential for cardiovascular disease. *Circulation*, Vol. 109, 47-58

Goldstein, J.L., & Brown, M.S. (2001). The cholesterol quartet. Science, Vol. 292, 1310-1312

Goodman, H. O. & Herndon, C. N. (1963). Genetic aspects of atherosclerosis in pigeons. Federation Proceedings Vol. 22, Abstract 1336, Atlantic City, April 1963

Gosselin, E. J. (1979). A morphological and ultrastructural study of spontaneous and cholesterol-aggravated atherosclerosis in susceptible and resistant pigeons. *M.S. Thesis*, University of New Hampshire, Durham

Gurr, M.I. (1992). Dietary lipids and coronary heart disease: old evidence, new perspective. *Progress in Lipid Research*, Vol. 31, 195-243

Hadjiisky, P., Bourdillon, M., & Grosgogeat, Y. (1991). Experimental models of atherosclerosis. Contribution, limits and trends. *Archive Mal Coeur Vaiss*, Vol. 84, 1593-1603

Hajjar, D., & Smith, S. (1980a). Focal differences in bioenergetic metabolism of atherosclerosis-susceptible and -resistant pigeon aortas. *Atherosclerosis*, Vol. 36, 209-22

Hajjar, D., Farber, I., & Smith, S. (1988). Oxygen tension within the arterial wall: relationship to altered bioenergetic metabolism and lipid accumulation. *Archives of Biochemistry and Biophysics*, Vol. 262, 375-380

Hajjar, D., Wight, T., & Smith, S. (1980b). Lipid accumulation and ultrastructural change within the aortic wall during early spontaneous atherogenesis. *American Journal of Pathology*, Vol. 100, 683-706

Hartman, J.L., IV, Garvik, B., & Hartwell, L. (2001). Principles for the buffering of genetic variation. *Science*, Vol. 291, 1001-1004

Herndon, C. N., Goodman, H. O., Clarkson, T. B., Lofland, H. B., & Prichard, R. W. (1962). Atherosclerosis resistance and susceptibility in two breeds of pigeons. Genetics, Vol. 47, 958

Hillier, L. W. 171 co-authors., (2004). International Chicken Genome Sequencing Consortium. Sequence and comparative analysis of the chicken genome provide unique perspectives on vertebrate evolution. Nature, Vol. 432, 695-716

Hiltunen, M., Tuomisto, T.T., Niemi, M., Brasen, J.H., Rissanen, T.T., P Toronen, P., Vajanto, I., & Yla-Herttuala, S. Changes in gene expression in atherosclerotic plaques analyzed using DNA array. *Atherosclerosis*, Vol. 165, 23-32 (2002).

Hulcher, F., & Margolis, R. (1982). Rate-limiting, diurnal activity of hepatic microsomal cholesterol-7 alpha-hydroxylase in pigeons with high serum cholesterol. *Biochimica et Biophysica Acta*, Vol. 712, 242-249

Inaba, T., Yamada, N., Gotoda, T., Shimano, H., Shimada, M., Momomura, K., Kadowaki, T., Motoyoshi, K., Tsukada, T., & Morisaki, N. (1992). Expression of M-CSF receptor encoded by c-fms on smooth muscle cells derived from arteriosclerotic lesion. *Journal of Biological Chemistry*, Vol. 267, 5693-5699

Jerome, W., & Lewis, J. (1984). Early atherogenesis in White Carneau pigeons. I. leukocyte margination and endothelial alterations at the celiac bifurcation. *American Journal of Pathology*, Vol. 116, 56-68

Jerome, W., & Lewis, J. (1985). Early atherogenesis in White Carneau pigeons. II. ultrastructural and cytochemical observations. *American Journal of Pathology* 119, 210-222

Johns Hopkins University, (2011). Apolipoprotein E, MIM ID +107741, In: Online Mendelian Inheritance in Man (OMIM), 5/23/2011, Available from: http://www.ncbi.nlm.nih.gov/omim

Jones, N., Jerome, W., & Lewis, J. (1991). Pigeon monocyte/macrophage lysosomes during beta VLDL uptake. induction of acid phosphatase activity. a model for complex arterial lysosomes. *American Journal of Pathology*, Vol. 139, 383-392

Julien P, Downar E, & Angel A. (1981). Lipoprotein composition and transport in the pig and dog cardiac lymphatic system. Circulation Research, Vol. 49, 248-54

Katsuda, S., & Okada, Y. (1994). Vascular smooth muscle cell migration and extracellular matrix. *Journal of Atherosclerosis and Thrombosis*, Vol. 1 Suppl 1, S34-38

Khosla, P., & Sundram, K. (1996). Effects of dietary fatty acid composition on plasma cholesterol. *Progress in Lipid Research*, Vol. 35, 93-132

Kjaernes, M., Svindland, A., Walloe, L., & Wille, S. (1981). Localization of early atherosclerotic lesions in an arterial bifurcation in humans. *Acta Pathologica Microbiologica Scandanavia [A]*, Vol. 89, 35-40

Knowles, J.W., & Maeda, N. (2000). Genetic modifiers of atherosclerosis in mice. *Arteriosclerosis, Thrombosis and Vascular Biology*, Vol. 20, 2336-2345

Kuriyama, M., Yoshida, H., Suzuki, M., Fujiyama, J., & Igata, A. (1990). Lysosomal acid lipase deficiency in rats: lipid analyses and lipase activities in liver and spleen. *Journal of Lipid Research*, Vol. 31, 1605-1642

Langelier, M., Connelly, P., & Subbiah, M. (1976). Plasma lipoprotein profile and composition in White Carneau and Show Racer breeds of pigeons. *Canadian Journal of Biochemistry*, Vol. 54, 27-31

Lofland, H. B., Jr. (1966). Irradiation and atherosclerosis in pigeons. Nutrition Reviews, Vol. 24, 178-179

Lohse, P., Maas, S., Lohse, P., Sewell, A.C., van Diggelen, O.P., & Seidel, D. (1999). Molecular defects underlying Wolman disease appear to be more heterogeneous than those resulting in cholesteryl ester storage disease. *Journal of Lipid Research*, Vol. Res 40, 221-228

Lusis, A.J. (2000). Atherosclerosis. *Nature*, Vol. 407, 233-241

Lusis, A.J., Fogelman, A.M., & Fonarow, G.C. (2004). Genetic basis of atherosclerosis: part I: new genes and pathways. *Circulation*, Vol. 110, 1868-1873

Moghadasian, M.H., Frohlich, J.J., & McManus, B. M. (2001). Advances in experimental dyslipidemia and atherosclerosis. *Laboratory Investigation*, Vol. 81, 1173-1183

Mosse, P., Campbell, G., & Campbell, J. (1986). Smooth muscle phenotypic expression in human carotid arteries. II. Atherosclerosis-free diffuse intimal thickenings compared with the media. *Arteriosclerosis, Thrombosis and Vascular Biology*, Vol. 6, 664-669

Mosse, P., Campbell, G., Wang, Z., & Campbell, J. (1985). Smooth muscle phenotypic expression in human carotid arteries. I. Comparison of cells from diffuse intimal thickenings adjacent to atheromatous plaques with those of the media. *Laboratory Investigation*, Vol. 53, 556-562

Mozes, G., Mohacsi, T., Gloviczki, P., Menawat, S., Kullo, I., Spector, D., Taylor, J., Crotty, T.B., & O'Brien, T. (1998). Adenovirus-mediated gene transfer of macrophage colony stimulating factor to the arterial wall in vivo. *Arteriosclerosis Thrombosis and Vascular Biology*, Vol. 18, 1157-1163

Munro, J., & Cotran, R. (1988). The pathogenesis of atherosclerosis: atherogenesis and inflammation. *Laboratory Investigation*, Vol. 58, 249-261

Nakashima, Y., Fujii, H., Sumiyoshi, S., Wight, T.N., & Sueishi, K. (2007). Early human atherosclerosis: accumulation of lipid and proteoglycans in intimal thickenings followed by macrophage infiltration. *Arteriosclerosis Thrombosis and Vascular Biology*, Vol. 27, 1159-1165

Napoli, C., deNigris, F., Welch, J.S., Calaria, F.B., Stuart, R.O., Glass C.K., & Palinski, W. (2002). Maternal hypercholesterolemia during pregnancy promotes early atherogenesis in LDL receptor-deficient mice and alters aortic gene expression determined by microarray. *Circulation*, Vol. 105, 1360-1367

Nicolosi, R. J., Santerre, R. F., & Smith, S. C. (1972). Lipid accumulation in muscular foci in White Carneau and Show Racer pigeon aortas. Experimental and Molecular of Pathology, Vol. 17, 29-37

Ordovas, J., & Shen, A. (2002). Genetics, the environment, and lipid abnormalities. *Current Cardiology Reports*, Vol. 4, 508-513

Overturf, M., Smith, S.A., Gotto, A.M., Jr., Morrisett, J.D., Tewson, T., Poorman, J., & Loose-Mitchell, D.S. (1990). Dietary cholesterol absorption, and sterol and bile acid excretion in hypercholesterolemia-resistant white rabbits. *Journal of Lipid Research*, Vol. 31, 2019-2027

Pagani, F., Garcia, R., Pariyarath, R., Stuani, C., Gridelli, B., Paone, G., & Baralle, F.E. (1996). Expression of lysosomal acid lipase mutants detected in three patients with cholesteryl ester storage disease. *Human Molecular Genetics*, Vol. 5, 1611-1617

Palinski, W., & Napoli, C. (2002). The fetal origins of atherosclerosis: maternal hypercholesterolemia and cholesterol-lowering or antioxidant treatment during pregnancy influence in utero programming and postnatal susceptibility to atherogenesis. *FASEB Journal*, Vol. 16, 1348-1360

Papaspyridonos, M., Smith, A., Burnand, K.G., Taylor, P., Padayachee, S., Suckling, K.E., James, C.H., Greaves, D.R., & Patel, L. (2006). Novel candidate genes in unstable areas of human atherosclerotic plaques. *Arteriosclerosis Thrombosis and Vascular Biology*, Vol. 26, 1837-1844

Peltonen, L., & McKusick, V.A. (2001). Genomics and medicine: dissecting human disease in the postgenomic era. *Science*, Vol. 291, 1224-1229

Pitman, W.A., Hunt, M.H., McFarland, C., & Paigen, B. (1998). Genetic analysis of the difference in diet-induced atherosclerosis between the inbred mouse strains SM/J and NZB/BlNJ. *Arteriosclerosis Thrombosis and Vascular Biology*, Vol. 18, 615-620

Prichard, R., Clarkson, T., Goodman, H., & Lofland, H. (1964). Aortic atherosclerosis in pigeons and its complications. *Archives of Pathology*, Vol. 77, 244-257

Qin, Z., & Nishimura, H. (1998). Ca2+ signaling in fowl aortic smooth muscle increases during maturation but is impaired in neointimal plaques. *Journal of Experimental Biology*, Vol. 201, 1695-1705

Rader, D.J., & Pure, E. (2000). Genetic susceptibility to atherosclerosis: insights from mice. Circulation Research, Vol. 86, 1013-1015

Randolph, R. & St. Clair, R. (1984). Pigeon aortic smooth muscle cells lack a functional low density lipoprotein receptor pathway. *Journal of Lipid Research*, Vol. 25, 888-902

Randolph, R., Smith, B., & St. Clair, R. (1984). Cholesterol metabolism in pigeon aortic smooth muscle cells lacking a functional low density lipoprotein receptor pathway. *Journal of Lipid Research*, Vol. 25, 903-912

Ridker, P. (2000). New clue to an old killer: inflammation and heart disease. *Nutrition Action* Vol. 27, 3-5

Roberts, J.C., Jr., & Straus, R., (Eds). (1965). *Comparative Atherosclerosis; the Morphology of Spontaneous and Induced Atherosclerotic Lesions in Animals and its Relation to Human Disease*, Harper & Row, New York

Ross, R., & Glomset, J.A. (1973). Atherosclerosis and the arterial smooth muscle cell. *Science*, Vol. 180, 1332-1339

Santamarina-Fojo, S., Remaley, A. T., Neufeld, E. B. & Brewer, H. B., Jr. (2001). Regulation and intracellular trafficking of the ABCA1 transporter. *Journal of Lipid Research*, Vol. 42, 1339-1345

Santerre, R., Nicolosi, R., & Smith, S. (1974). Respiratory control in preatherosclerotic susceptible and resistant pigeon aortas. *Experimental and Molecular of Pathology*, Vol. 20, 397-406

Santerre, R., Wight, T., Smith, S., & Brannigan, D. (1972). Spontaneous atherosclerosis in pigeons. A model system for studying metabolic parameters associated with atherogenesis. *American Journal of Pathology*, Vol. 67, 1-22

Schulz, J., Bermudez, A., Tomlinson, J., Firman, J., & He, Z. (2000). Blood plasma chemistries from wild mourning doves held in captivity. *Journal of Wildlife Diseases*, Vol. 36, 541-545

Scott, R., Kim, D., & Schmee, J. (1985). Endothelial and lesion cell growth patterns of early smooth-muscle cell atherosclerotic lesions in swine. *Archives of Pathology and Laboratory Medicine*, Vol. 109, 450-453

Seals, D.F., & Courtneidge, S.A. (2003). The ADAMs family of metalloproteases: multidomain proteins with multiple functions. *Genes and Development*, Vol., 17, 7-30

Shanahan, C.M., & Weissberg, P.L. (1998). Smooth muscle cell heterogeneity: patterns of gene expression in vascular smooth muscle cells in vitro and in vivo. *Arteriosclerosis, Thrombosis and Vascular Biology*, Vol. 18, 333-338

Shanahan, C.M., Carey, N.R., Osbourn, J.K., & Weissberg, P.L. (1997). Identification of osteoglycan as a component of the vascular matrix. *Arteriosclerosis Thrombosis and Vascular Biology*, Vol. 17, 2437-2447

Shao, B., Oda, M., Oram, J., & Heinecke, J. (2006). Myeloperoxidase: an inflammatory enzyme for generating dysfunctional high density lipoprotein. *Current Opinion in Cardiology*, Vol. 21, 322-328

Shi, W., Brown, M.D., Wang, X., Wong, J., Kallmes, D.F, Matsumoto, A.H., Helm, G.A., Drake, T.A., & Lusis, A.J. (2003). Genetic backgrounds but not sizes of atherosclerotic lesions determine medial destruction in the aortic root of apolipoprotein E-deficient mice. *Arteriosclerosis Thrombosis and Vascular Biology*, Vol. 23, 1901-1906

Shiomi, M., Ito, T., Yamada, S., Kawashima, S., & Fan, J. (2003). Development of an animal model for spontaneous myocardial infarction (WHHLMI Rabbit). *Arteriosclerosis Thrombosis and Vascular Biology*, Vol. 23, 1239-1244

Siekert, R., Dicke, B., Subbiah, M., & Kottke, B. (1975). Cholesterol balance in atherosclerosis-susceptible and atherosclerosis-resistant pigeons. *Research Communications in Chemical Pathology and Pharmacology*, Vol. 10, 181-184

Sigmund, C.D. (2000). Viewpoint: are studies in genetically altered mice out of control? *Arteriosclerosis Thrombosis and Vascular Biology*, Vol. 20, 1425-1429

Smith, J.D., Bhasin, J.M., Baglione, J., Settle, M., Xu, Y., & Barnard, J. (2006). Atherosclerosis susceptibility loci identified from a strain intercross of apolipoprotein E-deficient mice via a high-density genome scan. *Arteriosclerosis Thrombosis and Vascular Biology*, Vol. 26, 597-603

Smith, S. C., Smith, E. C. Gilman, M. L. Anderson, J. L., and Taylor, R. L., Jr. (2008). Differentially expressed soluble proteins in aortic cells from atherosclerosis-susceptible and resistant pigeons. *Poultry Science*, Vol. 87, 1328-1334

Smith, S.C., Smith, E.C., & Taylor, R.L., Jr. (2001). Susceptibility to spontaneous atherosclerosis in pigeons: an autosomal recessive trait. *Journal of Heredity*, Vol. 92, 439-442

Smith, S.C., Strout, R.G., Dunlop, W.R., & Smith, E.C. (1965). Fatty acid composition of cultured aortic smooth muscle cells from White Carneau and Show Racer pigeons. *Journal of Atherosclerosis Research*, Vol. 5, 379-387

St Clair, R. (1983). Metabolic changes in the arterial wall associated with atherosclerosis in the pigeon. *Federation Proceedings*, Vol. 42, 2480-2485

St Clair, R. (1998). The contribution of avian models to our understanding of atherosclerosis and their promise for the future. *Lab Animal Science*, Vol. 48, 565-568

St. Clair, R., Leight, M., & Barakat, H. (1986). Metabolism of low density lipoproteins by pigeon skin fibroblasts and aortic smooth muscle cells. comparison of cells from atherosclerosis- susceptible and atherosclerosis-resistant pigeons. *Arteriosclerosis Thrombosis and Vascular Biology*, Vol. 6, 170-177

Stary, H. (1989). Evolution and progression of atherosclerotic lesions in coronary arteries of children and young adults. *Arteriosclerosis, Thrombosis and Vascular Biology* Vol. 9, 19-32

Stein, O., Thiery, J., & Stein, Y. (2002). Is there a genetic basis for resistance to atherosclerosis? *Atherosclerosis*, Vol. 160, 1-10

Strong, J.P., Malcom, G.T., McMahon, C.A., Tracy, R.E., Newman, W.P., Herderick, E.E., & Cornhill, J.F. (1999). Prevalence and extent of atherosclerosis in adolescents and young adults: implications for prevention from the pathobiological determinants of atherosclerosis in youth study. *Journal of the American Medical Association*, Vol. 281, 727-735

Subbiah, M., & Connelly, P. (1976). Effect of dietary restriction on plasma cholesterol and cholesterol excretion in the White Carneau pigeon. *Atherosclerosis*, Vol. 24, 509-13

Subbiah, M., Schweiger, E., Deitmeyer, D., Gallon, L. & Sinzinger, H. (1980). Prostaglandin synthesis in aorta of atherosclerosis susceptible and atherosclerosis resistant pigeons. *Artery*, Vol. 8, 50-55

Suckling, K.E., & Jackson, B. (1993). Animal models of human lipid metabolism. *Progress in Lipid Research*, Vol. 32, 1-24

Sweetland, R. (1999). Lysosomal acid lipase activity in atherosclerosis susceptible and resistant pigeon aortas. *M.S. Thesis*, University of New Hampshire, Durham

Tall, A., Breslow, J.L., & Rubin, E.M. (2001). Genetic disorders affecting plasma high-density lipoproteins, In: *The Metabolic and Molecular Bases of Inherited Disease*, C.R. Scriver, A.L. Beaudet, W.S. Sly, & D. Valle, (Eds). pp 2915-2936, McGraw-Hill, ISBN 0079130356, New York

Thyberg, J., Hedin, U., Sjolund, M., Palmberg, L., & Bottger, B. (1990). Regulation of differentiated properties and proliferation of arterial smooth muscle cells. *Arteriosclerosis, Thrombosis and Vascular Biology*, Vol. 10, 966-990

Tovar, A. M. F., Cesar, D. C. F., Leta, G. C., & Mourao, P. A. S. (1998). Age-related changes in populations of aortic glycosaminoglycans : species with low affinity for plasma low-density lipoproteins, and not species with high affinity, are preferentially affected. *Arteriosclerosis Thrombosis and Vascular Biology*, Vol. 18, 604-614

Tsimikas, S., Willerson, J.T., & Ridker, P. M. (2006). C-Reactive protein and other emerging blood biomarkers to optimize risk stratification of vulnerable patients. *Journal of the American College of Cardiology*, Vol. 47, 19-31

Visvikis-Siest, S. & Marteau, J. (2006). Genetic variants predisposing to cardiovascular disease. *Current Opinion in Lipidology*, Vol. 17, 139-151

Wagner, W. D., Clarkson, T. B., Feldner, H. B., Lofland, H. B., & Prichard, R. W. (1973). The development of pigeon strains with selected atherosclerosis characteristics. *Experimental and Molecular Pathology*, Vol. 19, 304-319

Wagner, W. D., Conner, J., & Labutta, T. (1979). Blood pressure in atherosclerosis-susceptible and -resistant pigeons. *Proceedings of the Society for Experimental Biology & Medicine*, Vol. 162, 101-104

Wagner, W.D. (1978). Risk factors in pigeons genetically selected for increased atherosclerosis susceptibility. *Atherosclerosis*, Vol. 31, 453-463

Wang, S.S., Shi, W., Wang, X., Velky, L., Greenlee, S., Wang, M.T., Drake. T.A., & Lusis, A.J. (2007). Mapping, genetic isolation, and characterization of genetic loci that determine resistance to atherosclerosis in C3H mice. *Arteriosclerosis Thrombosis and Vascular Biology*, Vol. 27, 2671-2676

Warden, C.H., & Fisler, J.S. (1997). Integrated methods to solve the biological basis of common disease. *Methods in Enzymology*, Vol. 13, 347-357

Watanabe, Y., Ito, T., & Shiomi, M. (1985). The effect of selective breeding on the development of coronary atherosclerosis in WHHL rabbits. An animal model for familial hypercholesterolemia. *Atherosclerosis*, Vol. 56, 71-9

Weigensberg, B., Lough, J., & More, R. (1985). Modification of two types of cholesterol atherosclerosis in rabbits by blocking lipoprotein lysine epsilon-amino groups. *Atherosclerosis*, Vol. 57, 87-98

Wight, T. (1980). Differences in the synthesis and secretion of sulfated glycosaminoglycans by aorta explant monolayers cultured from atherosclerosis-susceptible and -resistant pigeons. *American Journal of Pathology*, Vol. 101, 127-142

Wight, T. (1985). Proteoglycans in pathological conditions: atherosclerosis. *Federation Proceedings*, Vol. 44, 381-385

Wight, T., Cooke, P., & Smith, S. (1977). An electron microscopic study of pigeon aorta cell cultures: cytodifferentiation and intracellular lipid accumulation. *Experimental and Molecular Pathology*, Vol. 27, 1-18

Wissler, R.W., Hiltscher, L., Oinuma, T., and the PDAY Research Group. (1996). The lesions of atherosclerosis in the young: from fatty streaks to intermediate lesions, In: *Atherosclerosis and Coronary Artery Disease*, V. Fuster, R. Ross, & E.J. Topol, (Eds). pp 475–489, Lippincott-Raven Press, ISBN 978-078-1702-66-9, New York

Worth, N., Rolfe, B., Song, J.& Campbell, G. (2001). Vascular smooth muscle cell phenotypic modulation in culture is associated with reorganisation of contractile and cytoskeletal proteins. *Cell Motility and Cytoskeleton*, Vol. 49, 130-145

Xu, Q. (2004). Mouse models of arteriosclerosis: from arterial injuries to vascular grafts. *American Journal of Pathology*, Vol. 165, 1-10

Yutzey, K.E., & Robbins, J. (2007). Principles of genetic murine models for cardiac disease. *Circulation*, Vol. 115, 792-799

Zemplenyi, T., & Rosenstein, A. (1975). Arterial enzymes and their relation to atherosclerosis in pigeons. *Experimental and Molecular of Pathology*, Vol. 22, 225-41

Zhang, S., Reddick, R., Burkey, B., & Maeda, N. (1994). Diet-induced atherosclerosis in mice heterozygous and homozygous for apolipoprotein E gene disruption. *Journal of Clinical Investigation*, Vol. 94, 937-945

Zhang, S., Reddick, R., Piedrahita, J., & Maeda, N. (1992). Spontaneous hypercholesterolemia and arterial lesions in mice lacking apolipoprotein E. *Science*, Vol. 258, 468-471

3

Mouse Models of Experimental Atherosclerosis as a Tool for Checking a Putative Anti-Atherogenic Action of Drugs

Jacek Jawien

Jagiellonian University School of Medicine, Chair of Pharmacology, Krakow,
Poland

1. Introduction

Studies concerning the pathogenesis of atherosclerosis entered a new phase at the turn of the 21st century. The 20th century was the age of cholesterol and lipoproteins, which has been concluded in a number of clinical studies carried out on a large scale, and they demonstrated unequivocally that normalization of hypercholesterolemia significantly decreased the incidence and mortality of coronary artery disease (Prevention of cardiovascular events and death with pravastatin in patients with coronary heart disease and a broad range of initial cholesterol levels. The Long-Term Intervention with Pravastatin in Ischaemic Disease (LIPID) Study Group. 1998; Scandinavian Simvastatin Survival Study Group. Randomised trial of cholesterol lowering in 4444 patients with coronary heart disease: The Scandinavian Simvastatin Survival Study (4S). 1994) Nearly to the end of the nineties, atherosclerosis had been assumed to develop as the so-called chronic response to injury (response-to-injury hypothesis) that resulted in the loss of endothelial cells which line the inner side of the vessels (Ross & Glomset, 1976).

Atherosclerosis had been considered first of all a degenerative disease (Ross et al., 1977; Ross et al. 1984; Ross, 1986). However, approximately 20 years ago, the trials started to focus to a large extent on another pathogenetic mechanism of atherosclerosis, not considered so far – the inflammatory process.

2. The first indications

In 1986, with the use of monoclonal antibodies, the small cells with round nucleus present in the atheromatous plaque, known before as "small monocytes", were demonstrated to be T lymphocytes (Jonasson et al., 1986). Several years later it was shown that these lymphocytes "recognize" as antigens the oxidized molecules of low-density lipoproteins (LDL) – oxLDL (Stemme et al., 1995). Moreover, the correlation between atherosclerosis and the presence of at least two types of infectious microorganisms: *Chlamydia pneumoniae* and *Herpes simplex virus* were observed (Thom et al., 1991; Hendrix et al., 1990). It raised the question if the inflammatory process participate in atherosclerosis. Speculations of this kind were initially received with great scepticism because there was no spectacular and unequivocal evidence of a significant role of inflammation in atherosclerosis.

This evidence was delivered by a new technique – gene targeting, for the invention of which Mario R. Capecchi (Italy), Martin J. Evans (United Kingdom) and Oliver Smithies (USA) received the Nobel Prize in Physiology or Medicine in 2007.

3. Additional evidence for the presence of inflammation in atherosclerosis

The newest model of atherosclerosis (described precisely at the end of the paper) enabled the investigators to create apoE-knockout mice, an ideal animal model to test the influence of singular proteins participating in the inflammatory response on the development of atherosclerosis. These studies showed, for example, that the absence of only one cytokine – interferon γ (IFN-γ), reduced atherosclerosis even by 60% (Gupta et al., 1997).

The overexpression of adhesive molecules (vascular adhesion molecule 1 and intercellular adhesion molecule 1) at sites with atheromatous changes was also observed in apoE-knockout mice (Nakashima et al., 1998). Monocyte chemotactic protein was shown to play an important part in the progression of atheromatous lesions (Aiello et al., 1999; Ni et al., 2001). Moreover, it was observed that interleukin-18 knockout decreased atherosclerosis by 35% (Elhage et al., 2003; Tenger et al., 2005).

Inhibition of CD40 signaling reduced atherosclerosis (Mach et al., 1998). This was explained by the fact that ligation of CD40 molecule (tumor necrosis factor α [TNF-α] receptor superfamily member) – found in the atheromatous plaque, on endothelial cells, vascular smooth muscle cells, antigen-presenting cells, platelets – with CD40L activates a number of transcription factors: NF-κB, AP-1, STAT-1 or Egr-1. Therefore, it influences, for example, the endothelial cell, which, in consequence, acquires proinflammatory and proatherosclerotic phenotype leading to the expression of adhesive molecules and tissue factor on its surface. It creates new possibilities of therapeutic approach, consisting in inhibition of the CD40–CD40L pathway (Welt et al., 2004; Alber et al., 2006; Tousoulis, et al. 2007). In mice the effect of CD40 is also antagonized by transforming growth factor β (Robertson et al., 2003).

Finally, in apoE-knockout mice with severe combined immunodeficiency (SCID) atherosclerosis was reduced by 70% in comparison to the control group, due to a significantly lower number of lymphocytes in mice with SCID. It was demonstrated that transfer of T cells to these mice aggravated atherosclerosis even by 164% (Zhou et al., 2000).

4. Atherosclerosis as an inflammatory process

These and other facts made the investigators realize unequivocally that inflammation was essential for atherogenesis. Therefore, in 1999, just before his death, Russell Ross (the author of the previous theory of atherosclerosis as a chronic response to injury) officially proclaimed that atherosclerosis was an inflammatory disease (Ross, 1999).

Whereas the deposition of atheromatous lipids and the accumulation of foam cells – macrophages filled with such lipids – in intima is the main morphological hallmark of atherosclerosis, the more subtle changes in the environment of the arterial wall, stimulated by the influx of inflammatory cells and local release of cytokines and other inflammatory mediators are currently recognized as the crucial causative factors of atherogenesis (Glass & Witztum, 2001; Binder et al., 2002).

Inflammation occurs in response to a factor that destabilizes the local homeostasis. The factors that cause Toll-like receptor dependent macrophage activation in the arterial wall include oxLDL, heat shock protein 60 (HSP60) and bacterial toxins (Hansson, 2005).

The first stage of atherogenesis consists in endothelial dysfunction (Ross, 1999). It involves first of all the regions of arterial bifurcations where the blood flow is not laminar. Hence, these localizations are prone to develop atherosclerosis. In such places LDL is stored in the subendothelial space. Low-density lipoprotein accumulation is increased if serum LDL level is elevated. Low-density lipoprotein is transported by passive diffusion and its accumulation in the vascular wall seems to depend on the interaction between apolipoprotein B of the LDL molecule and proteoglycans of the matrix (Boren et al., 1998).

There is evidence that unchanged LDL are "collected" by the macrophages too slowly to activate their transformation into foam cells. Therefore, it has been suggested that LDL molecule is "modified" in the vascular wall. The most significant modification is lipid oxidation, resulting in the formation of so-called "minimally oxidized" LDL (Gaut & Heinecke, 2001). The generation of these "aliens" for the body molecules leads to the development of inflammatory response, with participation of monocytes and lymphocytes in the first place (Fredrikson et al., 2003; Pentikäinen et al., 2000). The inflammation is triggered by accumulation of the minimally oxidized LDLs in the subendothelial space, thus stimulating the endothelial cells to produce a number of proinflammatory molecules (Lusis, 2000).

Before the "minimally oxidized" LDL have been phagocytised by the macrophages, they have to be modified into "highly oxidized" LDL. The scavenger receptors are responsible for the rapid uptake of the modified LDL (Suzuki et al., 1997).

During the following phase macrophages "present the antigen" to T lymphocytes. This antigen may be a fragment of oxidized LDL "digested" by the macrophages, HSP60, β2-glycoprotein I or the fragments of bacterial antigens (Hansson, 2001). The interaction between the immunological cells requires the presence of CD40 receptor on the surface of macrophages and its ligand CD40L on the surface of T lymphocytes (Schonbeck et al., 2000; Phipps et al., 2000). It is currently believed that the immunological response of Th1 type and its mediators: IFN-γ, TNF-α, interleukin-1, interleukin-12 as well as interleukin-18 accelerate atherosclerosis, whereas the response of Treg type and its mediators: interleukin-10 and TGF-β inhibit the development of atherosclerosis (Daugherty & Rateri, 2002; Laurat et al., 2001; Pinderski et al., 2002). Therefore, there has arisen an idea of vaccination as a future treatment against atherogenesis (Hansson, 2002).

The next phase of atherogenesis is the development of fibrous atheroma. The deposition of extracellular cholesterol and its esters is then intensified as well as the migration of smooth muscle cells from media to intima, proliferation of these cells and finally production of the extracellular matrix by the smooth muscles cells.

A stable atheromatous plaque is most commonly covered with a fairly thick fibrous layer, protecting the lipid nucleus from contact with the blood. In an unstable plaque there is a big lipid nucleus with a fairly thin fibrous layer. In atheromatous plaque, changed as described above, the proinflammatory factors produced by T lymphocytes (such as IFN-γ) seem to play a crucial role. They decrease production of the extracellular matrix by smooth muscles and at the same time increase production of the metalloproteinases by macrophages (Shishehbor & Bhatt, 2004).

5. Is atherosclerosis an autoimmunological disease?

The role of HSP60 as an initiator of atherogenesis is currently intensively investigated. Its "molecular mimicry" with HSP of *Chlamydia* has been observed (Wick et al., 1995).
Moreover, the anti-oxLDL antibodies resemble antiphospholipid antibodies, therefore the concept of atherosclerosis as an autoimmunological disease has been established (Hansson, 2001; Kobayashi K et al., 2007; Wick G et al., 2001). The investigators also emphasize a high pathogenetic similarity of atherosclerosis to rheumatoid arthritis (Shoenfeld et al., 2001).

6. The new experimental model of atherosclerosis

Since 1992 the mouse has become an excellent object for the studies on atherosclerosis, replacing the previous animal models. (Paigen et al., 1994; Moghadasian, 2002; Jawien et al., 2004).
Then, the first line of mice with a switched off gene for apolipoprotein E (apoE-knockout) was developed almost contemporaneously in two laboratories in the United States. (Piedrahita et al., 1992; Plump et al., 1992).
These mice were soon described as "reliable and useful, the best animal model of atherosclerosis in present times" (Meir & Leitersdorf, 2004).
During the generation of apoE-knockout mice (known also as apoE null or apoE deficient mice) the normal gene coding apolipoprotein E is replaced by a mutated gene which does not produce this molecule. Such mice are called apoE knockout because they have a knockout, switched-off, null or inactivated gene coding apolipoprotein E. For clarity, in the following sections of this paper we will use the most popular name: apoE-knockout mice.
The year 1992, in which apoE-knockout mice were invented by a homological exchange of genes, was a real breakthrough year in the studies on the pathogenesis of atherosclerosis (Savla, 2002).
The apoE-knockout mice were formed by homological recombination of embryonic stem cells. The changed cells were implanted into the blastocyst of a mouse of C57BL/6J strain which were subsequently implanted into the uterus. The offspring was a "chimera" that was next crossbred with a mouse of C57BL/6J strain (wild type), which led to the formation of apoE-knockout, homozygous mice in the second generation (Capecchi, 2001).
The inactivation of the gene coding apoE resulted in the formation of mice with a phenotype with a complete suppression of apoE, but with preservation of fertility and vitality (Breslow, 1996).
The apoE-knockout mice, in contrast to all of other animal models, develop atherosclerosis spontaneously, without high-cholesterol diet (Hansson et al., 2002).
The generation of such a model changed the nature of the studies on the pathogenesis of atherosclerosis and enabled the investigators to formulate a new definition of atherosclerosis as a chronic inflammation (Savla, 2002).
In a number of reports on atherogenesis published so far there has been a tendency to consider this process as the effect of dyslipidemia or inflammation alone. It is an erroneous dichotomy. It should be emphasized that atherosclerosis results from both lipid disorders and enhanced inflammation. Therefore, atherosclerosis is a chronic inflammatory disease, in most cases initiated and aggravated by hypercholesterolemia. In the review published in Nature Medicine hypercholesterolemia and inflammation were described as "partners in crime" (Steinberg, 2002).

The inflammatory concept of atherosclerosis has been formulated just in the recent years. However, it is currently an unquestionable achievement of science which also have specific therapeutic implications (Fan & Watanabe, 2003; Libby, 2000; Libby, 2002; Libby P et al., 2002; Jawien et al., 2006; Alpert & Thygesen, 2007).

7. Animal models of atherosclerosis

Atherosclerotic cardiovascular disease, the major cause of death in Western society, results from complex interactions among multiple genetic and environmental factors.

Numerous animal species have been used to study the pathogenesis and potential treatment of the lesions of atherosclerosis. The first evidence of experimental atherosclerosis came into view as early as in 1908 when Ignatowski (Ignatowski, 1908) reported thickening of the intima with formation of large clear cells in the aorta of rabbits fed with a diet rich in animal proteins (meat, milk, eggs). The most useful animal models have thus far been restricted to relatively large animals, such as nonhuman primates, swine, and rabbits. Hamsters and pigeons have been used occasionally but present problems peculiar to their species. Rats and dogs are not good models for atherosclerosis because they do not develop spontaneous lesions and require heavy modifications of diet to produce vascular lesion. Despite the fact that rabbits do not develop spontaneous atherosclerosis, they are useful because they are highly responsive to cholesterol manipulation and develop lesions in a fairly short time (Drobnik et al., 2000).

The lesions are much more fatty and macrophage-rich (inflammatory) than the human lesions and plasma cholesterol levels are extraordinarily high (very dissimilar to humans). Pigs and monkeys are better suited to model human atherosclerotic lesions. However, nowadays monkeys are not widely used due to obvious species - specific concerns (risk of extinction) and cost. The pig is a very good model - when fed with cholesterol, they reach plasma levels and atherosclerotic lesions that are quite similar to those seen in humans. Problems with the pig model are costs, the difficulties involved in maintaining the colonies and in their handling.

What has been traditionally lacking was a small, genetically reproducible, murine model of atherosclerosis. Such a model could help to overcome the many problems and deficiencies of larger animals and, in particular, would permit studies of possible therapies that require relatively large numbers of animals.

Until 1992, the majority of atherosclerotic research focused on mechanisms in rabbits, with a lesser number of studies in pigs and nonhuman primates. These large animal models have provided invaluable insight. The use of pig models of the disease initially revealed that monocyte infiltration was one of the primary cellular events in the atherogenic process (Gerrity, 1981).

Studies in monkeys and rabbits have been pivotal in defining the cellular events in the initiation and development of lesions (Faggiotto & Ross, 1984; Rosenfeld et al., 1987). In recent years, there has been an explosion in the number of *in vivo* studies that is largely attributable to the use of mouse models to study atherogenic mechanisms.

8. Mouse as a model of atherosclerosis

Mice are highly resistant to atherosclerosis. The only exception in mice is the C57BL/6 strain. When fed a very high cholesterol diet containing cholic acid, however, the vascular lesions in the C57BL/6 differ from the human condition in the histologic nature and location and are possibly attributed to a chronic inflammatory state rather than a genetic predisposition.

The earliest mouse model of atherosclerosis was the diet - induced model that was first characterized during the 1960s in Wissler's laboratory. Special diet contained 30% fat, 5% cholesterol, and 2% cholic acid led to atherosclerosis in C57BL/6 mice. However, this was a very toxic diet on which the mice lost weight and often got sick with morbid respiratory infections. Paigen et al. modified this diet by blending it one part to three parts with a 10% fat diet to yield what is called the "Paigen diet" which consists of 15% fat, 1.25% cholesterol, and 0.5% cholic acid (Paigen et al., 1985).

Although there were many uses of this model, there were also many disadvantages. The lesions are very small in mice at 4 to 5 months of age, in order of 200 to 1 000 square microns in the aortic root. The lesions are largely confined to the aortic root, and they usually do not develop beyond the early foam-cell, fatty-streak stage. The diet is also unphysiological with regard to its extremely high cholesterol content, 1.25%, and the presence of cholic acid. In addition, Lusis et al. have shown that this diet is in itself inflammatory, as leads to the induction of hepatic NF-kB activation and the expression of acute phase reactants, such as serum amyloid A (Liao et al., 1993).

Paigen et al. colleagues also developed assays that are widely used to quantify atherosclerosis in the mouse model. The most standard assay is the measurement of the cross-sectional lesion area in the aortic root (Paigen et al., 1987).

In this assay, freshly perfused and isolated hearts are fixed in formalin, embedded in gelatin, frozen, and cut into thin sections at anatomically defined sites in the aortic sinus and valve region. These sections are stained for lipids, and the lesion area is measured microscopically. Although this model has been widely employed and is of significant use in the study of atherosclerosis, the pathology of the lesions are not ideally suited as a model for human atherosclerosis. This shortcoming led many investigators to downplay the role of the mouse as a good model of atherosclerosis. Lesion formation in the diet - induced model is largely limited to the aortic root after feeding the Paigen - diet for periods of 14 weeks to 9 months. The lesions are quite small, only several hundred to a few thousand square micrometers, and they consist almost entirely of macrophage foam cells with little evidence for smooth muscle cell involvement. Thus, this model is largely limited to the fatty streak stage and does not progress to resemble human intermediate lesions.

For many years the mouse was not used as an experimental model for atherosclerosis research because of the beliefs that mice could not survive on high - fat atherogenic diets, that lesions were not reproducible, that most mice did not get lesions, and that lesion pathology did not resemble atherosclerosis in humans. However, the use of lower - fat diets solved the survival problem; the use of inbred strains rather than random - bred mice solved the reproducibility problem; the use of susceptible strains resulted in most mice getting lesions; and longer experimental times showed that lesions with fibrous caps were produced.

The following is a list of questions that can be used to judge the usefulness of animal models of atherosclerosis: 1) What is the nature of the experimental lesions and their similarity to human lesions; 2) is the plasma lipoprotein profile and metabolism similar to metabolism in humans; 3) what is the time frame necessary for lesions to form, and how long does it take to breed the animals for the studies; 4) what is the cost of acquiring and maintaining the animals; 5) what is the ability to perform in vivo manipulations and imaging; and 6) what is the ability of the model to take advantage of classical and molecular genetic approaches ?

The mouse as a model meets many of these criteria, but first it is important to acknowledge many important differences between mice and humans. The average lifespan of a mouse is about 2 years, compared to about 75 years in humans. Mice weigh much less, about 30 grams for the adult. The lipid profile in the mouse is very different from that in humans, who carry about 75% of their plasma cholesterol on LDL. Mice carry most of their cholesterol on high-density lipoprotein (HDL), which we know in humans is protective against atherosclerosis. Thus, mice fed their normal low-fat chow diet do not get atherosclerosis, while it is a common disease in humans. One difference, which is an advantage of all animal models, is the ability to control the environment and diet in mouse studies, which is impossible for long-term human studies. Human genetic studies are limited in range to various types of association studies. With mice, on the other hand, many additional kinds of genetic experiments are possible, including breeding and genetic engineering.

There are many advantages of using mice for experimental atherosclerosis research, including their relative ease and thriftiness to acquire and maintain. Their generation time is short, at about 9 weeks, 3 weeks for gestation and about 6 weeks until sexual maturity. It is easy to breed very large cohorts for experimental studies, and mice can develop atherosclerosis in a very short timeframe, as discussed below. Classical genetics in the mouse is very well established and is aided immensely by the availability of hundreds of inbred strains. Moreover, in 2002, The Mouse Genome Sequencing Consortium published the culmination of international efforts - a high quality sequence and analysis of the genome of the C57BL/6J mouse strain (Waterson et al., 2002).

With the coming of age of molecular genetics, it is now possible to add exogenous transgenes into mice, which can also be done in many other species. However, uniquely in mice, it is also possible to knock out or replace endogenous genes; this is one of the main advantages of working in the mouse model. The major disadvantage of the mouse model is their small size, which makes it difficult but not impossible to perform surgical manipulations and *in vivo* imaging. But there have been recent advances in these techniques that have overcome many of the size limitations, such as the ability to perform imaging of abdominal atherosclerotic lesions in living mice, cardiac catheterization to determine cardiovascular function in free-ranging mice, and surgical ligature of coronary arteries giving rise to myocardial ischemia.

9. Apolipoprotein E–knockout mice: A breakthrough

It has been a longstanding goal of many investigators around the world to create better mouse models for lipoprotein disorders and atherosclerosis and to identify genes that may modify atherogenesis and lesion progression. In 1992 apoE - deficient mice were generated by inactivating the apoE gene by targeting (Piedrahita et al., 1992).

They inactivated the apoE gene in mouse embryonic stem (ES) cells by homologous recombination. Two targeting plasmids were used, pJPB63 and pNMC109, both containing a neomycin-resistance gene that replaced a part of the apoE gene and disrupted its stucture. ES cell colonies targeted after electroporation with plasmids were identified by the polymerase chain reaction (PCR) followed by genomic Southern analysis. Chimeric mice were generated by blastocyst injection with targeted lines. They gave strong chimeras, which transmitted the disrupted apoE gene to their progeny. Mice homozygous for the disrupted gene were produced from the heterozygotes. The facts that homozygous animals have been born at the expected frequency and that they appeared to be healthy were important. They demonstrated that lack of apoE was compatible with normal development, and they also provided another tool for studies of the phenotypic consequences of apoE deficiency. At the same time another group created also apoE - deficient mice (Plump et al., 1992).

Mice homozygous or heterozygous for the disrupted apoE gene appeared healthy. No difference in their body weights compared to normal mice was observed. However, significant phenotypic differences between normal animals and the homozygous mutants were observed in their lipid and lipoprotein profiles. The apoE-knockout mice had markedly increased total plasma cholesterol levels, which were five times those of normal litter mates. These levels were unaffected by the age or sex of the animals. Although the total plasma cholesterol levels were greatly elevated in the mutants, the high density lipoprotein (HDL) cholesterol levels were only 45% the normal level. The triglyceride levels were 68% higher than those of normal animals. (These apoE-deficient mice have had a dramatic shift in plasma lipoproteins from HDL, the major lipoprotein in control mice, to cholesterol - enriched remnants of chylomicrons and VLDL.

Mice naturally have high levels of HDL and low levels of LDL, in contrast to humans who are high in LDL and low in HDL. In addition, mice apparently lack the cholesteryl ester transfer protein, en enzyme that transfers cholesterol ester from HDL to VLDL and LDL. Despite these differences, apoE - deficient mice have phenotypes remarkably similar to those of apoE - deficient humans.

A chronological analysis of atherosclerosis in the apoE - deficient mouse has shown that the sequential events involved in lesion formation in this model are strikingly similar to those in well - established larger animal models of atherosclerosis and in humans (Nakashima et al., 1994). Animals as young as 5-6 weeks of age have monocytic adhesions to the endothelial surface of the aorta that can be appreciated readily with electron microscopy (EM). EM also has demonstrated transendothelial migration of blood monocytes in similarly aged mice. By 6-10 weeks of age, most apoE - deficient mice have developed fatty - streak lesions comprised primarily of foam cells with migrating smooth muscle cells. These fatty - streak lesions rapidly progress to advanced lesions, which are heterogeneous but are typically comprised of a necrotic core surrounded by proliferating smooth muscle cells and varying amounts of extracellular matrix, including collagen and elastin.

These lesions have well - formed fibrous caps made up of smooth muscle cells and extracellular matrix that often have groups of foam cells at their shoulders. It is not uncommon for the inflammatory lesion to erode deep into the medial wall of the aorta, and some of these animals develop aortic aneurysms. Many of the lesions found in older mice develop calcified foci (Reddick et al., 1994).

Other characteristics of the lesions in the apoE - deficient mouse, such as indications of oxidative change, merit attention as well (Palinski et al., 1994).

The atherosclerotic lesions in this mouse contain oxidation - specific epitopes. In young lesions these epitopes are predominantly localized in macrophage - rich areas, whereas in advanced lesions they are localized in necrotic regions. In addition, high titers of antibodies against the oxidized epitopes are present in the plasma of the apoE - deficient mice.

The complexity of lesions in the apoE - deficient mouse, together with the benefits of using the mouse as a model of human disease, makes it a desirable system in which to study both environmental and genetic determinants of atherosclerosis. Initial studies examined the effects of grossly different diets on susceptibility to atherosclerosis in this animal. These studies confirmed the validity of this mouse as a model of human atherosclerotic disease and laid the groundwork for future dietary studies.

Hayek et al. developed a more physiological than Paigen diet - "western-type" diet for mouse studies, which is similar in composition to an average American diet of several years ago, consisting of 21% fat by weight, 0.15% cholesterol, and no cholic acid. When fed this diet, wild-type mice have a two-fold elevation in plasma cholesterol, while apoE-deficient mice have over a three-fold elevation, to about 2 000 mg/dl, again, mostly in βVLDL, but there is also an increase in LDL (Plump et al., 1992).

The post-prandial clearance of intestinally derived lipoproteins is dramatically impaired in apoE - deficient mice. The apoE - deficient mouse responds appropriately to a human - like western - type diet (Nakashima et al., 1994). On this diet, lesion formation is greatly accelerated and lesion size is increased. In 10-week old animals fed this diet for only 5 weeks, lesions are 3-4 times the size of those observed in mice fed a low - fat diet. In addition, monocytic adhesions and advanced lesions develop at a significantly earlier age. The results of this dietary challenge demonstrate that the mouse model responds in an appropriate manner, i.e. increased fat leads to increased plasma cholesterol, which in turn leads to increased atherosclerosis. Moreover, the data suggest that in addition to its histological similarity to humans, the mouse model exhibits a response to environmental cues resembling that of humans.

Lesions in the apoE-deficient mouse, as in humans, tend to develop at vascular branch points and progress from foam cell stage to the fibroproliferative stage with well-defined fibrous caps and necrotic lipid cores, although plaque rupture has not been observed in apoE - deficient mice or in any other mouse model. Progression of lesions appears to occur at a faster rate than in humans atherosclerosis; the rapidity of lesion progression can be advantageous in many experimental situations.

The genetic background has a major effect on atherosclerosis susceptibility in strains of apoE - deficient mice. For example, lesions from 16-week chow diet C57BL/6 apoE-KO were relatively larger than from FVB apoE-KO mice and in contrast to FVB mice there was evidence of early development of fibrous caps in these mice. In older mice, fibrous plaques from C57BL/6 apoE-KO mice were larger in size and had larger necrotic cores compared with FVB apoE-KO mice. Comparing humans and apoE - deficient mice, lesion progression and cell types are similar, as is the presence of oxidized lipoproteins. The major difference of this mouse model, as is the presence of oxidized lipoproteins. The major difference of this mouse model, as is the case for most of the other models of experimental atherosclerosis, is that plaque rupture is not observed, whereas plaque rupture is fairly common in humans and can lead to heart attacks. One potential reason for the lack of plaque rupture in mice is that the diameter of the aorta is less than 1 mm, which is even smaller than the diameter of the major coronary arteries in humans. As the vessel diameter decreases, the surface tension increases exponentially; thus, in the mouse there may be so much surface tension that plaque rupture would not be likely to occur.

ApoE-knockout mice are considered to be one of the most relevant models for atherosclerosis since they are hypercholesterolemic and develop spontaneous arterial lesions (Nakashima et al., 1994).

Heterozygous apoE-deficient mice do not exhibit elevated plasma cholesterol levels on the chow or Western-type diet, suggesting that when mice are fed a physiological diet, a 50% decrease in apoE is not sufficient to influence fasting plasma lipids (Van Ree et al., 1994).

The apoE-deficient mouse contained the entire spectrum of lesions observed during atherogenesis and was the first mouse model to develop lesions similar to those of humans. This model provided opportunity to study the pathogenesis and therapy of atherosclerosis in a small, genetically defined animal.

In 1995 Kashyap et al. (Kashyap et al., 1995) described the successful correction of apoE deficiency in apoE-deficient mice by using an alternative approach involving systemic delivery to mouse liver of recombinant adenovirus vectors expressing human apoE. Thus, the single genetic lesion causing apoE absence and severe hypercholesterolemia is sufficient to convert the mouse from a species that is highly resistant to one that is highly susceptible to atherosclerosis (Breslow, 1994).

The method of measure atherosclerosis by using the aortic root atherosclerosis assay was originally developed by Paigen et al. (Paigen et al., 1987). The aortic root cross sectioning assay is widely used in murine studies of atherosclerosis, allows for coincident inspection of lesion histology, and is amenable in studies using large numbers of mice. Alternative measures of atherosclerosis, such as the en face method, correlate with aortic root measurements. However, these methods are less amenable for studies using large numbers of mice and do not allow for inspection of lesion histology.

10. LDL receptor deficient mice

Gene targeting in embryonic stem cells has recently been used to create LDL receptor - knockout (LDLR-KO) mice, a model of familial hypercholesterolemia. LDL receptor - deficient mice was made in 1993 by Ishibashi et al. (Ishibashi et al.1993). These mice have a more modest lipoprotein abnormality than the apoE - deficient mice, with increases in LDL and VLDL cholesterol leading to a total plasma cholesterol of about 250 mg/dl on a chow diet. On this diet, and at that level of plasma cholesterol, LDL receptor - deficient mice do not get atherosclerosis. However, this is a very diet-responsive model. After these mice are fed the Paigen diet, their plasma cholesterol levels soar to about 1 500 mg/dl, and large atherosclerotic lesions form (Ishibashi et al., 1994). It has also been shown that feeding the less toxic western-type diet also leads to the development of large lesions, with plasma cholesterol levels of about 400 mg/dl. The lesion pathology in this model is not as well characterized as in the apoE - deficient model, but it does appear similar in that the lesions can progress beyond the foam - cell fatty-streak stage to the fibro-proliferative intermediate stage.

11. Other mouse models

Overexpression of human apoA-I in apoE - deficient mice increased HDL cholesterol levels twofold and substantially decreased fatty streak and advanced fibroproliferative lesion formation (Paszty et al. 1994; Plump et al., 1994).

By 4 months of age, all but 3-5% of apoE - deficient mice have had detectable fatty streaks that vary considerably in size; some are barely detectable, whereas others occlude as much as 8% of the aortic lumen. In apoE - deficient mice that overexpress human apoA-I, more than 50% of animals have no lesions by 4 months of age, and the animals that do develop atherosclerosis have lesions that are barley detectable. By 8 months of age, apoE - deficient mice have lesions that are highly organized and that occlude on average 25% of the aortic lumen. Those apoE - deficient mice that overexpress human apoA-I have mainly immature fatty - streak lesion that occlude on average only 5% of the aortic lumen. Collectively, these data suggest that overexpression of apoA-I can diminish lesion size and slow the initiation of fatty streak formation.

More recently, apoE and LDL-receptor (LDLr) double – knockout (apoE/LDLr-DKO) mice have been created (Ishibashi et al., 1994), representing a new mouse model that develops severe hyperlipidaemia and atherosclerosis (Bonthu et al., 1997).

It has been reported that, even on a regular *chow diet*, the progression of atherosclerosis is usually more marked in apoE/LDLr-DKO mice than in mice deficient for apoE alone (Witting et al., 1999).

Thus, the apoE/LDLr-DKO mouse is a suitable model in which to study the anti-atherosclerotic effect of compounds without having to feed the animals an atherogenic diet.

To study the contribution of endothelial nitric oxide synthase (eNOS) to lesion formation Kuhlencordt et al. (Kuhlencordt et al., 2001). created apoE / eNOS double - knockout mice. It has occured that chronic deficiency of eNOS increases atherosclerosis in apoE-KO mouse model. Furthermore, in the absence of eNOS, peripheral coronary disease, chronic myocardial ischemia, heart failure, and an array of vascular complications develop that have not been observed in apoE-KO animals.

Recently, Veniant et al. (Veniant et al., 2000) managed to even up the cholesterol levels in chow-fed apoE-KO mice and LDLR-KO mice. They did so by making both mouse models homozygous for the apolipoprotein B-100 allele, which ameliorates the hypercholesterolemia in the setting of apoE deficiency but worsens it in the setting of LDLR deficiency. Moreover, the LDLR-KO Apob100/100 mice developed extensive atherosclerosis even on a chow diet. So far this model seems to be the best as concerns the development of atherosclerosis in mice.

Therefore, gene - targeted mouse models has changed the face of atherosclerotic research (Savla U, 2002) and helped in creation of the new theory of atherosclerosis - as an inflammatory disease (Ross, 1999)

12. The experimental use of gene targeted mice

The apoE - deficient mouse model of atherosclerosis can then be used to: 1) identify atherosclerosis susceptibility modifying genes, by the candidate-gene and gene-mapping methods; 2) identify the role of various cell types in atherogenesis; 3) identify environmental factors affecting atherogenesis; and 4) assess therapies that might block atherogenesis or lesion progression.

ApoE-deficient mice have also been used to look for environmental and drug effects on atherosclerosis and to test novel therapies. One of the first observations was paradoxical effects of probucol on atherogenesis in both apoE-KO (Moghadasian et al., 1999) and LDL receptor deficient (Bird et al., 1998) mice. Probucol with strong antioxidant and cholesterol - lowering effects increased atherogenesis in apoE-KO mice by 3 folds (Moghadasian et al., 1999). Several other compounds reduced the extent and severity of atherosclerotic lesions without affecting plasma cholesterol levels in apoE–KO mice. For example, administration of antioxidant N,N'-diphenyl 1,4 - phenylenediamine (DPPD) to apoE-KO mice resulted in a significant decrease in atherosclerosis without reducing plasma cholesterol levels (Tangirala et al., 1995).

A marked reduction in atherosclerosis by dietary vitamin E was accompanied by no change in plasma cholesterol levels in apoE-KO mice (Pratico et al., 1998).

Likewise, antiatherogenic effects of the angiotensin - converting enzyme inhibitors (Hayek et al. 1998; Keidar et al. 2000; Hayek et al. 1999) or the angiotensin II receptor antagonist (Keidar et al. 1997) in apoE-KO mice were independent of plasma cholesterol lowering effects.

Since inflammation plays an important role in atherogenesis, during recent years it has become apparent that the 5-lipoxygenase (5-LO) pathway may take significant part in modifying the pathogenesis of atherosclerosis. Enzymes associated with the 5-LO pathway are abundantly expressed in arterial walls of patients afflicted with various lesion stages of atherosclerosis of the aorta and of coronary arteries. These data raised the possibility that antileukotriene drugs may be an effective treatment regimen in atherosclerosis (Mehrabian et al., 2002).

Of special interest for atherosclerosis is the arachidonate 5-LO which was originally identified in polymorphonuclear leukocytes, but which over-expression was recently demonstrated in macrophages, dendritic cells, foam cells, mast cells and neutrophils within atherosclerotic vessels. This enzyme generates an unstable epoxide intermediate compound leukotriene A4 (LTA4), which is an important precursor of LTB4, LTC4 and other cysteinyl leukotrienes. Initial observations and the use of drugs affecting the 5-LO metabolism were mainly connected with asthma and other inflammatory diseases (De Caterina & Zampolli, 2004).

However, a growing understanding of the role of inflammation in atherosclerosis has brought attention to the potential role of leukotrienes and their metabolism. In 2002 Mehrabian et al. identified the 5-LO as a crucial enzyme, contributing to atherosclerosis susceptibility in mice (Mehrabian et al., 2002; Spanbroek et al., 2003).

This observation, after a long pause (De Caterina R et al., 1988) has again focused the attention of researchers on the role of leukotrienes in the pathogenesis of atherosclerotic plaque (Radmark, 2003; Zhao & Funk, 2004; Zhao et al., 2004; Kuhn et al., 2005; Kuhn H, 2005; Lotzer et al., 2005; Back & Hansson, 2006; Radmark & Samuelsson, 2007). Therefore, the speculations have been risen that anti-asthmatic drugs could have beneficial effects on atherogenesis (Spanbroek & Habenicht, 2003; Wickelgren, 2004; Funk, 2005; Back, 2006).

Indeed, it has been recently demonstrated that the 5-LO substantially contribute to atherosclerosis in both mouse models and humans (Mehrabian & Allayee, 2003; Dwyer et al., 2004). Later Aiello et al. showed that LTB4 receptor antagonism reduced monocytic foam cells in mice (Aiello et al., 2002). Lotzer et al. pointed that macrophage-derived LTs differentially activate cysLT2-Rs via paracrine stimulation and cysLT1-Rs via autocrine and paracrine stimulation, during inflammation and atherogenesis (Lotzer et al., 2003).

Therefore, a hypothesis has been formulated that leukotriene-inhibiting drugs developed to treat asthma might protect the heart. There are numerous potential targets that could be useful in the intervention in leukotriene metabolism in atherosclerosis. Interestingly, the 18 kDa microsomal protein - five lipoxygenase activating protein (FLAP) was found to be critical for the regulation of 5-LO activity and biosynthesis of leukotrienes. The role of FLAP in atherosclerosis was additionally confirmed in humans by Helgadottir et al. (Helgadottir et al., 2004) who showed that genetic polymorphisms of FLAP are associated with myocardial infarction and stroke by increasing leukotriene production and inflammation in the arterial wall.

The 5-LO is abundantly expressed in atherosclerotic lesions of apoE and LDLR deficient mice, appearing to co-localize with a subset of macrophages but not with all macrophage-staining regions. Indeed, the results of our studies showed that the inhibition of FLAP by MK-886 or BAYx1005 can significantly prevent the development of atherosclerosis in gene-targeted apoE/LDLR-DKO mice (Jawien et al., 2006; Jawien et al., 2007).

Moreover, this study showed that cysteinyl leukotriene receptor blocker montelukast decreases atherosclerosis in apoE/LDLR-double knockout mice (Jawien et al., 2008). These results derived also from our numerous studies, concerned with atherosclerotic mice (Elhage et al., 2004; Elhage et al., 2005; Guzik et al., 2005; Jawien et al., 2005; Jawien et al., 2007).

The findings of the study concerning MK-886 were confirmed by Back et al. on their model of transgenic apoE-/- mice with the dominant negative transforming growth factor β type II receptor, which displays aggravated atherosclerosis (Back et al, 2007).

Colin D. Funk's research team questioned the hypothesis concerning leukotrienes, 5-LO and their role in atherogenesis in gene-targeted mice, stating that in mouse plaques there is no 5-LO overexpression detectable (Cao et al., 2008).

Finally, Poeckel & Funk in 2010, they tried to explain the whole complicated phenomenon.

13. Limitations of animal models

Animal models potentially bear the risk of compensatory mechanisms due to genetic modification of the target gene that render the results difficult to interpret. Another caveat is species differences between mice and humans. For instance, 5-LO expression in intimal atherosclerotic lesions varies between mice and humans; also, 5-LO and 12/15-LO appear to be differentially regulated in inflammatory cells of mice and humans with the murine 12/15-LO producing mainly 12-HPETE, while its human counterpart primarily synthesizes 15-HPETE. Notably, both products may have opposing effects in inflammation (Conrad DJ, 1999).

Moreover, atherogenesis in mice differs in several facets from the human pathology. Thus, T cells, whose presence in all stages of atherosclerotic lesions is acknowledged, are underrepresented in murine models of atherosclerosis (Daugherty & Hansson, as cited in Dean & Kelly, 2000; Roselaar et al., 1996).

Despite these shortcomings, animal models afford an invaluable means to study the effects of directed genetic overexpression, deletion or pharmacological inhibition of key enzymes of the LT cascade in a physiological setting that cannot be achieved in humans.

5-LO/LT pathway shows important disparities between murine and human atherosclerosis. Advanced human plaques show differences in 5-LO expression compared with mouse lesions. In human lesions, 5-LO (+) cells were identified in macrophages, DCs, mast cells, and neutrophils (Spanbroek et al, 2003) and notably, these 5-LO (+) cells are present in the neointimal region, whereas in mice, they are restricted to the adventitial layer (Zhao et al., 2004). With increasing age, these adventitial macrophages form clusters with T cells, independent of the severity of atherosclerosis. Intimal inflammatory reactions are connected to distinct adventitial inflammation responses, whereby B lymphocytes, plasma cells, and T cells conglomerate with macrophages. 5-LO (+) cells accumulate around new blood vessels, a common feature between mice and humans.

In human atherosclerotic plaque specimens, the quantity of 5-LO (+) cells even increased during progression from early to late phase coronary heart disease (Spanbroek et al., 2003).

Moreover, the elevated 5-LO activity was found to be associated with BLT1-mediated matrix metalloproteinase release from T cells, promoting plaque instability (Cipollone et al., 2005). Human lesions demonstrate detectable expression levels for all major components of the LT cascade, i.e., FLAP, LTA_4 hydrolase, and LTC_4 synthase, as well as BLT_1/BLT_2 and $CysLT_1/CysLT_2$ receptors.

Taken together, in advanced human atherosclerosis, a role for 5-LO is likely, which is distinct from its role in early atherogenesis. This presence of the 5-LO/LT pathway in advanced lesions is not found in mouse models, which might be due to: (i) rapid progression of atheroma growth in mice vs. slower, often interrupted progression in humans (i.e., initial fatty streaks might remain dormant for many years in humans, until certain factors promote the progression of some lesions into an advanced state) (Libby, 2006; Libby & Sasiela, 2006) (ii) advanced human plaques display a higher degree of instability and risk to rupture than murine plaques; (iii) temporal dissociation in the Th1/Th2 'balance' at distinct lesion stages between mice and humans (Kus et al., 2009; Toton-Zuranska et al., 2010; Smith et al. 2010).

14. Future directions

During the last few years there has been a resurgent focus on the 5-LO/LT pathway as a potential target in coronary vascular disease (CVD). The complexity of the 5-LO/LT pathway participation in mechanisms contributing to CVD is evident based on the many studies (Poeckel & Funk, 2010). Limitations of these studies often result from the 'snapshot' punctual nature of analysing a single time point in CVD pathogenesis that makes it difficult to gain systematic insight into 5-LO-driven or -independent processes.

Murine and human CVD etiology differ with respect to the 5-LO/LT pathway, and even within murine studies, the nature of the applied model (for atherosclerosis, abdominal aortic aneurysm (AAA), or ischemia/reperfusion injury) influences the conclusions. Whereas a role for 5-LO-derived LTs in early stages of murine and human atherosclerosis, AAA, and reperfusion injury is cogent based on their effects in chemotaxis and induction of pro-inflammatory responses, the 5-LO pathway appears to play a distinct role in advanced human atherosclerosis, but not in advanced murine disease. Targeting specific leukotriene G protein-coupled receptors rather than upstream targets involved in LT synthesis may be a superior strategy for future CVD therapeutic interventions, based on extensive past experience with other pathways (e.g., via angiotensin II and adrenergic receptors), although this remains to be determined. Conditional knockouts and comprehensive translational studies should serve better than the traditional, simplistic 'one model' approach to understand the complex effects exerted by 5-LO products. Understanding the cytokine milieu during distinct stages of CVD progression will be crucial to elucidate how the expression of members of the 5-LO/LT pathway is regulated. There is little doubt that 5-LO plays important roles in many facets of CVD, but the challenge for future studies will be to clearly dissect these activities in a temporal and cell- and tissue- specific context in order to provide a solid basis for potential therapeutic interventions.

15. Acknowledgments

This article was supported by the grant form Polish Ministry of Science and Higher Education nr: N N401548340 for the years 2011-2012.

16. References

Aiello R.J., Bourassa P.A., Lindsey S., et al. (1999). Monocyte chemoattractant protein-1 accelerates atherosclerosis in apolipoprotein E-deficient mice. *Arterioscler Thromb Vasc Biol*, 19, 1518-1525.

Aiello R.J., Bourassa P.A., Lindsey S., Weng W., Freeman A. & Showell HJ. (2002) Leukotriene B4 receptor antagonism reduces monocytic foam cells in mice. *Arterioscler Thromb Vasc Biol*, 22, 443-449.

Alber H.F., Frick M., Suessenbacher A., et al. (2006) Effect of atorvastatin on circulating proinflammatory T-lymphocyte subsets and soluble CD40 ligand in patients with stable coronary artery disease – a randomized, placebo-controlled study. *Am Heart J*, 151, 139.

Back M. (2006) Leukotrienes: potential therapeutic targets in cardiovascular diseases. *Bull Acad Natl Med*, 190, 1511-1518.

Back M. & Hansson G.K. (2006) Leukotriene receptors in atherosclerosis. *Ann Med*, 38, 493-502.

Back M., Sultan A., Ovchinnikova O. & Hansson GK. (2007) 5-lipoxygenase-activating protein. A potential link between innate and adaptive immunity in atherosclerosis and adipose tissue inflammation. *Circ Res*, 100, 946-949.

Binder CJ, Chang MK, Shaw PX, et al. (2002) Innate and acquired immunity in atherogenesis. *Nat Med*, 8, 1218-1226.

Bird D.A., Tangirala R.K., Fruebis J., Steinberg D., Witztum J.L., & Palinski W. (1998) Effect of probucol on LDL oxidation and atherosclerosis in LDL receptor - deficient mice. *J Lipid Res*, 39: 1079-1090.

Bonthu S., Heistad D.D., Chappell D.A., Lamping K.G., & Faraci F.M. (1997) Atherosclerosis, vascular remodeling, and impairment of endothelium - dependent relaxation in genetically altered hyperlipidemic mice. *Arterioscler Thromb Vasc Biol*, 17, 2333-2340

Boren J., Olin K., Lee I., et al. (1998) Identification of the principal proteoglycan-binding site in LDL. A single-point mutation in apo-B100 severly affects proteoglycan interaction without affecting LDL receptor binding. *J Clin Invest*, 101, 2658-2664.

Breslow J.L. (1994) Lipoprotein metabolism and atherosclerosis susceptibility in transgenic mice. *Curr Opin Lipidol*, 5: 175-184.

Breslow J.L. (1996) Mouse models of atherosclerosis. *Science*, 272, 685-688.

Cao R.Y., St Amand T., Grabner R., Habenicht A.J., & Funk C.D. (2008) Genetic and pharmacological inhibition of the 5-lipoxygenase/leukotriene pathway in atherosclerotic lesion development in apoE deficient mice. *Atherosclerosis*, 203, 395-400.

Capecchi M.R. (2001) Generating mice with targeted mutations. *Nature Med*, 7, 1086-1090.

Cipollone F., Mezzetti A., Fazia M.L., et al. (2005) Association between 5-lipoxygenase expression and plaque instability in humans. *Arterioscler Thromb Vasc Biol*, 25, 1665-1670.

Conrad D.J. (1999) The arachidonate 12/15 lipoxygenases. A review of tissue expression and biologic function. *Clin Rev Allergy Immunol*, 17, 71-89.

Daugherty A. & Hansson G.K. (2000) Lymphocytes in atherogenesis, In: *Atherosclerosis*, RT Dean R.T & Kelly D., pp. 230-249, New York, Oxford Press.

Daugherty A., & Rateri D.L. (2002) T lymphocytes in atherosclerosis. The Yin-Yang of Th1 and Th2 influence on lesion formation. *Circ Res*, 90, 1039-1040.

De Caterina R., Mazzone A., Giannessi D., Sicari R., Pelosi W., Lazzerini G., Azzara A., Forder R., Carey F. & Caruso D. (1988) Leukotriene B4 production in human atherosclerotic plaques. *Biomed Biochim Acta*, 47, S182-S185.

De Caterina R. & Zampolli A. (2004) From asthma to atherosclerosis - 5-lipoxygenase, leukotrienes, and inflammation. *N Engl J Med*, 350, 4-7.

Dwyer J.H., Allayee H., Dwyer K.M., et al. (2004) Arachidonate 5-lipoxygenase promoter genotype, dietary arachidonic acid, and atherosclerosis. *N Engl J Med*, 350, 29-37.

Elhage R., Jawien J., Rudling M., et al. (2003) Reduced atherosclerosis in interleukin-18 deficient apolipoprotein E-knockout mice. *Cardiovasc Res*, 59, 234-240.

Elhage R., Gourdy P., Brouchet L., et al. (2004) Deleting TCR alpha beta+ or CD+ T lymphocytes leads to opposite effects on site-specific atherosclerosis in female apolipoprotein E - deficient mice. *Am J Pathol*, 165, 2013-2018.

Elhage R., Gourdy P., Jawien J., et al. (2005) The atheroprotective effect of 17-estradiol depends on complex interactions in adaptive immunity. *Am J Pathol*, 167, 267-274.

Faggiotto A. & Ross R. (1984) Studies of hypercholesterolemia in the nonhuman primate. II. Fatty streak conversion to fibrous plaque. *Arteriosclerosis*, 4, 341-356.

Fan J. & Watanabe T. (2003) Inflammatory reaction in the pathogenesis of atherosclerosis. *J Atheroscler Thromb*, 10, 63-71.

Fredrikson G.N., Soderberg I., Lindholm M., et al. (2003) Inhibition of atherosclerosis in apoE null mice by immunization with apoB-100 peptide sequences. *Arterioscler Thromb Vasc Biol*, 23, 879-884.

Funk C.D. (2005) Leukotriene modifiers as potential therapeutics for cardiovascular disease. *Nature*, 4, 664-672.

Gaut J.P. & Heinecke J.W. (2001) Mechanisms for oxidizing low-density lipoprotein. Insights from patterns of oxidation products in the artery wall and from mouse models of atherosclerosis. *Trends Cardiovasc Med*, 11, 103-112.

Glass C.K. & Witztum J.L. (2001) Atherosclerosis: the road ahead. *Cell*, 104, 503-516.

Gupta S., Pablo A.M., Jiang X., et al. (1997) IFN-gamma potentiates atherosclerosis in ApoE knock-out mice. *J Clin Invest*, 99, 2752-2761.

Hansson G.K. (2001) Immune mechanisms in atherosclerosis. *Arterioscler Thromb Vasc Biol*, 21, 1876-1890.

Hansson G.K. (2002) Vaccination against atherosclerosis: science or fiction? *Circulation*, 106, 1599-1601.

Hansson G.K. (2005) Inflammation, atherosclerosis, and coronary artery disease. *N Engl J Med*, 352, 1685-1695.

Hansson G.K., Libby P., Schonbeck U., & Yan ZQ. (2002) Innate and adaptive immunity in the pathogenesis of atherosclerosis. *Circ Res*, 91, 281-291.

Hayek T., Attias J., Coleman R. et al. (1999) The angiotensin - converting enzyme inhibitor, fosinopril, and the angiotensin II receptor antagonist, losartan, inhibit LDL oxidation and attenuate atherosclerosis independent of lowering blood pressure in apolipoprotein E deficient mice. *Cardiovasc Res*, 44, 579-587.

Helgadottir A., Manolescu A., Thorleifsson G., et al. (2004) The gene encoding 5-lipoxygenase activating protein confers risk of myocardial infarction and stroke. *Nat Genet*, 36, 233-239.

Hendrix M.G., Salimans M.M., van Boven C.P., & Bruggeman CA. (1990) High prevalence of latently present cytomegalovirus in arterial walls of patients suffering from grade III atherosclerosis. *Am J Pathol*, 136, 23-28.

Ignatowski A.C. (1908) Influence of animal food on the organism of rabbits. *S Peterb Izviest Imp Voyenno-Med. Akad*, 16, 154-173.

Ishibashi S., Brown M.S., Goldstein J.L., Gerard R.D., Hammer R.E., & Herz J. (1993) Hypercholesterolemia in low density lipoprotein receptor knockout mice and its reversal by adenovirus – mediated gene delivery. *J Clin Invest*, 92, 883-893.

Ishibashi S., Herz J., Maeda N., Goldstein J.L., & Brown MS. (1994) The two-receptor model of lipoprotein clearance: tests of the hypothesis in "knockout" mice lacking the low density lipoprotein receptor, apolipoprotein E, or both proteins. *Proc Natl Acad Sci USA*, 91, 4431-4435.

Jawien J., Nastalek P. & Korbut R. (2004) Mouse models of experimental atherosclerosis. *J Physiol Pharmacol*, 55, 503-517.

Jawień J., Gajda M., Mateuszuk L., et al. (2005) Inhibition of nuclear factor-kappaB attenuates artherosclerosis in apoE/LDLR - double knockout mice. *J Physiol Pharmacol*, 56, 483-489.

Jawien J., Gajda M., Rudling M., et al. (2006) Inhibition of five lipoxygenase activating protein (FLAP) by MK-886 decreases atherosclerosis in apoE/LDLR double knockout mice. *Eur J Clin Invest*, 36, 141-146.

Jawien J., Gajda M., Olszanecki R. & Korbut R. (2007) BAYx1005 attenuates atherosclerosis in apoE/LDLR - double knockout mice. *J Physiol Pharmacol* 58: 583-538.

Jawien J., Csanyi G., Gajda M., et al. (2007) Ticlopidine attenuates progression of atherosclerosis in apolipoprotein E and low density lipoprotein receptor double knockout mice. *Eur J Pharmacol*, 556, 129-135.

Jawien J., Gajda M., Wolkow P.P., Zuranska J., Olszanecki R. & Korbut R. (2008) The effect of montelukast on atherogenesis in apoE/LDLR - double knockout mice. *J Physiol Pharmacol*, 59, 633-639.

Jawień J. (2008) New insights into immunological aspects of atherosclerosis. *Pol Arch Med Wewn*, 118, 127-131.

Jawień J. (2009) The putative role of leukotrienes in experimental atherogenesis. *Pol Arch Med Wewn*, 119, 90-93.

Jawień J. & Korbut R. (2010) The current view on the role of leukotrienes in atherogenesis. *J Physiol Pharmacol*, 61: 647-650.

Jonasson L., Holm J., Skalli O., et al. (1986) Regional accumulations of T cells, macrophages, and smooth muscle cells in the human atherosclerotic plaque. *Arteriosclerosis*, 6, 131-138.

Kashyap V.S., Samantarina-Fojo S., Brown D.R. et al. (1995) Apolipoprotein E deficiency in mice: gene replacement and prevention of atherosclerosis using adenovirus vectors. *J Clin Invest*, 96, 1612-1620.

Keidar S., Attias J., Smith J., Breslow J.L, & Hayek T. (1997) The angiotensin-II receptor antagonist, losartan, inhibits LDL lipid peroxidation and atherosclerosis in apolipoprotein E – deficient mice. *Biochem Biophys Res Comm*, 236, 622-625.

Keidar S., Attias J., Coleman R., Wirth K., Scholkens B., & Hayek T. (2000) Attenuation of atherosclerosis in apolipoprotein E - deficient mice by ramipril is dissociated from its antihypertensive effect and from potentiation of bradykinin. *J Cardiovasc Pharmacol* 35, 64-72.

Kobayashi K., Tada K., Itabe H., et al. (2007) Distinguished effects of antiphospholipid antibodies and anti-oxidized LDL antibodies on oxidized LDL uptake by macrophages. *Lupus*, 16: 929-938.

Kuhlencordt P.J., Gyurko R., Han F. et al. (2001) Accelerated atherosclerosis, aortic aneurysm formation, and ischemic heart disease in apolipoprotein E/endothelial nitric oxide synthase double knockout mice. *Circulation* 104: 448-454.

Kuhn H. (2005) Biologic relevance of lipoxygenase isoforms in atherogenesis. *Expert Rev Cardiovasc Ther*, 3, 1099-1110.

Kuhn H., Romisch I. & Belkner J. (2005) The role of lipoxygenase isoforms in atherogenesis. *Mol Nutr Food Res*, 49, 1014-1029.

Kus K., Gajda M., Pyka-Fosciak G., et al. (2009) The effect of nebivolol on atherogenesis in apoE - knockout mice. *J Physiol Pharmacol*, 60, 163-165.

Laurat E., Poirier B., Tupin E., et al. (2001) In vivo downregulation of T helper cell 1 immune responses reduces atherogenesis in apolipoprotein E-knockout mice. *Circulation*, 104, 197-202.

Liao F., Andalibi A., deBeer F.C. et al. (1993) Genetic control of inflammatory gene induction and NF kappa B-like transcription factor activation in response to an atherogenic diet in mice. *J Clin Invest*, 91, 2572-2579.

Libby P. (2000) Changing concepts of atherogenesis. *J Intern Med*, 247, 349-358.

Libby P. (2002) Inflammation in atherosclerosis. *Nature*, 420, 868-874.

Libby P., Ridker P.M., & Maseri A. (2002) Inflammation and atherosclerosis. *Circulation*, 105, 1135-1143.

Libby P. (2006) Atherosclerosis: disease biology affecting the coronary vasculature. *Am J Cardiol*, 98, 3Q-9Q.

Libby P. & Sasiela W. (2006) Plaque stabilization: can we turn theory into evidence? *Am J Cardiol*, 98, 26P-33P.

Lotzer K., Spanbroek R., Hildner M., et al. (2003) Differential leukotriene receptor expression and calcium responses in endothelial cells and macrophages indicate 5-lipoxygenase dependent circuits of inflammation and atherogenesis. *Arterioscler Thromb Vasc Biol*, 23, e32-e36.

Lotzer K., Funk C.D. & Habenicht A.J. (2005) The 5-lipoxygenase pathway in arterial wall biology and atherosclerosis. *Biochim Biophys Acta*, 1736, 30-37.

Lusis A.J. (2000) Atherosclerosis. *Nature*, 407, 233-241.

Mach F., Schönbeck U., Sukhova G.K., et al. (1998) Reduction of atherosclerosis in mice by inhibition of CD40 signalling. *Nature*, 394, 200-203.

Mehrabian M., Allayee H., Wong J., Shi W., Wang X.P., Shaposhnik Z., Funk C.D. & Lusis A.J. (2002) Identification of 5-lipoxygenase as a major gene contributing to atherosclerosis susceptibility in mice. *Circ Res*, 91, 120-126.

Mehrabian M. & Allayee H. (2003) 5-lipoxygenase and atherosclerosis. *Curr Opin Lipidol*, 14, 447-457.

Meir K.S., Leitersdorf E. (2004) Atherosclerosis in the apolipoprotein E – deficient mouse. A decade of progress. *Arterioscler Thromb Vasc Biol*, 24, 1006-1014.

Moghadasian M.H., McManus B.M., Godin D.V., Rodrigues B., & Frohlich J.J. (1999) Proatherogenic and antiatherogenic effects of probucol and phytosterols in apolipoprotein E - deficient mice. Possible mechanisms of action. *Circulation*, 99, 1733-1739.

Moghadasian M.H. (2002) Experimental atherosclerosis: a historical overview. *Life Sci*, 70, 855-865.

Nakashima Y., Plump A.S., Raines E.W., Breslow J.L., & Ross R. (1994) ApoE - deficient mice develop lesions of all phases of atherosclerosis throughout the arterial tree. *Arterioscler Thromb*, 14: 133-140.

Nakashima Y., Raines E.W., Plump A.S., et al. (1998) Upregulation of VCAM-1 and ICAM-1 at atherosclerosis-prone sites on the endothelium in the ApoE-deficient mouse. *Arterioscler Thromb Vasc Biol*, 18, 842-851.

Ni W., Egashira K., Kitamoto S., et al. (2001) New anti-monocyte chemoattractant protein-1 gene therapy attenuates atherosclerosis in apolipoprotein E-knockout mice. *Circulation*, 103, 2096-2101.

Olszanecki R., Jawień J., Gajda M., et al. (2005) Effect of curcumin on atherosclerosis in apoE/LDLR – double knockout mice. *J Physiol Pharmacol*, 56, 627-635.

Paigen B., Morrow C., Brandon C., et al. (1985) Variation in susceptibility to atherosclerosis among inbtred strains of mice. *Atherosclerosis* 57: 65-73.

Paigen B., Morrow A., Holmes P.A., Mitchell D., & Williams R.A. (1987) Quantitative assessment of atherosclerotic lesions in mice. *Atherosclerosis*, 68, 231-240.

Paigen B., Plump A.S. & Rubin E.M. (1994) The mouse as a model for human cardiovascular disease and hyperlipidemia. *Curr Opin Lipidol*, 5, 258-264.

Palinski W., Ord V.A., Plump A.S., Breslow J.L., Steinberg D., & Witztum J.L. (1994) ApoE - deficient mice are a model of lipoprotein oxidation in atherogenesis. Demonstration of oxidation – specific epitopes in lesions and high titers of autoantibodies to malondialdehyde - lysine in serum. *Arterioscler Thromb*, 14, 605-616.

Paszty C., Maeda N., Verstuyft J., & Rubin E.M. (1994) Apolipoprotein AI transgene corrects apolipoprotein E deficiency - induced atherosclerosis in mice. *J Clin Invest*, 94, 899-903.

Pentikäinen M.O., Öörni K., Ala-Korpela M., & Kovanen P.T. (2000) Modified LDL-trigger of atherosclerosis and inflammation in the arterial intima. *J Intern Med*, 247, 359-370.

Piedrahita J.A., Zhang S.H., Hagaman J.R., Oliver P.M. & Maeda N. (1992) Generation of mice carrying a mutant apolipoprotein E gene inactivated by gene targeting in embryonic stem cells. *Proc Natl Acad Sci USA*, 89, 4471-4475.

Phipps R.P. (2000) Atherosclerosis: the emerging role of inflammation and the CD40-CD40L system. *Proc Natl Acad Sci*, 97, 6930-6932.

Pinderski L.J., Fischbein M.P., Subbanagounder G., et al. (2002) Overexpression of interleukin-10 by activated T lymphocytes inhibits atherosclerosis in LDL receptor-deficient mice by altering lymphocyte and macrophage phenotypes. *Circ Res*, 90, 1064-1071.

Plump A.S., Smith J.D., Hayek T., et al. (1992) Severe hypercholesterolemia and atherosclerosis in apolipoprotein E – deficient mice created by homologous recombination in ES cells. *Cell*, 71, 343-353.

Plump A.S., Scott C.J., & Breslow J.L. (1994) Human apolipoprotein A-I gene expression increases high density lipoprotein and suppresses atherosclerosis in the apolipoprotein E - deficient mouse. *Proc Natl Acad Sci USA*, 91, 9607-9611.

Poeckel D. & Funk CD. (2010) The 5-lipoxygenase/leukotriene pathway in preclinical models of cardiovascular disease. *Cardiovasc Res*, 86, 243-253.

Pratico D., Tangirala R.K., Rader D.J., Rokach J., & Fitzgerald G.A. (1998) Vitamin E suppresses isoprostane generation in vivo and reduces atherosclerosis in apoE - deficient mice. *Nature Med*, 4, 1189-1192.

Prevention of cardiovascular events and death with pravastatin in patients with coronary heart disease and a broad range of initial cholesterol levels. The Long-Term Intervention with Pravastatin in Ischaemic Disease (LIPID) Study Group. (1998) *N Engl J Med*, 339, 1349-1357.

Radmark O. (2003) 5-lipoxygenase-derived leukotrienes. Mediators also of atherosclerotic inflammation. *Arterioscler Thromb Vasc Biol*, 23, 1140-1142.

Radmark O. & Samuelsson B. (2007) 5-lipoxygenase: regulation and possible involvement in atherosclerosis. *Prostaglandins Other Lipid Mediat*, 83, 162-174.

Reddick R.L., Zhang S.H., & Maeda N. (1994) Atherosclerosis in mice lacking apoE. Evaluation of lesional development and progression. *Arterioscler Thromb*, 14, 141-147.

Robertson A.K., Rudling M., Zhou X., et al. (2003) Disruption of TGF-beta signaling in T cells accelerates atherosclerosis. *J Clin Invest*, 112, 1342-1350.

Roselaar S.E., Kakkanathu P.X. & Daugherty A. (1996) Lymphocyte populations in atherosclerotic lesions of apoE -/- and LDL receptor -/- mice. Decreasing density with disease progression. *Arterioscler Thromb Vasc Biol*, 16, 1013-1018.

Rosenfeld M.E., Tsukada T., Chait A. et al. (1987) Fatty streak expansion and maturation in Watanabe heritable hyperlipidemic and comparably hypercholesterolemic fat-fed rabbits. *Arteriosclerosis* 1987, 7, 24-34.

Ross R. & Glomset J.A. (1976) The pathogenesis of atherosclerosis. *N Engl J Med*, 295, 369-377.

Ross R., Glomset J., & Harker L. (1977) Response to injury and atherogenesis. *Am J Pathol*, 86, 675-684.

Ross R., Faggiotto A., Bowen-Pope D., & Raines E. (1984) The role of endothelial injury and platelet and macrophage interactions in atherosclerosis. *Circulation*, 70, 77-82.

Ross R. (1986) The pathogenesis of atherosclerosis – an update. *N Engl J Med*, 314, 488-500.

Ross R. (1999) Atherosclerosis – an inflammatory disease. *N Eng J Med*, 340, 115-126.

Savla U. (2002) At the heart of atherosclerosis. *Nat Med*, 8, 1209.

Scandinavian Simvastatin Survival Study Group. Randomised trial of cholesterol lowering in 4444 patients with coronary heart disease: The Scandinavian Simvastatin Survival Study (4S). 1994. *Lancet* 344: 1383-1389.

Schonbeck U., Sukhova G.K., Shimizu K., et al. (2000) Inhibition of CD40 signaling limits evolution of established atherosclerosis in mice. *Proc Natl Acad Sci USA*, 97, 7458-7463.

Shishehbor M.H. & Bhatt D.L. (2004) Inflammation and atherosclerosis. *Curr Atheroscler Rep*, 6: 131-139.

Shoenfeld Y., Sherer Y., & Harats D. (2001) Atherosclerosis as an infectious, inflammatory and autoimmune disease. *TRENDS Immunol*, 22, 293-295.

Smith D.D., Tan X., Tawfik O., Milne G., Stechschulte D.J. & Dileepan K.N. (2010) Increased aortic atherosclerotic plaque development in female apolipoprotein E-null mice is associated with elevated thromboxane A2 and decreased prostacyclin production. *J Physiol Pharmacol*, 61, 309-316.

Spanbroek R., Grabner R., Lotzer K., et al. (2003) Expanding expression of the 5-lipoxygenase pathway within the arterial wall during human atherogenesis. *Proc Natl Acad Sci USA*, 100, 1238-1243.

Spanbroek R. & Habenicht A.J. (2003) The potential role of antileukotriene drugs in atherosclerosis. *Drug News Perspect*, 16, 485-489.

Steinberg D. (2002) Atherogenesis in perspective: hypercholesterolemia and inflammation as partners in crime. *Nat Med*, 8, 1211-1217.

Stemme S., Faber B., Holm J., et al. (1995) T lymphocytes from human atherosclerotic plaques recognize oxidized low density lipoprotein. *Proc Natl Acad Sci USA*, 92, 3893-3897.

Suski M., Olszanecki R., Madej J., et al. (2011) Proteomic analysis of changes in protein expression in liver mitochondria in apoE knockout mice. *J Proteomics*, 74, 887-893.

Suzuki H., Kurihara Y., Takeya M., et al. (1997) A role for macrophage scavenger receptors in atherosclerosis and susceptibility to infection. *Nature*, 386, 292-296.

Tangirala R.K., Casanada F., Miller E., Witztum J.L., Steinberg D., & Palinski W. (1995) Effect of the antioxidant N,N' - diphenyl 1,4-phenylenediamine (DPPD) on atherosclerosis in apoE - deficient mice. *Arterioscler Thromb Vasc Biol*, 15, 1625-1630.

Tenger C., Sundborger A., Jawien J., & Zhou X. (2005) IL-18 accelerates atherosclerosis accompanied by elevation of IFN-gamma and CXCL16 expression independently of T cells. *Arterioscler Thromb Vasc Biol*, 25, 791-796.

Thom D.H., Wang S.P., Grayston J.T., et al. (1991) Chlamydia pneumoniae strain TWAR antibody and angiographically demonstrated coronary artery disease. *Arterioscler Thromb*, 11, 547-551.

Toton-Zuranska J., Gajda M., Pyka-Fosciak G., et al. (2010) AVE 0991 - angiotensin-(1-7) receptor agonist, inhibits atherogenesis in apoE-knockout mice. *J Physiol Pharmacol*, 61, 181-183.

Tousoulis D., Antoniades C., Nikolopoulou A., et al. (2007) Interaction between cytokines and sCD40L in patients with stable and unstable coronary syndromes. *Eur J Clin Invest*, 37, 623-628.

Van Ree J.H., van der Broek W., Dahlmans V. et al. (1994) Diet-induced hypercholesterolemia and atherosclerosis in heterozygous apolipoprotein E - deficient mice. *Atherosclerosis*, 111, 25-37.

Veniant M.M., Withycombe S., & Young SG. (2000) Lipoprotein size and atherosclerosis susceptibility in Apoe-/- and Ldlr-/- mice. *J Clin Invest*, 106, 1501-1510.

Waterson R.H., Lindblad-Toh K., Birney E., et al. (2002) Initial sequencing and comparative analysis of the mouse genome. *Nature*, 420, 520-562.

Welt F.G., Rogers S.D., Zhang X., et al. (2004) GP IIb/IIIa inhibition with eptifibatide lowers levels of soluble CD40L and RANTES after percutaneous coronary intervention. *Catheter Cardiovasc Interv*, 61, 185-189.

Wick G., Schett G., Amberger A., et al. (1995) Is atherosclerosis an immunologically mediated disease? *Immunol Today*, 16: 27-33.

Wick G., Perschinka H., & Millonig G. (2001) Atherosclerosis as an autoimmune disease: an update. *TRENDS Immunol*, 22, 665-669.

Wickelgren I. (2004) Gene suggests asthma drugs may ease cardiovascular inflammation. *Science*, 303: 941.

Witting P.K., Pettersson K., Ostlund-Lindqvist A.M., Westerlund C., Eriksson A.W., & Stocker R. (1999) Inhibition by a coantioxidant of aortic lipoprotein lipid peroxydation and atherosclerosis in apolipoprotein E and low density lipoprotein receptor gene double knockout mice. *FASEB J*, 13, 667-675.

Zhang S.H., Reddick R.L., Piedrahita J.A., & Maeda N. (1992) Spontaneous hypercholesterolemia and arterial lesions in mice lacking apolipoprotein E. *Science*, 258, 468-471.

Zhao L. & Funk C.D. (2004) Lipoxygenase pathways in atherogenesis. Trends Cardiovasc Med, 14, 191-195.

Zhao L., Moos M.P., Gräbner R., Pédrono F., Fan J., Kaiser B., John N., Schmidt S., Spanbroek R., Lötzer K., Huang L., Cui J., Rader D.J., Evans J.F., Habenicht A.J. & Funk C.D. (2004) The 5-lipoxygenase pathway promotes pathogenesis of hyperlipidemia dependent aortic aneurysm. Nat Med, 10, 966-973.

Zhou X., Nicoletti A., Elhage R., Hansson G.K. (2000) Transfer of CD4(+) T cells aggravates atherosclerosis in immunodeficient apolipoprotein E knockout mice. *Circulation*, 102, 2919-2922.

4

Parametric Determination of Hypoxic Ischemia in Evolution of Atherogenesis

Lawrence M. Agius
Department of Pathology, Mater Dei Hospital, Tal-Qroqq,
University Of Malta Medical School, Msida,
Malta

1. Introduction

Atherosclerosis constitutes a primarily destructive phenomenon inherently arising from dynamics of pathobiologic effect within the intima of elastic and muscular arteries. It is significant to view the development of elevated intimal lesions within dimensions of ongoing further injury to the endothelium.

Considerable interactivity evolves within plaques in consequence to neovascularization in particular. The outline evolution of individual atherosclerotic plaques would considerably modulate the dynamics of migration of smooth muscle cells to the intima and as a consequence of various agonists such as hypoxia, growth factors and coagulation-anticoagulation-fibrinolysis systems. Also, insulin appears to exert toxicity on the vascular wall and possibly promote atherogenesis (Nandish et al., 2011).

2. System pathways of injury

System pathways constitute a representative sequence of events that depend on dysfunctional activation of endothelial cells. It is within scope of parameters of permeability and loss of endothelial cells that a full plethora of forms of injury converge as intimal cell proliferation and as deposition of protein matrix proteoglycans. Oxidative stress and chronic inflammation promote diabetes, hypertension and atherosclerosis (Sewon et al., 2011).

The individual roles played by various agonist actions in the definition of the atherosclerotic plaque would evolve within the specificity of focal injury to the intima in particular. The convergence of such injuries appears a constitutive attribute of the variable expression of sequence prototypes in lesion demarcation.

Developmental parameters of modelling include the delineation of individual pathogenic events in terms that integrally reconstitute the modified anatomy of the individual atherosclerotic plaque. In this regard, Ghrelin improves endothelial function, lowers blood pressure and regulates atherosclerosis (Zhang et al., 2011).

Significance in terms of complicated plaques as constitutive pathways in modelling of plaques includes the essential interactivity of endothelium with smooth muscle cell trophic effect. Macrophages in particular implicate a series of converging events that sequentially re-define in repetitive form the dynamics of atherogenesis. Dyslipidemmia increases lipid content in foam cells found in atherosclerotic plaques (Wong et al., 2011).

Growth factors are instrumental in terms of the emerging morphologic features of the early atherosclerotic plaque and as derivative phenomena of endothelial injury and permeability. The constitutive parameters of re-distribution of trophic effect particularly interact with neovascularization within the plaque core.

Developmental sequences of multifactorial type in atherogenesis are particularly prone to a staged outline evolution that permeates the intima and sustains injury to the endothelium. Such significant interactivity contributes to outline emergence of new sequences in trophic effect and as proliferation and migration of smooth muscle cells.

The macrophage is central to such interactivity and operates primarily in chemotaxis and trophism, and also in terms that dominantly influence in significant fashion the attributes of lipid foam cells. Plant-derived alpha-linolenic acid, for example, restricts plaque T-cell proliferation, differentiation and inflammatory activity (Winnik et al., 2011).

3. Focality of inflammation

The inflammatory infiltrates include a representative response to injury as atherogenesis further compounds injury to the vascular intima. The role of endothelium is implicated as dysfunctional response with increased permeability to monocytes in particular. Proteoglycans retain lipoproteins subendothelially (Anggraeni et al., (2011).

Such recruitment of novel forms of injury includes the transforming ability of protein matrix proteoglycans as integral constitution of the injurious agents. It is within the dimensional redistribution of such injury that the endothelium plays a prominent role in sequence selectivity and in modulation of parameters of redefinition of activated dysfunctional states of inflammatory cells within the plaque.

The focality of injury is particularly significant within the neovascularized core of the individual plaque and as parameters in the growth and maturation of smooth muscle cells. Reparative processes allow for a sequential remodelling within such system pathways as coagulation and cellular migration within the vascular intima.

The variability of delineation of injurious agents indicates an activation of new parameters as the plaque evolves. The overall confines further extend parameters in plaque modelling that permits responsive elements in the creation of multiple sequence pathways that evolve in their own right; for example, deletion of microsomal prostaglandin E2 synthase-1 retards atherogenesis (Wang et al., 2011).

4. The individual smooth muscle cell/macrophage

The secretory dynamics of smooth muscle cells and of macrophages attribute a central pathogenic role to foam cells within the intima. Both smooth muscle cells and macrophages are recognized source for foam cells that, in turn, predominate in the mature atheromatous plaque. On the other hand, the matrix proteoglycans are also central players in re-defining attributes of the injured endothelium.

The reactivity of macrophages within the protein matrix that accumulate within the intima allows for the emergence of multiple converging agonists that characterize endothelial cell activation. The development of subsequent new forms of injury transforms such endothelial dysfunctionality as parameters of maturation of the plaque. Interleukin 18 is involved in plaque destabilization and regulates the innate immune response (Yamaoka-Tojo et al., 2011).

The central core of the plaque is one dominated by influences exerted by transformations in terms of neovascularization and as compounded maturation leading to lipid core formation within the plaque. Insulin resistance and cardiovascular pathology may share a common genetic background (Bacci et al., 2011).

It is highly significant to view the trophic attributes of injury to the endothelium as source of the evolutionary traits of emerging atherosclerotic plaques; indeed, Insulin-like growth factor-1 stabilizes the atherosclerotic plaque by altering smooth muscle phenotype (von der Thusen et al., 2011). Stages in sequence pathway maturation are central to the outline demarcation of individual plaques in a manner that depends integrally on dynamics of neovascularization of the plaque core.

Hemodynamic shear stress contributes to a redistribution of actin microfilaments within endothelial cells in a manner that modulates dysfunctional issues of activated endothelium.

5. Cellular proliferative kinetics

A proliferative smooth muscle cellular response is further significant in the maturation of the atherosclerotic plaque within such sequence steps as redefined injury to the endothelium.

Stages in preparation for subsequent events in the outline of the atherogenesis process would include the delivery of injurious agents to the intima. The sequence pathways are significant parametric factors in defining the dimensions of the endothelial participation in atherogenesis. Endoplasmic reticulum stress and the unfolded protein response characterize endothelial susceptibility to atherogenesis (Civelek et al., 2011).

It is further to the evolving forms of agonist action that atherogenesis modifies in repeatedly staged sequence the pathways of dysfunctional activation of the endothelium.

6. Low-density lipoproteins

Neovascularization proves to be a centrally operative agonist in the modified development of atheroma formation and deposition. The added parameters of consequence appear to implicate a primarily evolutionary role for hypoxia and ischemia as plaque re-definition, both morphologically and in dysfunctional forms of endothelial activation.

The inflammatory nature of the intimal deposits elicits a responsive panorama that implicates derivative attributes of low density lipoproteins and cholesterol and as extended participation of the neovascularization of the plaque. MicroRNA-29a targets lipoprotein lipase in oxidized low density lipoprotein and modulates cytokines and scavenger receptors (Chen et al., 2011)

Hypoxia is itself essential for the formation of new vessels within the plaque with the production of growth factors and would additionally contribute to the intimal thickening as further evidence for staged representation of injury to the intima.

Directional re-orientation of active dysfunctional states of endothelial cells compounds hypoxia and ischemia within the vascular intima. By-products of matrix proteoglycans and of lipid metabolism indicate the essential staging events in plaque maturation and as derivative phenomenon to further atherogenesis. Chemokines produced by endothelial cells are associated with leukocyte recruitment and angiogenesis in atherosclerosis (Speyer & Ward, 2011).

7. Intimal remodeling

It is as remodelling of the injury to the intima that hypoxia and ischemia further modulate the migration of smooth muscle cells within the intima. The increased permeability of the endothelium is significant as a redefined series of further injuries to the underlying intima.

The orientational redistribution of the agonists in atherogenesis redefine a central plaque contribution to increasing profiles of further hypoxia/ischemia and as evidential remounting of parameters of sequence effect. The multi-factorial injurious events are converging agonists in hypoxic/ischemic core regions of the individual atherosclerotic plaque. In such manner, the multi-staged evolution of plaques correlates with interactive dynamics of further injury within the intima.

Dynamics of action of oxidized lipids correlate closely with emerging new roles for agonist action in developing plaques. The interaction of variably participating agonists contrast with the intimal emergence of incremental hypoxia/ischemia in terms of increasing matrix proteoglycan deposition and cellular proliferation of smooth muscle cells in particular. Atherosclerosis affecting different topographic sites correlate with the type of hyperlipidemia (Van Craeyveld et al., 2011).

The platelet/coagulation systems are incremental sequence events as trophic influence in staged convergence of multiple agonists in intimal injury.

Distributional parameters are particularly significant in the dimensional targeting of the intima in terms of the vasa vasorum supplying the arterial wall.

Component systems of sequential impact would contribute to the emergence of positive feedback effect in agonist action. The endothelial cells participate by the production of various agents such as growth factors, in particular Platelet-Derived Growth Factor. The semblance of such influence dominantly re-characterizes the atherosclerotic plaque that trophically redefines the form of hypoxic/ischemic injury to the intima. miRNA –mediated epigenetic regulation may be implicated in atherogenesis, involving oxidized low-density lipoproteins (Chen et al., 2011).

8. Hemodynamics

Hemodynamics within the neovascularized core of the plaque allows for a developmental evolution in terms of so-called complications such as hemorrhage and rupture of the plaque and as staged representation of the endothelial cell injury. Consequential pathways of significance would confirm the agonist nature of hypoxia/ischemia in terms of further emergence of intimal deposition and of cellular proliferation and migration.

A response to injury permits role redefinition as emerging parameters in pathogenesis of the deposition of proteoglycans within the vascular intima. Matrix metalloproteinases participate in plaque destabilization and rupture. Their overexpression is an independent factor in the pathogenesis of acute coronary syndromes (Kulach et al., 2010). A proliferative response in particular illustrates the nature of the vascular wall injury that incrementally progresses as gradients of hypoxia and ischemia within the vessel wall.

9. Gradient parameters

Consequential involvement of the lipid deposition phenomenon integrally permits the establishment of gradient parameters of hypoxia/ischemia within the operative fields of emerging neovascularization in the plaque core.

Procedural and technical specificity of individual plaques illustrate dynamic turnover within plaques in terms particularly of agonists and cellular parameters in redefinition of atherogenesis. In this regard, Interferon-alpha upregulates expression of scavenger-A in monocytes/macrophages with foam cell formation (Li et al., 2011).

The specificity of the inflammatory response is sequentially consequent to the inter-changeability of agonist-induced parameters in creating a microenvironment of hypoxia and ischemia centered on the intima.

10. Cellular endothelial injury

The contributing roles of endothelium especially in cases of trauma to the vessel wall would indicate the prototypical attributes in lesion emergence and of subsequent maturation of the atherogenesis phenomenon. Atherogenesis is contributory phenomenon to an ongoing migratory involvement of the intima. This is well-testified by smooth muscle cells that synthesize and secrete matrix proteoglycans, and oxidative stress also induces production of superoxide by endothelial cells with nitric oxide synthase uncoupling (Zweier et al., 2011).

Significant participation in atherogenesis involves mirror-imaged targeting of multiple component systems within the vessel wall that developmentally integrate as regions of hypoxia and ischemia, including the thioredoxin system that correlates with cellular apoptosis in endothelial cell lines in hypoxic stress (Park et al., 2011). Neovascularization proves a permissive phenomenon in development of gradients of ischemia that redefine the individual plaque as compounding parameters of progression to further injury to the vascular wall.

Permissive dynamics are characteristic of oxidation of lipids and particularly of low-density lipoproteins and as evolution of deposition within the intima. Targeting of subsets of cells indicates a selectivity process of progression within sequential pathways of incremental further injury to the vessel wall. Disrupted endoplasmic reticulum equilibrium engages the unfolded protein response in such cells as monocytes (Carroll et al., 2011).

11. Vulnerability issues

System reproduction indicates vulnerability selectivity in the evolution of atheromatous plaques in terms ranging from cell kinetics to proliferative migration of smooth muscle cells directed to the intima and a sensitivity of endothelial cells to responsive pathway generation and trophic factor production. The macrophage system is especially representative of novel pathway events that induce a sequential series of models in manipulative further compromise of viability of the endothelial cells.

Within such scopes of pathogenic representation, there would emerge a parametric remodelling based on aberrant reconstitution of injury as further projected by responses to injury to the intima and endothelium. Within such context, the unfolded protein response is implicated in all stages of atherogenesis and plaque progression (Lhotak et al., 2011).

12. Pathway activation

The operative essentiality of the intimal involvement in atheroma formation calls into operation the developmental dimensions of both endothelium and also of medial smooth muscle cells. The sequence attributes of multiple different pathways contribute to the subsequent emergence of activation phenomena as well represented by the macrophage and foam cell systems. Mast cells, macrophages and neutrophils release TNF-alpha, IFN-gamma and IL-6 with expression of adhesion molecules and leukocyte recruitment (Zhang et al., 2011). Synthetic and contractile phenotypes of the individual smooth muscle cell indicate specialized forms of series determination in reconstitution of the damaged or injured subintima and also modelled parametric fashioning of the overlying endothelium. Hemodynamics of blood flow localizes such injured endothelium as representative and constitutive foci of persistent pathway activation that delivers dysfunctional attributes to the multi-components of the early atheromatous plaque.

13. Eventual sequence emergence

Contrasting sequentiality is triggered by an aberrant selectivity for trophic effect reproduction in terms of ongoing creation of hypoxia/ischemic gradients across both the endothelium lining the vascular lumen and also within critical regions of operative effect in the involved vascular intima. Such representation calls into evidence gradient pathways of projected reproduction that specifically induce focality of involvement of the plaque within systems of cascade effect. A complex interaction of genetic and environmental factors operates (Chyu & Shah, 2011)

The platelet and coagulation systems conclusively demonstrate a participating series of roles culminating in organization of adherent thrombus within the plaque as incorporated dynamics of trophic potential.

Incremental attributes of further compromise of the viability of the intima are demonstrable as evidential pathways of increasing impact in terms of enhanced intimal thickness. In this regard, cells proliferate in atherosclerotic lesions and also in vascular tissue bordering the plaque (Zettler et al., 2010).

Scope of representative projection is conclusively constituted by the end-stage plaque with a central atheromatous core that consists of cholesterol lipid, lipoprotein and oxidized molecular entities of variable derivation. Increasing representation of inflammatory dynamics is largely dependent on initiating events within the foci of intima underlying dysfunctionally activated endothelium. The dynamics of spread and of replication of individual endothelial cells constitutes a further pathway model for gradient creation between flowing blood and vascular wall intima. Pancoronary arterial instability implicates multifocal disease in acute coronary syndromes (Puri et al., 2011).

14. Concluding remarks

Re-distribution and retargeting events are primary modelling systems in sequence pathways and as multi-staged involvement of the intima of arterial vessel walls. The intimal thickness and remodelling of pathways allow for incremental redistribution of agonists that target differential systems such as endothelium and smooth muscle cells. Macrophages are constitutive systemic parameters that focally re-orientate the targeting dynamics of hypoxia and ischemia in intimal lesion creation. Oxidation-specific epitopes present on apoptotic cells induce the selection of Pattern Recognition Receptors and damage-associated molecular patterns that may be targeted by innate immunity (Miller et al., 2011).

Only in terms of ensuing neovascularization of the individual atherosclerotic plaque can system specificity in atherogenesis permit the emergence of converging pathways of injury and attempted reconstitution of the vessel wall and endothelium.

Macrophages induce transformational events within micro-environmental conditions of propagated susceptibility patterns that relate in particular to selective sites of vascular involvement such as near-arterial branch points of exit. It is such representation that illustrates the evolving vulnerability of focal sites of intima and endothelium in the generation of multiple atheromatous plaques; these subsequently promote self-involvement in dynamic transformation to the so-called complicated plaque.

Regional pathways of spread and further expansion contrast with the maturation of plaque morphology within such systems as macrophage and endothelial cell activation, with the creation of the synthetic/secretory phenotype of the individual smooth muscle cell within the intima.

Distributional dynamics in generation of the atheromatous plaque are developmental issues as indicated by activation of the proto-oncogenes c-fos and c-myc. The considerable heterogeneity of component cell subpopulations within any atheromatous plaque also permits the emergence of monoclonal groups of smooth muscle cells that trophically sustain growth of the plaque within dimensional confines of the involved intima and of injured overlying endothelium.

Hypoxia-ischemia is a powerful component series of systems in evolution of the susceptibility pattern determination of plaque localization and remodelling, as well-typified by the marked eventual thickening of the involved intima.

Gradient generation is a key mechanistic system in generation of projected effects of hypoxia-ischemia that coordinate the convergence of injurious agonists in terms of trophic and destructive elements within the intima of the arterial wall.

15. References

Anggraemi VY, Emoto N, Yagi K, Mayasari DS, Nakayama K, Izumikawa T et al. "Correlation of C4ST-1 and ChGn-2 expression with chondroitin sulphate chain elongation in atherosclerosis" Biochem Biophys Res Commun 2011 Jan 29.

Bacci S, Rizza S, Prudente S, Spoto B, Powers C, Facciorusso A et al. "The ENPPI Q121 variant predicts major cardiovascular events in high-risk individuals: evidence for interaction with obesity in diabetic patients" Diabetes 2011 Jan31.

Carroll TP, Greene CM, McEloaney NG "Measurement of the unfolded protein response (UPR) in monocytes" Methods Enzymol 2011;489:83-95.

Chen KC, Wang YS, Hu CY, Chang WC, Liao YC, Dai CY et al. "OxLDL up-regulates microRNA-29b, leading to epigenetic modifications of MMP-2/MMP-9 genes: a novel mechanism for cardiovascular diseases" FASEB J 2011 Jan25.

Chen T, Li Z, Tu J, Zhu W, Ge J, Zheng X et al. "MicroRNA-29a regulates pro-inflammatory cytokine secretion and scavenger receptor expression by targeting LPL in oxLDL-stimulated dendritic cells" FEBS Lett 2011 Jan27.

Chyu KY, Shah PK "Emerging therapies for atherosclerosis prevention and management" Cardiol Clin 2011 Feb;29(1):123-35.

Civelek M, Manduchi E, Grant GR, Stoeckert CJ Jr, Davies PF "Discovery approaches to UPR in athero-susceptible endothelium in vivo" Methods Enzymol 204;489:109-26.

Kulach A, Dabek J, Glogowska-Ligus J, Garczorz W, Gasior Z "Effects of standard treatment on the dynamics of matrix metalloproteinases gene expression in patients with acute coronary syndromes" Pharmacol Rep 2010 Nov-Dec;62(6):1108-16.

Lee S, Park Y, Zuidema MY, Hannink M, Zhang C "Effects of interventions on oxidative stress and inflammation of cardiovascular diseases" World J Cardiol 2011 Jan 26;3(1):18-24.

Lhotak S, Zhou J, Austin RC "Immunohistochemical detection of the unfolded protein response in atherosclerotic plaques" Methods Enzymol 2011;489:23-46.

Li J, Fu Q, Cui H, Qu B, Pan W, Shen N et al. "Interferon-alpha priming promotes lipid uptake and macrophage-derived foam cell formation: A novel link between interferon-alpha and atherosclerosis in lupus" Arthritis Rheum 2011 Feb;63(2):492-502.

Miller YI, Choi SH, Wiesner P, Fang L, Harkewicz R, Hartvigsen K et al. "Oxidation-specific epitopes are danger-associated molecular patterns recognized by pattern recognition receptors of innate immunity" Circ Res 2011 Jan21; 108(2):235-48.

Nandish S, Barlon O, Wyatt J, Smith J, Stevens A, Lujan M et al. "Vasculotoxic effects of insulin and its role in atherosclerosis: what is the evidence?" Curr Atheroscler Rep 2011 Feb2.

Park KJ, Kim YJ, Choi EJ, Park NK, Kim GH, Kim SM et al. "Expression pattern of the thioredoxin system in human endothelial progenitor cells and endothelial cells under hypoxic injury" Korean Circ J 2010 Dec;40(12):651-8.

Puri R, Worthley MI, Nicholls SJ "Intravascular imaging of vulnerable coronary plaque: current and future concepts" Nat Rev Cardiol 2011 Jan25.

Speyer CL, Ward PA "Role of endothelial chemokines and their receptors during inflammation" J Invest Surg 2011;24(1):18-27.

Van Craeyveld E, Gordts SC, Jacobs F, DeGeest B "Correlation of atherosclerosis between different topographic sites is highly dependent on the type of hyperlipidemia" Heart Vessels 2011 Jan26.

Von der Thusen JH, Borensztajn KS, Mormas S, van Heiningen S, Teeling P, van Berkel TJ et al. "IGF-1 has plaque stabilizing effects in atherosclerosis by altering vascular smooth muscle cell phenotype" Am J Pathol 2011 Feb;178 | (2):924-34.

Wang M, Ihida-Stansbury K, Kothapalli D, Tamby MC, Yn Z, Chen L et al. "Microsomal prostaglandin E2 synthase-1 modulates the response to vascular injury" Circulation 2011 Jan31.

Winnik S, Lohmann C, Richter EK, Schafer N, Song WL, Leiber F etal., „Dietary {alpha}-linolenic acid diminishes experimental atherogenesis and restricts T-cell-driven inflammation" Eur Heart J 2011 Jan31.

Wong BX, Kyle RA, Croft KD, Quinn CM, Jessup W, Yeap BB "Modulation of macrophage fatty acid content and composition by exposure to dyslipidemia serum in vitro" Lipids 2011 Feb1.

Yamaoka-Tojo M, Tojo T, Wakaume K, Kameda R, Nemoto S et al. "circulating interleukin-18: A specific biomarker for atherosclerosis-prone patients with metabolic syndrome" Nutr Metab (Lond) 2011 Jan20;8(1):3.

Zettler ME, Merchant MA, Pierce GN « Augmented cell cycle protein expression and kinase activity in atherosclerotic rabbit vessels » Exp Clin Cardiol 2010 Winter ;15(4) :e139-44.

Zhang G, Yin X, Qi Y, Pendyale L, Chen J, Hou D et al. «Ghrelin and cardiovascular diseases «

Zhang J, Alcaide P, Liu L, Sun J, He A, Luscinskas FV et al. « Regulation of endothelial cell adhesion molecule expression by mast cells, macrophages, and neutrophils » PLoS One 2011 Jan14 ;6(1) :e14525.

Zweier J, Chen CA, Druhan LJ "S-Glutathionylation reshapes our understanding of eNOS uncoupling and NO/ROS mediated signaling" Antioxid Redox Signal 2011 Jan24.

5

Endothelial and Vascular Smooth Cell Dysfunctions: A Comprehensive Appraisal

Luigi Fabrizio Rodella and Rita Rezzani
Anatomy Section, Department of Biomedical Sciences and Biotechnology,
University of Brescia,
Italy

1. Introduction

Cardiovascular disease (CvDs) such as coronary artery disease, hypertension, congestive heart failure and stroke are the leading causes of death and disability in the Western World (Madamanchi et al., 2005; Thom, 1989). The majority of CvDs results from complication of atherosclerosis. Prevention of cardiovascular events is therefore urgently needed and is one of the major recent challenges of medicine. New molecular imaging approaches featuring the assessment of inflammatory processes in the vascular wall (on top of existing anatomic and functional vessel imaging procedures) could emerge as decisive tools for the understanding and prevention of cardiovascular events (Schafers et al., 2010).

2. Atherosclerosis

Atherosclerosis is a progressive disease, affecting medium and large-sized arteries, characterized by patchy intramural thickening of the subintimal that encroaches on the arterial lumen (Bonomini et al., 2008). The atherosclerosis plaque is characterized by an accumulation of lipid in the artery wall, together with infiltration of macrophages, T cells and mast cells, and the formation by vascular smooth muscle cells (VSMCs) of a fibrous cap composed mostly of collagen. Early lesions called "fatty streaks" consist of sub-endothelial deposition of lipid, macrophage foam cells loaded with cholesterol and T cells. Over time, a more complex lesion develops, with apoptotic as well as necrotic cells, cell debris and cholesterol crystals forming a necrotic core in the lesion. This structure is covered by a fibrous cap of variable thickness, and its "shoulder" regions are infiltrated by activated T cells, macrophages and mast cells, which produce proinflammatory mediators and enzymes (Hansson et al., 2006). Plaque growth can cause stenosis (narrowing of the lumen) that can contribute to ischemia in the surrounding tissue (Hansson & Hermansson, 2011).

Although the pathophysiological mechanisms underlying atherosclerosis are not completely understood, it is widely recognized that both inflammation and oxidative stress play important roles in all of the phases of atherosclerosis evolution (Cipollone et al., 2007).

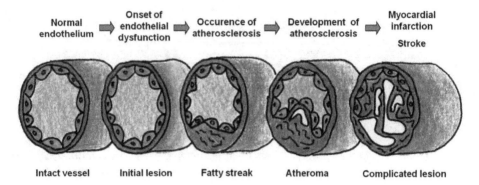

Fig. 1. Steps involved in atherosclerosis progression from endothelial dysfunction to cardiovascular complication.

2.1 Atherosclerosis and oxidative stress

Oxidative stress can be defined as an "imbalance between oxidants and antioxidants in favor of the oxidants, potentially leading to damage" (Sies, 1991). Age, gender, obesity, cigarette smoking, hypertension, diabetes mellitus and dyslipidemia are known atherogenic risk factors that promote the impairment of endothelial function, smooth muscle function and vessel wall metabolism. These risk factors are associated with an increased production of reactive oxygen species (ROS) (Antoniades et al., 2003). ROS play a physiological role in the vessel wall and participate as second messengers in endothelium-dependent function, in smooth muscle cells and endothelial cells (ECs) growth and survival, and in remodelling of the vessel wall. Each of these responses, when uncontrolled, contributes to vascular diseases (Fortuño et al., 2005; Griendling & Harrison, 1999; Irani, 2000; Taniyama & Griendling, 2003).

In the vasculature wall, ROS are produced by all the layers, including tunica intima, media and adventitia. ROS include superoxide anion radical (O_2^-), hydrogen peroxide (H_2O_2), hydroxyl radical (OH), nitric oxide (NO), and peroxynitrite ($ONOO^-$) (Lakshmi et al., 2009). The major vascular ROS is O_2^-, which inactivates NO, the main vascular relaxing factor, thus impairing relaxation (Cai & Harrison, 2000; Kojda & Harrison, 1999). Dismutation of O_2^- by superoxide dismutase (SOD) produces H_2O_2, a more stable ROS, which, in turn, is converted to water by catalase and glutathione peroxidase. H_2O_2 and other peroxides appear to be important in the regulation of growth-related signalling in VSMCs and inflammatory responses in vascular lesions (Irani, 2000; Li, P.F. et al., 1997). High levels of O_2^-, the consequent accumulation of H_2O_2 and diminished NO bioavailability play a critical role in the modulation of vascular remodelling. Finally, $ONOO^-$, resulting from the reaction between O_2^- and NO, constitutes a strong oxidant molecule, which is able to oxidize proteins, lipids and nucleic acids and then causes cell damage (Beckman & Koppenol, 1996; Fortuño et al., 2005).

There are several potential sources of ROS production. In cardiovascular disease the sources include xanthine oxidase, cyclooxygenase, lipooxygenase, mitochondrial respiration, cytochrome P450, uncoupled nitric oxide synthase (NOS) and NAD(P)H oxidase. They have been identified as sources of ROS generation in all type of vasculature. These sources may contribute to ROS formation, depending on cell type, cellular activation site and disease context. Numerous studies have shown that various physiological stimuli that contribute to pathogenesis of vascular disease can induce the formation of ROS (Lakshmi et al., 2009). ROS have detrimental effects on vascular function through several mechanisms. First, ROS, especially hydroxyl radicals, directly injure cell membranes and nuclei. Second, by interacting with endogenous vasoactive mediators formed in ECs, ROS modulate vasomotion and the atherogenic process. Third, ROS peroxidize lipid components, leading to the formation of oxidized lipoproteins (LDL), one of the key mediators of atherosclerosis (Bonomini et al., 2008).

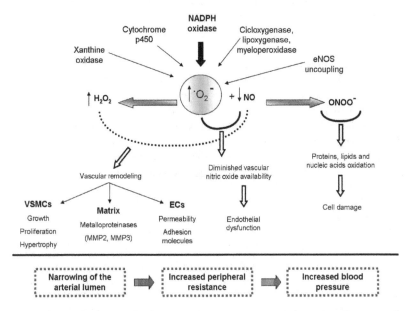

Fig. 2. Potential sources of ROS production in atherosclerosis progression.

Cholesterol is transported in the blood by LDL. These particles contain esterified cholesterol and triglycerides surrounded by a shell of phospholipids, free cholesterol and apolipoprotein B100 (ApoB100). Circulating LDL particles can accumulate in the intimal, the innermost layer of the artery. Here ApoB100 binds to proteoglycans of the extracellular matrix (ECM) through ionic interactions (Tabas et al., 2007). This is an important initiating factor in early atherogenesis (Skålen et al., 2002; Steinberg, 2009; Witztum & Steinberg, 2001). As a consequence of this subendothelial retention, LDL particles are trapped in the tunica intima, where they are prone to oxidative modifications caused by enzymatic attack of myeloperoxidase (Heinecke, 2007) and lipoxygenases, or by ROS such as hypoclorous acid (HOCl), phenoxyl radical intermediates or ONOO- generated in the intimal during inflammation and atherosclerosis (Hansson & Hermansson, 2011).

Oxidized LDL (Ox-LDL) has several biological effects (Madamanchi et al., 2005); it is pro-inflammatory; it causes inhibition of endothelial NOS (eNOS); it promotes vasoconstriction and adhesion; it stimulates cytokines such as interleukins (ILs) and increases platelet aggregation. Ox-LDL-derived products are cytotoxic and induce apoptosis. Ox-LDL can adversely affect coagulation by stimulating tissue factor and plasminogen activator inhibitor-1 (PAI-1) synthesis. Another atherogenic property of Ox-LDL is its immunogenicity and its ability to promote retention of macrophages in the arterial wall by inhibiting macrophage motility (Singh & Jialal, 2006). In addiction, Ox-LDL stimulates VSMCs proliferation (Stocker & Keaney, 2004). Thus, intimal thickening further reduces the lumen of blood vessels, leading to further potentation of hypertension and atherosclerosis (Singh & Jialal, 2006). With ongoing oxidation, the physicochemical properties gradually change, including alterations in charge, particle size, lipid content and other features. The precise nature of each of these alterations obviously depends on the oxidizing agent. For all these reasons, Ox-LDL is not a defined molecular species but is instead a spectrum of LDL particles that have undergone a variety of physicochemical changes (Hansson & Hermansson, 2011).

2.2 Atherosclerosis and inflammation

Inflammation participates in atherosclerosis from its inception onwards. Fatty streaks do not cause symptoms, and may either progress to more complex lesions or involute. Fatty streaks have focal increases in the content of lipoproteins within regions of the intimal, where they associate with components of the ECM such as proteoglycans, slowing their egress. This retention sequesters lipoproteins within the intimal, isolating them from plasma antioxidants, thus favoring their oxidative modification (Kruth, 2002; Packard & Libby, 2008; Skålen et al., 2002). Oxidatively modified LDL particles comprise an incompletely defined mixture, because both the lipid and protein moieties can undergo oxidative modification. Constituents of such modified lipoprotein particles can induce a local inflammatory response (Miller et al., 2003; Packard & Libby, 2008).

Vascular ECs function to prevent clotting of blood and adhesion of blood cells to the endothelial cells, in addition to playing the role of a barrier, as a cell monolayer, to prevent blood constituents from invading the vascular wall. When ECs are injured or activated by various coronary risk factors, infections or physical stimuli, adhesion molecules become expressed in ECs, and peripheral monocytes adhere to the endothelial cell surface. Adhesion molecules are broadly divided into three molecular families: integrin family, immunoglobulin family, and selectin family (L-selectin, Eselectin, P-selectin) (Yamada, 2001).

Chemoattractant factors, which include monocyte chemoattractant protein-1 (MCP-1) produced by vascular wall cells in response to modified lipoproteins, direct the migration and diapedesis of adherent monocytes (Boring et al., 1998; Packard & Libby, 2008). Monocytic cells, directly interacting with human ECs, increase several fold monocyte matrix metalloproteinase (MMP) 9 production, allowing for the subsequent infiltration of leukocytes through the endothelial layer and its associated basement membrane (Amorino & Hoover, 1998; Packard & Libby, 2008) Within the intima, monocytes mature into macrophages under the influence of macrophage colony stimulating factor (M-CSF), which is overexpressed in the inflamed intima. M-CSF stimulation also increases macrophage expression of scavenger receptors, members of the pattern-recognition receptor superfamily, which engulf modified lipoproteins through receptor-mediated endocytosis. Accumulation of cholesteryl esters in the cytoplasm converts macrophages into foam cells, i.e., lipid-laden macrophages characteristic of early-stage atherosclerosis. In parallel, macrophages proliferate and amplify the inflammatory response through the secretion of numerous growth factors and cytokines, including tumor necrosis factor α (TNFα) and IL-1β. Recent evidence supports selective recruitment of a proinflammatory subset of monocytes to nascent atheroma in mice (Packard & Libby, 2008).

A number of proinflammatory cytokines have been shown to participate in atherosclerotic plaque development, growth and rupture (Dabek, 2010; Libby et al., 2002). Nuclear factor kappa-light-chain-enhancer of activated B cells (NF-kB) seems to be a crucial transcription factor in the cross-talk among cytokines, adhesion molecules and growth factors. On one hand, NF-kB is a major transcription factor leading to cytokine synthesis, and on the other hand, the above mentioned factors keep NF-kB persistently activated in acute coronary syndromes (Dabek, 2010). In atherogenesis, NF-kB before regulates the expression of cyclooxygenases, lipooxygenases, cytokines, chemokines (i.e., MCP-1) and adhesion molecules (Dabek, 2010; Kutuk & Basaga, 2003). Later in the progression of the atherosclerotic lesion, NF-kB regulates gene expression of M-CSF, a factor stimulating infiltrating monocyte differentiation and transformation into "foamy cells", and other genes participating in the transformation (Brach et al., 1991; Dabek, 2010). As stated, atherosclerosis is an inflammatory reaction of the arterial wall. The factors IL-1β, TNF-α, IL-6, IL-12 and interferon γ (IFNγ) are involved in this reaction and their expression is coregulated by NF-kB.

Intracellular matrix degradation is an important process in both plaque development and rupture. The vital factors involved include MMPs, particularly those that are able to break down the vascular base membrane. It has been shown that NF-kB is an essential regulator of MMP gene expression, especially MMP-2 and MMP-9, which are critical in plaque rupture (Bond et al., 1998; Dabek, 2010). Thus, NF-kB regulates the expression of a wide spectrum of atherosclerosis mediating factors. On the other hand, most of these factors also up-regulate NF-kB activity. Increased NF-kB activity was found in unstable regions of atherosclerotic plaques (Brand et al., 1997; Dabek, 2010). The significance of NF-kB activity has been confirmed in some clinical studies as well. Li and colleagues reported significantly increased NF-kB activity in white blood cells from unstable angina patients *vs.* stable angina patients and *vs.* control patients (the lowest activity in the latter) (Li, J.J. et al., 2004).

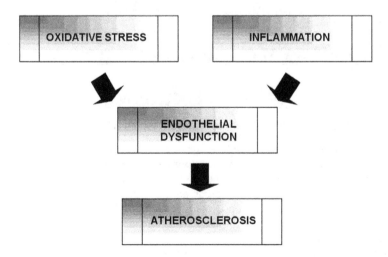

Fig. 3. Role of oxidative stress and inflammation in the early atherosclerosis.

3. Endothelial cells dysfunction in atherosclerosis

The endothelium is responsible for the regulation of vascular tone, the exchange of plasma and cell biomolecules, inflammation, lipid metabolism and modulation of fibrinolysis and coagulation (Andrews et al., 2010). Aging affects many pathways involved in cardiovascular functions and particularly of ECs (Barton, 2010; Virdis et al., 2010). In fact, endothelial-aging is associated with anatomical disruption, morphological abnormalities in ECs size and shape (Haudenschild et al., 1981), susceptibility to apoptosis and abnormal release of EC-derived factors (Barton, 2010). These factors, which are synthetized not only by ECs, but also by VSMCs, are now known to contribute to pathogenetic mechanisms of CVDs (Higashi et al., 2009).

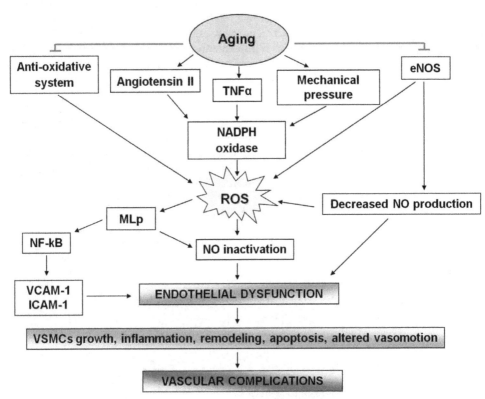

Fig. 4. Central role of ROS in inducing endothelial dysfunction in vascular diseases.

ECs dysfunction, inflammation, oxidative stress and dyslipidaemia are known to play prominent and vital roles not only in the development of atherosclerotic lesions, but also in their progression. (Andrews et al., 2010; Bai et al., 2010; Higashi et al., 2009 ; Virdis et al., 2010). Number of factors and modalities are available to interfere with age related changes in EC function (Barton, 2010; Jensen-Urstad et al., 1999). When endothelial damage compromises the normal vascular function, the intracellular dynamic balance probably leans on an athero-prone phenotype.

Growing evidence indicates that chronic and acute overproduction of ROS activates ECs as pivotal early event in atherogenesis. Oxidative stress induces cell proliferation, hypertrophy, apoptosis and inflammation through activation of various signaling cascades, redox-sensitive transcriptional factors and expression of pro-inflammatory phenotype (Higashi et al., 2009). ECs dysfunction has been shown to be associated with an increase of ROS in atherosclerotic animal models and in human subjects with atherosclerosis (Dai, D.Z. & Dai, Y., 2010; Davies et al., 2010; Higashi et al., 2009). Moreover, in APOE-deficient mice, a widely used animal model of atherosclerosis (Xu, 2009; Zhang, S.H. et al., 1992), studies have demonstrated that aged-ECs are more sensitive to apoptosis than younger ones. ECs in the areas of the artery resistant to atherosclerosis have a life span of about 12 months, whereas cells at lesion-prone sites live for few weeks and even shorter in aged animals (Xu, 2009).

3.1 Endothelial cell-factors

The vascular endothelium is nowadays considered to be a paracrine organ responsible for the secretion of several substances exerting atherogenic effects. The reduced bioavailability of NO as an indirect result of the effects of those factors, leads to atherosclerosis and its clinical manifestations (Muller & Morawietz, 2009; Tousoulis et al., 2010). Under normal conditions, ECs constantly produce a number of vasoactive and trophic substances that control inflammation, VSMC growth, vasomotion, platelet function and plasmatic coagulation (Barton & Haudenschild, 2001; Traupe et al., 2003).

Normal vascular activity is essential for maintaining normal function of organs, dependent on a balance of vasoconstrictive and vasodilative substances derived from the endothelium, which mainly include NO to dilate and endothelin-1 (ET-1) to constrict the cells of tunica media. Furthermore, ECs activated by ROS can regulate vascular function via the release of inflammatory mediators, such as intercellular adhesion molecule-1 (ICAM-1), vascular cell adhesion molecule (VCAM-1), MCP-1, ILs, angiotensin-II (A-II), TNFα, NF-kB and E- and P-selectin, or the release of haemostatic regulators, such as von Willebrand factor, tissue factor inhibitor and plasminogen activator, fibrinogen and NO (Sima et al., 2009; Vanhoutte, 2009).

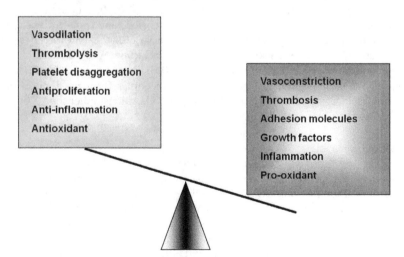

Fig. 5. Regulatory functions of the endothelium maintaining the equilibrium between antiatherogenic and atherogenic properties.

The purpose of the following paragraphs will be to provide a brief description and characterization of the main EC-factors that are synthesize and secrete after ROS stimulus during endothelial athero-susceptibility.

3.1.1 Angiotensin-II

A-II, a causal factor to the dysfunction of vascular endothelium, adversely stimulates the activity of the cardiovascular system (Dai, D.Z. & Dai, Y., 2010). A-II increases blood pressure by vasoconstriction and sodium and fluid retention and produces overt oxidative stress resultant from the activation of NADPH oxidase, a source of ROS in blood vessels, that promotes endothelial dysfunction, inducing cytokines, chemokines and adhesion molecules secretion and contributes to vascular remodeling (Dai, D.Z. & Dai, Y., 2010; Ferrario, 2009; Partigulova & Naumov, 2010). The A-II effects on gene expression are mediated, at least in part, through the cytoplasmic NF-kB transcription factor. Through these actions, A-II augments vascular inflammation, induces EC dysfunctions and, in so doing, enhances the atherogenic process (Sprague & Khalil, 2009).

3.1.2 Endothelial nitric oxide synthase

Endothelium-derived NO, formed by eNOS, (isoform 3 of NO shynthase) is known as a potent vasodilator (Barton, 2010). eNOS is also the master gene regulator used by ECs to orchestrate their own phenotype, function and survival. eNOS is modulated by shear stress (Rodella et al., 2010, a) and agonists acting on cell surface receptors; its activity is dependent on many mechanisms, including substrate availability, phosphorylation, Ca^{2+} flux and protein–protein interactions (Andrews et al., 2010).

With age, a number of changes occur in the cardiovascular system that can be considered pro-atherogenic (Barton, 2010). It is widely accepted that the most important mechanism leading to endothelial dysfunction is the reduced bioavailability of NO; so the decreased bioavailability of NO is consequently regarded a critical precursor to the development of atherosclerotic plaque and has been considered as one of the factors contributing to the higher incidence of atherosclerosis, arterial hypertension and renal disease in aged individuals (Barton, 2005). Together with its role as a vasodilator, NO impedes processes that are vital for atherosclerotic progression, including vasoconstriction, VSMCs proliferation and monocyte adhesion (Napoli et al., 2006). Furthermore, with atherosclerotic conditions, eNOS can become dysfunctional as it uncouples from its dimeric state to a monomeric state, in which it is able to produce superoxide anions rather than NO (Andrews et al., 2010; Vàsquez-Vivar et al., 1998).

3.1.3 Endothelin-1

Endothelins are EC-derived vasoactive peptides. Since its discovery, ET-1 has been demonstrated as one of the most potent known vasoconstrictors (Barton, 2010). ET-1 is synthesized in bulk by ECs and VSMCs (Rodella et al., 2010,a) as well as by macrophages, cardiomiocytes, neurons, renal medulla and Kupffer cells (Piechota et al., 2010). Factors that stimulate the release of ET-1 include endotoxins, TNFα, IL-1, adrenaline, insulin, thrombin and A-II. ROS are involved in the modulation and activation of ET-1 that induced various signaling pathways; in fact, during the inflammation process, atherosclerosis and hypertension there are elevated levels of ET-1 (Piechota et al., 2010; Skalska et al., 2009; Teplyakov, 2004).

3.1.4 Tumor necrosis factor α

TNFα is crucially involved in the pathogenesis and progression of atherosclerosis, myocardial ischemia/reperfusion injury and heart failure. The TNFα-mediated vascular dysfunction involves alterations in EC metabolism and function, platelet aggregation, EC-blood cell interaction, VSMC function and proliferation (McKellar et al., 2009). It increases the expression of many pro-inflammatory, pro-coagulant, proliferative and pro-apoptotic genes involved in initiation and progression of atherosclerosis (Bergh et al., 2009). TNFα induces the rapid expression of cellular adhesion molecules (CAMs), such as VCAM-1 and ICAM-1, and E-selectin at the endothelial surface (Chandrasekharan et al., 2007; Kleinbongard et al., 2010). Endothelial dysfunction associated with TNFα during atherogenesis is linked to an excess in production of ROS and a decrease in NO bioavailability. The production of ROS can stimulate a cytokine cascade through NF-κB-induced transcriptional events, which then induce the expression of TNFα (Zhang, H. et al., 2009).

3.1.5 Cellular adhesion molecules (ICAM-1 and VCAM-1)

When ECs undergo inflammatory activation, an increase in the expression of CAMs promotes the adherence of inflammatory cells (monocytes, neutrophils, lymphocytes and macrophages) and the recruitment of additional cytokines, growth factors and MMPs into the vascular wall (Sprague & Khalil, 2009). ICAM-1 and VCAM1 are immunoglobulin-like CAMs expressed by several cell types including ECs and leukocytes. They are present in atherosclerotic lesions during their progression, because they are involved in the transendothelial migration of leukocytes, lymphocytes and antigen presenting cells to sites of inflammation (Blankenberg et al., 2001; Ho et al., 2008; Lawson & Wolf, 2009; Rodella et al., 2010,b). Nevertheless their pathological role remain still uncertain. An important stimulus for CAMs expression is the fluid shear stress, which exerts both pro-inflammatory and protective effects, depending on the type of shear.

3.2 Shear stress

As the regulator of vascular tone, ECs are highly sensitive to different types of shear stress caused by the complex structure of artery geometry. It is clearly observed that atherogenesis generally occurs at curved or branching points with disturbed flow. Endothelium in the regions of flow disturbances near arterial branches, bifurcations and curvatures shows an athero-prone phenotype, while laminar flow regions exhibit an athero-protective phenotype (Bai et al., 2010; Traub & Berk, 1998). When endothelial monolayer is stimulated by laminar flow, rapidly cellular responses occur, included opening of ion channels, release of vasoactive NO and activation of transcription factors and cell cycle regulators (Foteinos et al., 2008). In particular, laminar flow induces NO production through both the transcriptional up-regulation of eNOS gene expression and the posttranslational modification of eNOS protein (Jin et al., 2003; Xu, 2009). Compared with ECs under laminar flow, cells at disturbed flow show an atherogenic phenotype as altered alignment, deformation of luminal ECs surface, accelerated proliferation and apoptosis (Bai et al., 2010; Zeng et al., 2009), higher permeability, immunoinflammation responses and more athero-prone gene expression which are proportional to risk factor severity (Foteinos et al., 2008; Xu, 2000). Oscillatory shear stress leads to continuous O^{2-}

production in an NADPH-oxidase-dependent manner, resulting in NF-kB-mediated monocyte adhesion.

NF-kB is an inducible transcription factor present at increased levels in the thickened intima-media of atherosclerotic lesions, whereas little or no activated NF-kB has been detected in healthy vessels (Andrews et al., 2010; Rodella et al., 2010,b). The NF-kB pathway have been implicated in athero-susceptibility for more than a decade. NF-kB is normally held inactive in the cytosol as a complex with IkB, a family of inhibitors of NF-kB. Oxidative stress by ROS production induces IkB degradation, releases of NFkB for translocation to the nucleus where it regulates pro-inflammatory genes (Davies et al., 2010). Several pro-inflammatory cytokines and growth factors found in atherosclerotic lesions, such as TNFα, ILs, MCP-1 and tissue factors, activate NF-kB signaling pathway in cultured ECs (Pennathur & Heinecke, 2007). NF-κB plays a central role in the development of inflammation through further regulation of genes encoding pro-inflammatory cytokines, CAMs, chemokines, growth factors and inducible enzymes (Andrews et al., 2010; Sprague & Khalil, 2009).

3.3 EC-foam cells

The formation of foam cells as a result of the lipid loading in ECs is a late event in atherosclerosis. Since the atherogenesis process is gradual, it is known that plasma hypercholesterolemia is associated with increased transcytosis of lipoproteins (Lps), leading to their accumulation within the ECs. At this location, Lps interact with proteoglycans and other matrix proteins and carry on their conversion to oxidatively modified and reassembled Lps (MLps). MLps have been identified in early intimal thickenings of human aorta and in the late atheroma (Sima et al., 2009; Tirziu et al., 1995).

It is known that, in the initial stage of atherogenesis, upon the accumulation and retention of MLp within intima, the EC lining the plaque take up MLp, which are either degraded within the cell or exocytosed into the lumen; in time, the non-regulated uptake of MLp by the EC-scavenger receptor is overwhelmed, leading to the accumulation of numerous large lipid droplets within the ECs. Concurrently, the EC shifts to a secretory phenotype, characterized by an increased number of biosynthetic organelles that correlates with the appearance of a multilayer, hyperplastic basal lamina in meshes of which MLp in accumulate large numbers. These insults lead to a dysfunctional endothelium and inflammatory process in which the EC-derived foam cells express more of new CAM and synthesize EC-factors that attract and induce migration of plasma inflammatory cells, such as monocytes and T lymphocytes to the subendothelium (Simionescu & Antohe, 2006); however, ECs maintain some of their specific attributes, such as Weibel-Palade bodies, intercellular junctions and caveolae (Sima et al., 2009). Infiltration of atherogenic Lps, monocytes and T lymphocytes within the subendothelium start the atherogenetic process both in animal models and in humans (Lawson & Wolf, 2009; Simionescu & Antohe, 2006; Williams & Tabas, 2005). In late stages of atherosclerosis, all cellular components of the plaque, ECs, VSMCs and macrophages, accumulate considerable number of lipid droplets and exhibit the foam cell characteristics (Sima et al., 2009). In the subendothelium, the monocytes become macrophage-derived foam cells, which release cytokines and factors that, within the oxidative stress process, change the cross-talk between ECs and the neighbouring VSMCs and induce migration of VSMCs from media to the developing neointima (Lawson & Wolf, 2009; Simionescu & Antohe, 2006).

4. The role of vascular smooth muscle cells in atherosclerosis

VSMCs are important actors in the pathogenesis of atherosclerosis. The classical *"response to injury"* hypothesis of atherosclerosis suggests that one of the major events in the development of this pathology is the intimal thickening caused by hyperplasia and migration of VSMC in the tunica intima (Ross & Glomset, 1973): the combined action of growth factors, proteolytic agents, and ECM proteins, produced by a dysfunctional endothelium and/or inflammatory cells, induces proliferation and migration of VSMCs from the tunica media into the intima (Clowes et al., 1983; Hao et al., 2003). Finally, progression of atherosclerotic lesions in the intima is characterized by the accumulation of alternating layers of dedifferentiated VSMCs and lipid-laden macrophages (Sobue et al., 1999). This model focuses on the central role of activated and proliferating VSMCs that are histologically observed in the early and late stages of atherosclerosis, thus being a key event in atherosclerosis (Dzau et al., 2002; Owens, 1995). Because of their involvement in atherosclerosis, intimal VSMCs, their origin and the mechanisms that regulate their phenotype have been the subject of numerous studies and much debate over recent years.

4.1 Origin of intimal VSMCs in atherosclerosis
4.1.1 Phenotypic modulation of VSMCs
The long-standing dogma in the field has been that the majority of intimal VSMCs are derived from preexisting mature medial VSMCs that undergo phenotypic modulation on moving from the media to the intima (Owens et al., 2004). This hypothesis, proposed for the first time by Chamley-Campbell and colleagues (Chamley-Campbell et al., 1979) arose from a limited number of studies showing that in primary human cell cultures derived from different sources (e.g. medial cells or cells derived from atherosclerotic plaques) stable differences in phenotype could be identified. This dogma implies the potential for marked plasticity of the VSMC phenotype, with the ultimate phenotype being determined by a variety of extracellular stimuli (Bochaton-Piallat et al., 1996): numerous studies of cells cultured from different species have demonstrated that cytokines, matrix components, and mechanical stimuli can influence VSMC phenotype and behavior (Shanahan et al., 1993; Topouzis & Majesky, 1996).

VSMCs are the predominant cellular elements of the medial layer of the vascular wall, essential for good performance of the vasculature. VSMCs perform many different functions in maintaining vessel's health (Rensen et al., 2007). The VSMC is the only cell populating the normal vascular media, wherein it is uniquely responsible for maintaining vascular tone and hemodynamic stability: it is a highly specialized cell whose principal function is vasoconstriction and dilation in response to normal or pharmacologic stimuli to regulate blood vessel tone, blood pressure, and blood flow (Rzucidlo et al., 2007). Moreover, except in unusual circumstances when the adventitia may be involved, the VSMC is also the only vascular cell capable of repairing the injured vessel wall by migrating, proliferating, and elaborating an appropriate ECM. It is therefore equally essential that, when it is necessary, the VSMC can also adopt a phenotype capable of these synthetic functions (Shanahan & Weissberg, 1998). So, it is important that VSMCs retain remarkable plasticity and can undergo rather intense and reversible changes in phenotype in response to changes in local environmental cues, particularly under the influence of growth factors (Li, S. et al., 1999; Owens, 1995). In the pathogenesis of atherosclerotic lesions it is now accepted that VSMC can display at least two different phenotypes, the first characteristic of the media and the second typical of the cells invading the intima (Shanahan & Weissberg, 1999). These phenotypes are also seen *in vitro*: an elongated spindle-shaped phenotype, with the classic "hill-and-valley" growth pattern typical of cultured contractile normal medial VSMCs and an epithelioid or rhomboid phenotype, with cells growing in a monolayer with a cobblestone morphology at confluence typical of the cells from neointima (Hao et al., 2003). In the medial layer of a mature blood vessel, VSMCs exhibit a low rate of proliferation, low synthetic activity and ECM proteins secretion, and express a unique repertoire of contractile proteins (e.g. intracellular myofilaments bundles are abundant), ion channels, and signalling molecules required for the cell's contractile function that is clearly unique compared with any other cell type (Rzucidlo et al., 2007). The dense body, the dense membrane and myofibrils (composed of thin filaments and myosin thick filaments) are well developed in differentiated VSMCs, whereas organelles (e.g. rough endoplasmic reticulum (RER), Golgi and free ribosomes) are few in number (Owens, 1995). This "contractile" state (referred also as "differentiated phenotype"), is required for the VSMC to perform its primary function. The gene expression pattern in end-differentiated VSMCs is well characterized and comprised a number of proteins involved in contraction, membrane-skeletal markers specific to smooth muscle and cell adhesion molecules and their receptors (integrins), which are important either as a structural component of the contractile apparatus or as a regulator of contraction (Owens, 1995; Rensen et al., 2007). Their expressions are regulated at the gene levels, such as at transcription and splicing: caldesmon, smooth muscle myosin heavy chain (SMM-HC), α-smooth muscle actin (α-SMA), h-caldesmon, calponin, SM22, α- and β-tropomyosins and α1 integrin genes are transcriptionally regulated; transcription of these genes (except for the α-smooth muscle actin gene) is upregulated in differentiated VSMCs, but is downregulated in dedifferentiated VSMCs (Stintzing et al., 2009). It's important to note that, although α-SMA is permanently expressed in VSMCs, it is more abundant in contractile VSMCs than in synthetic VSMCs (Lemire et al., 1994). Isoform changes of caldesmon, α-tropomyosin, vinculin/metavinculin, and SMM-HC are instead regulated by alternative splicing in a VSMC phenotype-dependent manner (Sobue et al., 1999). At present, the two marker proteins that provide the best definition of a mature contractile VSMC phenotype are SM-MHC and smoothelin. SM-MHC expression has never been detected in non-VSMCs *in vivo*, and is the only marker protein that is also VSMCs-specific during embryogenesis (Miano et al., 1994). Smoothelin complements SM-MHC as a contractile VSMC marker in that it appears to be more sensitive.

On the contrary, intimal VSMCs associated with vascular disease (as well as VSMCs involved in blood vessel formation) are phenotypically distinct from their medial counterparts (Campbell, G.R. & Campbell, J.H., 1985; Mosse et al., 1985): they resemble immature and show a typical "synthetic" state (referred also as "dedifferentiated phenotype"), characterized by an increased rate of proliferation, migration and ECM protein synthesis. Several studies by Aikawa and coworkers (Aikawa et al., 1997, 1998) demonstrated that intimal VSMCs show a synthetic phenotype including: *1)* increased DNA synthesis and expression of proliferation markers and cyclins (Gordon et al., 1990); *2)* decreased expression of smooth muscle-specific contractile markers (Layne et al., 2002); *3)* alterations in calcium handling and contractility (Hill et al., 2001); *4)* alterations in cell ultrastructure, including a general loss of myofilaments, which is replaced largely by synthetic organelles such as RER and large Golgi complex (Sobue et al., 1999), supporting its function in production and secretion of ECM components that, leading to intimal thickening and fibrosis of the vascular wall, may contribute to lesion development and/or stability (Schwartz et al., 1986, 1995). The preceding studies have been extended by Geary and colleagues (Geary et al., 2002), who completed microarray-based profiling of gene expression patterns of SMCs in the neointima. A total of 147 genes were differentially expressed in neointimal VSMCs versus normal aorta VSMCs, most genes underscoring the importance of matrix production during neointimal formation. Therefore, these VSMCs assume the proliferative activity in response to mitogens, while lose contractile ability. Markers that are upregulated in the synthetic phenotype are rare. SMemb/non-muscle myosin heavy chain isoform B (MHC-B) represents a suitable synthetic VSMCs marker, since this protein is quickly and markedly upregulated in proliferating VSMCs (Neuville et al., 1997). At last, an interesting correlation has been demonstrated, albeit occasionally, between dedifferentiated VSMC phenotype and increased LDL uptake (Thyberg, 2002) or decreased HDL binding sites (Dusserre et al., 1994). Nevertheless, the role of LDL and HDL processes in atheromatous plaque formation with respect to VSMC heterogeneity should be further investigated.

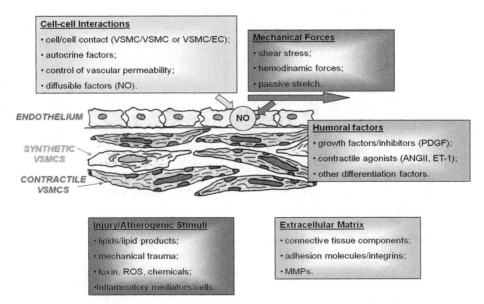

Fig. 6. Factors involved in VSMCs development, differentiation and phenotypic modulation

However, it is now recognized that a simple two-state model, based on "contractile" and "synthetic" states only, is inadequate to explain the diverse range of phenotypes that can be exhibited by the VSMCs under different physiological and pathological circumstances (Owens et al., 2004). In particular, the environmental cues that exist within atherosclerotic lesions are without doubts very different from those that exist within a normal healthy blood vessel and these change at different stages of lesion development and progression and thereby are likely to contribute to continued phenotypic switching of VSMC within the lesion. So, an heterogeneity of VSMC phenotype, ranging from contractile to synthetic, which represent the two ends of a spectrum of VSMCs with intermediate phenotypes, is nowadays considered. Not surprisingly, as the repertoire of VSMC markers has expanded, the picture that has emerged is that there is likely a wide spectrum of possible VSMC phenotypes that might exist such that it may be very artificial to assign cells to distinct subcategories. So the distinction between "contractile" and "synthetic" state of the VSMC become very difficult. The complexity of different phenotypes that may be manifested by VSMC is clearly evident not only between VSMCs of different vessels or among VSMCs within the same vessel, but there is very clear evidence that the properties of the VSMCs vary also at different stages of atherosclerosis, within different lesion types, and between VSMCs located in different regions within a given lesion (Owens et al., 2004).

4.1.2 Monoclonality of atheromatous lesion and heterogeneity of proliferating VSMCs

Alternative to the predominant hypothesis that all VSMCs of the media can undergo phenotypic modulation, is the concept that a predisposed VSMCs subpopulation is responsible for the production of intimal thickening. This possibility has been raised on the basis of original work by Benditt and Benditt (Benditt, E.P. & Benditt, J.M., 1973) who reported that VSMC accumulation in the atheromatous plaques is monoclonal or, at least, oligoclonal (Chung et al., 1998), implying that only a small number of "immature" cells in the vessels media and/or adventitia undergo proliferation (Holifield et al., 1996). More recent studies have questioned the origin of VSMCs comprising atherosclerosis and neointima formation. Intimal VSMCs have been proposed to originate from diverse sources, including fibroblasts of the adventitia (Zalewski et al., 2002), ECs (Gittenberger-de Groot et al., 1999) and/or circulating bone marrow–derived cells (Hillebrands et al., 2003). Whereas the gene expression pattern of differentiated VSMC is pretty well characterized (Shanahan & Weissberg, 1999), many *in vivo* and *in vitro* studies dealing with proliferating VSMC showed heterogeneous cell marker expressions of multilineage differentiation (Tintut et al., 2003). A possible explanation of the heterogeneity of VSMCs in adult vessels can be found in embryologic vascular development (Gittenberger-de Groot et al., 1999): interestingly, similar to atherosclerosis, processes of multilineage differentiation with transition states could be observed during vascular development (Slomp et al., 1997). During vasculogenesis, VSMCs originate from different sources via transdifferentiation (Liu et al., 2004) (a highly conserved phenomenon of transdifferentiation is proved by a stable cytokeratins expression in atherosclerotic lesions as well as it happens during development (Neureiter et al., 2005)) depending on the vessel type, including mesoderm, neurectoderm, epicardium (for coronary arteries) and, more rarely, endothelium (Orlandi & Bennett, 2010). It is thus possible that the various VSMC phenotypes can arise from distinct lineages. Another possibility is that local VSMC of the contractile phenotype re-obtain the embryonic potential of proliferation and migration (Bar et al., 2002) via transdifferentiation and dedifferentiation processes as a response to injury. Looking at atherosclerosis and VSMC, there is a lot of evidence that VSMC progenitor cells are essentially involved in the progression of atherosclerosis (Roberts et al., 2005).

The origin of such VSMC progenitor cells is under debate. VSMC progenitor cells have been identified in the bone marrow (multipotent vascular stem cell progenitors and mesenchymal stem cells), in the circulation (circulating VSMC progenitor cells), in the vessel wall (resident VSMC progenitor cells and mesangioblasts) and various extravascular sites (extravascular, non-bone marrow progenitor cells) (Orlandi & Bennett, 2010).

BONE MARROW-DERIVED PROGENITOR CELLS

Multipotent vascular stem cell progenitors and mesenchimal stem cells (MSCs)

EXTRAVASCULAR NON-BONE MARROW PROGENITOR CELLS

(liver, adipose tissue, gut, spleen)

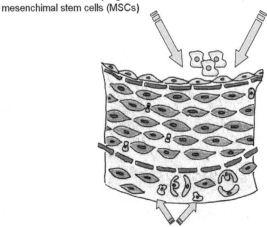

VASCULAR PROGENITOR CELLS

Resident VSMCs and mesangioblasts

Fig. 7. Different origins of VSMCs progenitor cells.

4.1.2.1 Bone marrow-derived VSMCs

Several studies have suggested that circulating bone marrow-derived cells contribute to neointima formation: one possibility is that circulating smooth muscle precursor cells of myeloid or hematopoietic lineage relocate from the blood into the neointima following vascular injury (Metharom et al., 2008) and start to proliferate giving rise to cells that express at least some properties of VSMCs (Simper et al., 2002).

Other studies, on the other hand, report no evidence for a contribution of bone marrow derived VSMCs in the neointimal layer (Hu et al., 2002; Li, J. et al., 2001). Alternatively, these circulating cells may fuse with resident VSMCs and thus show co-localization of VSMC markers and bone marrow lineage markers, although to date, no direct evidence for cell fusion in the vasculature has been shown (Owens et al., 2004).

4.1.2.2 Resident VSMC progenitor cells and mesangioblasts

Inside normal vessel walls the existence of resident progenitor cells (expressing stem cell antigens) capable of contributing to neointima formation has been recently shown (Orlandi et al., 2008; Torsney et al., 2007): the number of these resident VSMCs progenitors has been shown to increase in atherosclerotic lesions (Torsney et al., 2007). These progenitor cells are different from marrow-derived smooth muscle progenitor cells, since they lack the ability to differentiate into erythroid, lymphoid, or myeloid tissue (Jackson et al., 1999). Subsequent studies examining telomere loss indicate that fibrous cap VSMCs have undergone more population doublings than cells in the normal media (Matthews et al., 2006), suggesting the existence of a resident arterial subpopulation predisposed to clonally contribute to arterial healing in response to injury (Hirschi & Majesky, 2004), so that plaques arise by selective expansion of a preexisting 'patch' of progenitor cells.

Unfortunately, against this theory, there is very limited evidence for the presence of vessel wall stem cells in human vessels. A population of CD34$^+$/CD31$^-$ cells has been identified in the space between the media and adventitia of large and medium-sized human arteries and veins (Pasquinelli et al., 2007), but the capacity of these cells to give rise to VSMCs was low (Zengin et al., 2006). Few other studies showed that the adventitial layer potentially harbours a population of stem cells that can also contribute to vascular remodelling. In particular, Hu and colleagues demonstrated that abundant progenitor cells in the adventitia can differentiate in VSMCs (Hu et al., 2004).

Moreover, satellite-like cells named 'mesoangioblasts' express both myogenic and EC markers (Drake et al., 1997), which can give rise to both hematopoietic and endothelial progenies (Cossu & Bianco, 2003). Gene expression profiles reveal that mesoangioblasts express genes belonging to developmental signaling pathways (such as β-catenin/Wnt signaling pathway) and are able to differentiate very efficiently into VSMCs (Tagliafico et al., 2004).

In summary, there is evidence for several distinct resident progenitor cells in different layers of the normal adult arterial wall capable of proliferating and differentiating into VSMCs. What has not yet been established is how many of these cells contribute to formation of vascular lesions and whether clonality reflects selective proliferation of one or more of these populations.

4.2 VSMCs: Friend or foe in atherosclerosis?

It is important to note that the exact role of VSMCs, in the progression of atherosclerosis is not clear. The functional role of VSMCs likewise is likely to vary depending on the stage of the disease. For example, at the early onset of atherosclerosis, these cells presumably plays a maladaptive role, because of their involvement in neointima formation (Rodella et al., 2011): mobilisation of these cells would therefore be predicted to promote, as a "foe", vascular disease (van Oostrom et al., 2009). On the other hand, over recent years, there has been an increasing recognition of the role played by intimal VSMCs in the formation and maintaining of a protective fibrous cap over the atherosclerotic plaque, desirable for plaque stability in the advanced atherosclerotic process (Weissberg et al., 1996). In particular, IFN-γ released by activated macrophages induces collagen synthesis by VSMCs, which is important for the stabilization of the fibrous cap (Shah et al., 1995). Moreover, injection of smooth muscle progenitor cells in a mouse model of advanced atherosclerosis reduced the progression of early atherosclerotic plaques (Zoll et al., 2008), confirming the potential benefit of VSMCs at advanced stages of atherosclerosis. Therefore, VSMCs could be beneficial in atherogenesis as a factor promoting plaque stability and can thus be considered a "friend" in vascular disease (van Oostrom et al., 2009).

Since the VSMC is the only cell capable of synthesizing the fibrous cap, failure of this vascular repair response leads to weakening of the cap and plaque rupture, with potentially fatal consequences (Weissberg et al., 1996). In diseased tissue many factors are present that substantially alter the normal balance of proliferation and apoptosis, and the apoptosis may predominate (Bennett, 2002). In particular, in plaque VSMCs an elevated level of spontaneous apoptosis and enhanced susceptibility to apoptosis induced by ROS (Li, W.G. et al., 2000) has been recently described both *in vivo* and *in vitro* (Ross, 1999). Apoptosis of VSMCs, bringing a plaque with reduced number of VSMCs, could participate in the rupture of the stability of the plaque (Rudijanto, 2007). Rupture of atherosclerotic plaques is associated with a thinning of VSMC-rich fibrous cap overlying the core (atrophic fibrous cap lesion), due to rapid replicative senescence and apoptosis of VSMCs (Schwartz et al., 2000). Rupture occurs particularly at the plaque shoulders, which exhibits lack of VSMCs and the presence of inflammatory cells (Newby et al., 1999). So, VSMCs may later contribute to plaque destabilization through apoptosis and/or activation of various protease cascades (Galis & Khatri, 2002).

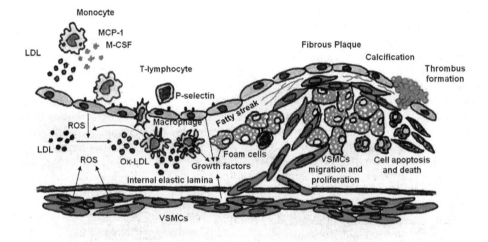

Fig. 8. Involvement of VSMCs apoptosis in fibrous plaque rupture.

However, detailed studies demonstrating whether VSMC progenitors either protect or promote vessel disease are needed before cell-based or pharmacological approaches aimed at regulating progenitor cell trafficking can be recommended.

4.3 VSMCs can auto-regulate their replication/migration
The contemporary paradigm explaining smooth muscle replication in the vessel wall is that dysfunctional endothelium and/or inflammatory cells produce growth factors and ECM proteins that can induce replication and migration of VSMCs from the media to the intima (van Oostrom et al., 2009). In his "response-to injury" hypothesis, Ross proposed that VSMCs in the wall normally exist in a quiescent state, but, when the endothelium is injured, platelets release factors that stimulate VSMCs movement into and replication within the arterial intima (Ross, 1981-1982).

Growth factors have been known to influence the differentiated state of VSMCs (Willis et al., 2004). An interesting possibility is that smooth muscle replication may be controlled by factors intrinsic to the vessel wall. One possibility comes from evidence that normal endothelium contains inhibitors of smooth muscle proliferation (Haudenschild & Schwartz, 1979). The principal factor involved in VSMCs replication is the platelet derived growth factor (PDGF), which is a potent VSMC mitogen linked to vascular homeostasis and atherogenesis (Majesky et al., 1992). This peptide not only is mitogenic for VSMCs, but is chemotactic as well (Schwartz et al., 1986): the data on PDGF and its receptor subunits suggest, infact, a role in migration/localization of primordial VSMCs to the endothelium. This growth factor consists of two chain types, A and B, giving rise to three different PDGF subtypes (AA, AB, BB): PDGF-BB and -AB are known VMSCs chemoattractans, whereas PDGF-AA is associated with inhibition of chemotaxis (Zachary et al., 1999). PDGF binds to specific dimeric receptors (α and β) found on smooth muscle cells (Bowen-Pope & Ross, 1982) where initiates a series of events leading to DNA synthesis: receptor α can bind all PDGF subtypes, while receptor β binds only subtypes -AB and -BB. VSMCs have been determined to upregulate expression of receptor β in response to vascular injury, inducing their chemotaxis; at the same time, these cells are able to increase the PDGF-AA, acting as a paracrine or autocrine regulator of their chemotaxis. This represents the first described autoregulation pathway of VSMCs on their own proliferation/migration (Willis et al., 2004). The second known requirement for cell cycle progression is availability of insulin-like growth factor (IGF-1), a co-factor that VSMCs require for completion of the cell cycle following stimulation with PDGF (Clemmons, 1984). Perhaps more surprising is that, as reported above, VSMCs may be able to stimulate their own growth by synthesis of both PDGF and IGF-1 (PDGF is able to stimulate smooth muscle cells to produce IGF-1).

Moreover, those VSMCs that, once migrated into the intima, retained the ability to produce mitogen, due to their dedifferentiated state (Schwartz et al., 1986), are able to sustain proliferation also after the initial stimulation of platelet and PDGF release during vascular injury. Selection of such a proliferogenic subpopulation could account for both the monoclonal phenotype of chronic human atherosclerotic lesions (Gown & Benditt, E.P., 1982) and the suggestion that monoclonality arises gradually as the human lesion evolves (Lee et al., 1985). In summary, the emerging picture of growth control in arterial smooth muscle is a complex balance of forces. In addition to exogenous stimuli to cell growth, the vessel wall is capable of synthesis of endogenous growth inhibitors (including heparin sulfates, nitric oxide (NO), and transforming growth factor (TGF)-β) and growth stimulants (such as PDGF, IGF-1, ET-1, thrombin, FGF, IFNγ, and IL-1) (Berk, 2001).

5. Conclusions

Atherosclerosis and its associated complications remain the primary cause of death of the 21st century in humans. Recently it has been suggested that atherosclerosis is a multifactorial, multistep disease. Clinical and histopathological studies of atherosclerotic patient groups have identified inflammatory and oxidative stress-linked mechanisms as being pathogenetically important in atherosclerosis at every step from initiation to progression. Endothelial damage is also crucial for the progress of atherosclerosis and risk factors for atherosclerosis represent crucial factors associated with endothelial dysfunction. Studies have shown that patients with cardiovascular disease are characterized by impaired endothelial function, being vascular endothelium responsible for the secretion of several substances exerting proved anti-atherogenic effects. Finally, VSMCs are an important component of atherosclerotic plaques, responsible for promoting plaque stability in advanced lesions. In contrast, VSMC apoptosis has been implicated in a number of deleterious consequences of atherosclerosis, including plaque rupture, vessel remodelling, coagulation, inflammation and calcification. A better understanding of the pathogenesis of atherosclerosis will aid in for reducing mortality. An in-depth knowledge of the various pathogenic mechanisms involved in atherosclerosis can help in formulating preventive and therapeutic strategies and devising pharmaceutical and lifestyle modifications for reducing mortality.

6. Acknowledgments

The Authors want to thank Dr. Favero Gaia, Dr. Foglio Eleonora and Dr. Rossini Claudia for their excellent work in writing and improving this chapter and for their contribution in realizing the figures. Moreover, the Authors thank Peroni Michele for his help in editing this chapter.

7. References

Aikawa, M.; Sakomura, Y.; Ueda, M.; Kimura, K.; Manabe, I.; Ishiwata, S.; Komiyama, N.; Yamaguchi, H.; Yazaki, Y. & Nagai, R. (1997). Redifferentiation of smooth muscle cells after coronary angioplasty determined via myosin heavy chain expression. *Circulation*, Vol.96, No.1, (July 1997), pp. 82-90, ISSN 0009-7322.

Aikawa, M.; Rabkin, E.; Voglic, S.J.; Shing, H.; Nagai, R.; Schoen, F.J. & Libby, P. (1998). Lipid lowering promotes accumulation of mature smooth muscle cells expressing smooth muscle myosin heavy chain isoforms in rabbit atheroma. *Circulation Research*, Vol.83, No.10, (November 1998), pp. 1015-1026, ISSN 0009-7330.

Amorino, G.P. & Hoover, R.L. (1998). Interactions of monocytic cells with human endothelial cells stimulate monocytic metalloproteinase production. *The American Journal of Pathology*, Vol.152, No.1, (January 1998), pp. 199-207, ISSN 0002-9440.

Andrews, K.L.; Moore, X.L. & Chin-Dusting, J.P. (2010). Anti-atherogenic effects of high-density lipoprotein on nitric oxide synthesis in the endothelium. *Clinical and Experimental Pharmacology and Physiology*, Vol.37, No.7, (July 2010), pp. 736-742, ISSN 0305-1870.

Antoniades, C.; Tousoulis, D.; Tentolouris, C.; Toutouzas, P. & Stefanadis, C. (2003). Oxidative stress, antioxidant vitamins, and atherosclerosis. From basic research to clinical practice. *Herz*, Vol.28, No.7, (November 2003), pp. 628-638, ISSN 0340-9937.

Bai, X.; Wang, X. & Xu, Q. (2010). Endothelial damage and stem cell repair in atherosclerosis. *Vascular Pharmacology*, Vol.52, No.5-6, (May-June 2010), pp. 224-229, ISSN 1537-1891.

Bär, H.; Wende, P.; Watson, L.; Denger, S.; van Eys, G.; Kreuzer, J. & Jahn, L. (2002). Smoothelin is an indicator of reversible phenotype modulation of smooth muscle cells in balloon-injured rat carotid arteries. *Basic Research in Cardiology*, Vol.97, No.1, (January 2002), pp. 9-16, ISSN 0300-8428.

Barton, M. (2005). Ageing as a determinant of renal and vascular disease: role of endothelial factors. *Nephrology, Dialysis, Transplantation*, Vol.20, No.3, (March 2005), pp. 485-490, ISSN 0931-0509.

Barton, M. (2010). Obesity and aging: determinants of endothelial cell dysfunction and atherosclerosis. *Pflugers archiv*, Vol.460, No.5, (October 2010), pp. 825-837, ISSN 0031-6768.

Barton, M. & Haudenschild C.C. (2001). Endothelium and atherogenesis: endothelial therapy revisited. *Journal of Cardiovascular Pharmacology*, Vol.38, No.S2, (November 2001), pp. S23-25, ISSN 0160-2446.

Beckman, J.S. & Koppenol, W.H. (1996). Nitric oxide, superoxide, and peroxynitrite: the good, the bad, and ugly. *The American Journal of Physiology*, Vol.271, No. 5Pt1, (November 1996), pp. C1424-1437, ISSN 0363-6143.

Benditt, E.P. & Benditt, J.M. (1973). Evidence for a monoclonal origin of human atherosclerotic plaques. *Proceedings of the National Academy of Sciences of the United States of America*, Vol.70, No.6, (June 1973), pp. 1753-1756, ISSN 0027-8424.

Bennett, M. (2002). Apoptosis in the cardiovascular system. *Heart*, Vol.87, No.5, (May 2002), pp. 480-487, ISSN 1355-6037.

Bergh, N.; Ulfhammer, E.; Glise, K.; Jern, S. & Karlsson, L. (2009). Influence of TNF-alpha and biomechanical stress on endothelial anti- and prothrombotic genes. *Biochemical and Biophysical Research Communications*, Vol.385, No.3, (July 2009), pp. 314-318, ISSN 0006-291X.

Berk, B.C. (2001). Vascular smooth muscle growth: autocrine growth mechanisms. *Physiological Reviews*, Vol. 81, No.3, (July 2001), pp. 999-1030, ISSN 0031-9333.

Blankenberg, S.; Rupprecht, H.J.; Bickel, C.; Peetz, D.; Hafner, G.; Tiret, L. & Meyer, J. (2001). Circulating cell adhesion molecules and death in patients with coronary artery disease. *Circulation*, Vol.104, No.12, (September 2001), pp. 1336-1342, ISSN 0009-7322.

Bochaton-Piallat, M.L.; Ropraz, P.; Gabbiani, F. & Gabbiani, G. (1996). Phenotypic heterogeneity of rat arterial smooth muscle cell clones. Implications for the development of experimental intimal thickening. *Arteriosclerosis, Thrombosis, and Vascular Biology*, Vol.16, No.6, (June 1996), pp. 815-820, ISSN 1079-5642.

Bond, M.; Fabunmi, R.P.; Baker, A.H. & Newby, A.C. (1998). Synergistic upregulation of metalloproteinase-9 by growth factors and inflammatory cytokines: an absolute requirement for transcription factor NF-kB. *FEBS Letters*, Vol.435, No.1, pp. 29–34, ISSN 0014-5793.

Bonomini, F.; Tengattini, S.; Fabiano, A.; Bianchi, R. & Rezzani, R. (2008). Atherosclerosis and oxidative stress. *Histology and Histopathology*, Vol.23, No.3, (March 2008), pp. 381-390, ISSN 1699-5848.

Boring, L.; Gosling, J.; Cleary, M. & Charo, I.F. (1998). Decreased lesion formation in CCR2-/- mice reveals a role for chemokines in the initiation of atherosclerosis. *Nature*, Vol.394, No.6696, (August 1998), pp. 894-897, ISSN 0028-0836.

Bowen-Pope, D.F. & Ross, R. (1982). Platelet-derived growth factor. II. Specific binding to cultured cells. *Journal of Biological Chemistry*, Vol.257, No.9, (May 1982), pp. 5161-5171, ISSN 0021-9258.

Brach, M.A.; Henschler, R.; Mertelsmann, R.H. & Herrmann, F. (1991). Regulation of M-CSF expression by M-CSF: role of protein kinase C and ranscription factor NF kappa B. *Pathobiology*, Vol.59, No.4, pp. 284–288, ISSN 1015-2008.

Brand, K.; Eisele, T.; Kreusel, U.; Page, M.; Page, S.; Haas, M.; Gerling, A.; Kaltschmidt, C.; Neumann, F.J.; Mackman, N.; Baeurele, P.A.; Walli, A.K. & Neumeier, D. (1997). Dysregulation of monocytic nuclear factor-kappa B by oxidized low-density lipoprotein. *Arteriosclerosis, Thrombosis and Vascular Biology*, Vol.17, No.10, (October 1997), pp. 1901–1909, ISSN 1079-5642.

Cai, H. & Harrison, D.G. (2000). Endothelial Dysfunction in Cardiovascular Diseases: The Role of Oxidant Stress. *Circulation Research*, Vol. 87, No.10, (September 2000), pp.840-844, ISSN 0009-7330.

Campbell, G.R. & Campbell, J.H. (1985). Smooth muscle phenotypic changes in arterial wall homeostasis: implications for the pathogenesis of atherosclerosis. *Experimental and Molecular Pathology*, Vol.42, No.2, (April 1985), pp. 139-162, ISSN 0014-4800.

Chamley-Campbell, J.; Campbell, G.R. & Ross, R. (1979). The smooth muscle cell in culture. *Physiological Reviews*, Vol.59, No.1, (January 1979), pp. 1-61, ISSN 0031-9333.

Chandrasekharan, U.M.; Siemionow, M.; Unsal, M.; Yang, L.; Poptic, E.; Bohn, J.; Ozer, K.; Zhou, Z.; Howe, P.H.; Penn, M. & DiCorleto, P.E. (2007). Tumor necrosis factor alpha (TNF-alpha) receptor-II is required for TNF-alpha-induced leukocyte-endothelial interaction in vivo. *Blood,* Vol.109, No.5, (March 2007), pp. 1938-1944, ISSN 0006-4971.

Chung, I.M.; Schwartz, S.M. & Murry, C.E. (1998). Clonal architecture of normal and atherosclerotic aorta: implications for atherogenesis and vascular development. *American Journal of Pathology,* Vol.152, No.4, (April 1998), pp. 913-923, ISSN 0002-9440.

Cipollone, F.; Fazia, M.L. & Mezzetti, A. (2007). Oxidative stress, inflammation and atherosclerosis plaque development. *International Congress Series,* Vol.1303, (August 2007), pp. 35-40, ISSN 0531-5131.

Clemmons, D.R. (1984). Interaction of circulating cell-derived and plasma growth factors in stimulating cultured smooth muscle cell replication. *Journal of Cellular Physiology,* Vol.121, No.2, (November 1984), pp. 425-430, ISSN 0021-9541.

Clowes, A.W.; Reidy, M.A. & Clowes, M.M. (1983). Kinetics of cellular proliferation after arterial injury. I. Smooth muscle growth in the absence of endothelium. *Laboratory Investigation,* Vol.49, No.3, (September 1983), pp. 327-333, ISSN 0023-6837.

Cossu, G. & Bianco, P. (2003). Mesoangioblasts--vascular progenitors for extravascular mesodermal tissues. *Current Opinion in Genetics and Development,* Vol.13, No.5, (October 2003), pp. 537-542, ISSN 0959-437X.

Dabek, J.; Kułach, A. & Gąsior, Z. (2010). Nuclear factor kappa-light-chain-enhancer of activated B cells (NF-κB): a new potential therapeutic target in atherosclerosis? *Pharmacological Reports,* Vol.62, No.5, (September-October 2010), pp. 778-783, ISSN 1734-1140.

Dai, D.Z. & Dai, Y. (2010). Role of endothelin receptor A and NADPH oxidase in vascular abnormalities. *Journal of Vascular Health and Risk Management,* Vol.6, (September 2010), pp. 787-794, ISSN 1178-2048.

Davies, P.F.; Civelek, M.; Fang, Y.; Guerraty, M.A. & Passerini, A.G. (2010). Endothelial heterogeneity associated with regional athero-susceptibility and adaptation to disturbed blood flow in vivo. *Seminars in Thrombosis and Hemostasis,* Vol.36, No.3, (April 2010), pp. 265-275, ISSN 0094-6176.

Drake, C.J.; Brandt, S.J.; Trusk, T.C. & Little, C.D. (1997). TAL1/SCL is expressed in endothelial progenitor cells/angioblasts and defines a dorsal-to-ventral gradient of vasculogenesis. *Developmental Biology,* Vol.192, No.1, (December 1997), pp. 17-30, ISSN 0012-1606.

Dusserre, E.; Bourdillon, M.C.; Pulcini, T. & Berthezene, F. (1994). Decrease in high density lipoprotein binding sites is associated with decrease in intracellular cholesterol efflux in dedifferentiated aortic smooth muscle cells. *Biochimica et Biophysica Acta,* Vol.1212, No.2, (May 1994), pp. 235-244.

Dzau, V.J.; Braun-Dullaeus, R.C. & Sedding, D.G. (2002). Vascular proliferation and atherosclerosis: new perspectives and therapeutic strategies. *Nature Medicine,* Vol.8, No.11, (November 2002), pp. 1249-1256, ISSN 1078-8956.

Ferrario, C. (2009). Effect of angiotensin receptor blockade on endothelial function: focus on olmesartan medoxomil. *Vascular Health and Risk Management,* Vol.5, No.1, pp. 301-314, ISSN 1176-6344.

Fortuño, A.; San José, G.; Moreno, M.U.; Díez, J. & Zalba, G. (2005). Oxidative stress and vascular remodelling. *Experimental physiology*, Vol.90, No.4, (July 2005), pp. 457-462, ISSN 0958-0670.

Foteinos, G.; Hu, Y.; Xiao, Q.; Metzler, B. & Xu, Q. (2008). Rapid Endothelial Turnover in Atherosclerosis-Prone Areas Coincides With Stem Cell Repair in Apolipoprotein E–Deficient Mice. *Circulation*, Vol.117, No.14, (March 2008), pp. 1856-1863, ISSN 0009-7322.

Galis, Z.S. & Khatri, J.J. (2002). Matrix metalloproteinases in vascular remodeling and atherogenesis: the good, the bad, and the ugly. *Circulation Research*, Vol.90, No.3, (February 2002), pp. 251-262, ISSN 0009-7330.

Geary, R.L.; Wong, J.M.; Rossini, A.; Schwartz, S.M. & Adams, L.D. (2002). Expression profiling identifies 147 genes contributing to a unique primate neointimal smooth muscle cell phenotype. *Arteriosclerosis, Thrombosis, and Vascular Biology*, Vol.22, No.12, (December 2002), pp. 2010-2016, ISSN 1079-5642.

Gittenberger-de Groot, A.C.; DeRuiter, M.C.; Bergwerff, M. & Poelmann, R.E. (1999). Smooth muscle cell origin and its relation to heterogeneity in development and disease. *Arteriosclerosis, Thrombosis, and Vascular Biology*, Vol.19, No.7, (July 1999), pp. 1589-1594, ISSN 1079-5642.

Gordon, D.; Reidy, M.A.; Benditt, E.P. & Schwartz, S.M. (1990). Cell proliferation in human coronary arteries. *Proceedings of the National Academy of Sciences of the United States of America*, Vol.87, No.12, (June 1990), pp. 4600-4604, ISSN 0027-8424.

Gown, A.M. & Benditt, E.P. (1982). Lactate dehydrogenase (LDH) isozymes of human atherosclerotic plaques. *The American Journal of Pathology*, Vol.107, No.3, (June 1982), pp. 316-321, ISSN 0002-9440.

Griendling, K.K. & Harrison, D.G. (1999). Dual role of reactive oxygen species in vascular growth. *Circulation Research*, Vol.85, No.6, (September 1999), pp.562-563, ISSN 0009-7330.

Hansson, G.K.; Robertson, A.K. & Söderberg-Nauclér, C. (2006). Inflammation and atherosclerosis. *Annual Review of Pathology*, Vol.1, pp. 297-329.

Hansson, G.K. & Hermansson, A. (2011). The immune system in atherosclerosis. *Nature Immunology*, Vol.12, No.3, (March 2011), pp. 204-212, ISSN 1529-2908.

Hao, H.; Gabbiani, G. & Bochaton-Piallat, M.L. (2003). Arterial smooth muscle cell heterogeneity: implications for atherosclerosis and restenosis development. *Arteriosclerosis, Thrombosis, and Vascular Biology*, Vol.23, No.9, (September 2003), pp. 1510-1520, ISSN 1079-5642.

Haudenschild, C.C.; Prescott, M.F. & Chobanian A.V. (1981). Aortic endothelial and subendothelial cells in experimental hypertension and aging. *Hypertension*, Vol.3, No.3 Pt 2, (May-June 1981), pp. I148-153, ISSN 0194-911X.

Haudenschild, C.C. & Schwartz, S.M. (1979). Endothelial regeneration. II. Restitution of endothelial continuity. *Laboratory Investigation*, Vol.41, No.5, (November 1979), pp. 407-418, ISSN 0023-6837.

Heinecke, J.W. (2007). The role of myeloperoxidase in HDL oxidation and atherogenesis. *Current Atherosclerosis Reports*, Vol.9, No.4, (October 2007), pp. 249-251, ISSN 1523-3804.

Higashi, Y.; Noma, K.; Yoshizumi, M. & Kihara, Y. (2009). Endothelial function and oxidative stress in cardiovascular diseases. *Circulation Journal*, Vol.73, No.3, (March 2009), pp. 411-418, ISSN 1346-9843.

Hill, B.J.; Wamhoff, B.R. & Sturek, M. (2001). Functional nucleotide receptor expression and sarcoplasmic reticulum morphology in dedifferentiated porcine coronary smooth muscle cells. *Journal of Vascular Research*, Vol.38, No.5, (September- October 2001), pp. 432-443, ISSN 1018-1172.

Hillebrands, J.L.; Klatter, F.A. & Rozing, J. (2003). Origin of vascular smooth muscle cells and the role of circulating stem cells in transplant arteriosclerosis. *Arteriosclerosis, Thrombosis, and Vascular Biology*, Vol.23, No.3, (March 2003), pp. 380-387, ISSN 1079-5642.

Hirschi, K.K. & Majesky, M.W. (2004). Smooth muscle stem cells. *The Anatomical Record. Part A, Discoveries in Molecular, Cellular, and Evolutionary Biology*, Vol.276, No.1, (January 2004), pp. 22-33, ISSN 1552-4884.

Ho, A.W.; Wong, C.K. & Lam, C.W. (2008). Tumor necrosis factor-alpha up-regulates the expression of CCL2 and adhesion molecules of human proximal tubular epithelial cells through MAPK signaling pathways. *Immunobiology*, Vol.213, No.7, pp. 533-544, ISSN 0171-2985.

Holifield, B.; Helgason, T.; Jemelka, S.; Taylor, A.; Navran, S.; Allen, J. & Seidel, C. (1996). Differentiated vascular myocytes: are they involved in neointimal formation?. *The Journal of Clinical Investigation*, Vol.97, No.3, (February 1996), pp. 814-825, ISSN 0021-9738.

Hu, Y.; Davison, F.; Ludewig, B.; Erdel, M.; Mayr, M.; Url, M.; Dietrich, H. & Xu, Q. (2002). Smooth muscle cells in transplant atherosclerotic lesions are originated from recipients, but not bone marrow progenitor cells. *Circulation*, Vol.106, No.14, (October 2002), pp. 1834-1839, ISSN 0009-7322.

Hu, Y.; Zhang, Z.; Torsney, E.; Afzal, A.R.; Davison, F.; Metzler, B. & Xu, Q. (2004). Abundant progenitor cells in the adventitia contribute to atherosclerosis of vein grafts in ApoE-deficient mice. *The Journal of Clinical Investigation*, Vol.113, No.9, (May 2004), pp. 1258-1265, ISSN 0021-9738.

Irani, K. (2000). Oxidant signaling in vascular cell growth, death, and survival : a review of the roles of reactive oxygen species in smooth muscle and endothelial cell mitogenic and apoptotic signaling. *Circulation Research*, Vol.87, No.3, (August 2000), pp.179-183, ISSN 0009-7330.

Jackson, K.A.; Mi, T. & Goodell, M.A. (1999). Hematopoietic potential of stem cells isolated from murine skeletal muscle. *Proceedings of the National Academy of Sciences of the United States of America*, Vol.96, No.25, (December 1999), pp. 14482-14486, ISSN 0027-8424.

Jensen-Urstad, K.; Bouvier, F. & Jensen-Urstad, M. (1999). Preserved vascular reactivity in elderly male athletes. *Scandinavian Journal of Medicine and Science in Sports*, Vol.9, No.2, (April 1999), pp. 88-91, ISSN 0905-7188.

Jin, Z.G.; Ueba, H.; Tanimoto, T.; Lungu, A.O.; Frame, M.D. & Berk, B.C. (2003). Ligand-independent activation of vascular endothelial growth factor receptor 2 by fluid shear stress regulates activation of endothelial nitric oxide synthase. *Circulation Research*, Vol.93, No.4, (August 2003), pp. 354-363, ISSN0009-7330.

Kleinbongard, P.; Heusch, G. & Schulz, R. (2010). TNFalpha in atherosclerosis, myocardial ischemia/reperfusion and heart failure. *Pharmacology & Therapeutics*, Vol.127, No.3, (September 2010), pp. 295-314, ISSN 0163-7258.

Kojda, G. & Harrison, D. (1999). Interactions between NO and reactive oxygen species: pathophysiological importance in atherosclerosis, hypertension, diabetes and heart failure. *Cardiovascular Research*, Vol.43, No.3, (August 1999), pp. 562-571, ISSN 0008-6363.

Kruth, H.S. (2002). Sequestration of aggregated low-density lipoproteins by macrophages. *Current Opinion in Lipidology*, Vol.13, No.5, (October 2002), pp.433-438, ISSN 0957-9672.

Kutuk, O. & Basaga, H. (2003). Inflammation meets oxidation: NF-kB as a mediator of initial lesion development in atherosclerosis. *Trends in Molecular Medicine*, Vol.9, No.12, pp. 549-557, ISSN 1471-4914.

Lakshmi, S.V.; Padmaja, G.; Kuppusamy, P. & Kutala, V.K. (2009). Oxidative stress in cardiovascular disease. *Indian Journal of Biochemistry & Biophysics*, Vol.46, No.6, (December 2009), pp. 421-440, ISSN 0301-1208.

Lawson, C. & Wolf, S. (2009). ICAM-1 signaling in endothelial cells. *Pharmacological Reports*, Vol.61, No.1, (January-February 2009), pp. 22-32, ISSN 1734-1140.

Layne, M.D.; Yet, S.F.; Maemura, K.; Hsieh, C.M.; Liu, X.; Ith, B.; Lee, M.E. & Perrella, M.A. (2002). Characterization of the mouse aortic carboxypeptidase-like protein promoter reveals activity in differentiated and dedifferentiated vascular smooth muscle cells. *Circulation Research*, Vol.90, No.6, (April 2002), pp. 728-736, ISSN 0009-7330.

Lee, K.T.; Janakidevi, K.; Kroms, M.; Schmee, J. & Thomas, W.A. (1985). Mosaicism in female hybrid hares heterozygous for glucose-6-phosphate dehydrogenase. VII. Evidence for selective advantage of one phenotype over the other in ditypic samples from aortas of hares fed cholesterol oxidation products. *Experimental and Molecular Pathology*, Vol.42, No.1, (February 1985), pp. 71-77, ISSN 0014-4800.

Lemire, J.M.; Covin, C.W.; White, S.; Giachelli, C.M. & Schwartz, S.M. (1994). Characterization of cloned aortic smooth muscle cells from young rats. *The American Journal of Pathology*, Vol.144, No.5, (May 1994), pp. 1068-1081, ISSN 0002-9440.

Li, P.F.; Dietz, R. & von Harsdorf, R. (1997). Differential effect of hydrogen peroxide and superoxide anion on apoptosis and proliferation of vascular smooth muscle cells. *Circulation*, Vol.96, No.10, (November 1997), pp.3602-3609, ISSN 0009-7322.

Li, J.; Han, X.; Jiang, J.; Zhong, R.; Williams, G.M.; Pickering, J.G. & Chow, L.H. (2001). Vascular smooth muscle cells of recipient origin mediate intimal expansion after aortic allotransplantation in mice. *The American Journal of Pathology*, Vol.158, No.6, (June 2001), pp. 1943-1947, ISSN 0002-9440.

Li, J.J.; Fang, C.H.; Chen, M.Z.; Chen, X. & Lee, S.W. (2004). Activation of nuclear factor-kappaB and correlation with elevated plasma c-reactive protein in patients with unstable angina. *Heart, Lung and Circulation*, Vol.13, No.2, (June 2004), pp.173–178, ISSN 1443-9506.

Li, S.; Sims, S.; Jiao, Y.; Chow, L.H. & Pickering, J.G. (1999). Evidence from a novel human cell clone that adult vascular smooth muscle cells can convert reversibly between non-contractile and contractile phenotypes. *Circulation Research*, Vol.85, No.4, (August 1999), pp. 338-348, ISSN 0009-7330.

Li, W.G.; Miller, F.J. Jr.; Brown, M.R.; Chatterjee, P.; Aylsworth, G.R.; Shao, J.; Spector, A.A.; Oberley, L.W. & Weintraub, N.L. (2000). Enhanced H_2O_2-induced cytotoxicity in "epithelioid" smooth muscle cells: implications for neointimal regression. *Arteriosclerosis, Thrombosis, and Vascular Biology*, Vol.20, No.6, (June 2000), pp. 1473-1479, ISSN 1079-5642.

Libby, P.; Ridker, P.M. & Maseri, A. (2002). Inflammation and atherosclerosis. *Circulation*, Vol.105, No.9, (March 2002), pp.1135–1143, ISSN 0009-7322.

Libby, P.; DiCarli, M. & Weissleder, R. (2010). The vascular biology of atherosclerosis and imaging targets. *Journal of Nuclear Medicine*, Vol.51, No.S1, (May 2010), pp. 33S-37S, ISSN 2159-662X.

Liu, C.; Nath, K.A.; Katusic, Z.S. & Caplice, N.M. (2004). Smooth muscle progenitor cells in vascular disease. *Trends in Cardiovascular Medicine*, Vol.14, No.7, (October 2004), pp. 288-293, ISSN 1050-1738.

Madamanchi, NR.; Vendrov, A. & Runge, MS. (2005). Oxidative stress and vascular disease. *Arteriosclerosis, Thrombosis, and Vascular Biology*, Vol.25, No.1, (January 2005), pp.29-38, ISSN 1079-5642.

Majesky, M.W.; Giachelli, C.M.; Reidy, M.A. & Schwartz, S.M. (1992). Rat carotid neointimal smooth muscle cells reexpress a developmentally regulated mRNA phenotype during repair of arterial injury. *Circulation Research*, Vol.71, No.4, (October 1992), pp. 759-768, ISSN 0009-7330.

Matthews, C.; Gorenne, I.; Scott, S.; Figg, N.; Kirkpatrick, P.; Ritchie, A.; Goddard, M. & Bennett, M. (2006). Vascular smooth muscle cells undergo telomere-based senescence in human atherosclerosis: effects of telomerase and oxidative stress. *Circulation Research*, Vol.99, No.2, (July 2006), pp. 156-164, ISSN 0009-7330.

McKellar, G.E.; McCarey, D.W.; Sattar, N. & McInnes, I.B. (2009). Role for TNF in atherosclerosis? Lessons from autoimmune disease. *Nature Reviews Cardiology*, Vol.6, No.6, (June 2009), pp. 410-417, ISSN 1759-5002.

Metharom, P.; Liu, C.; Wang, S.; Stalboerger, P.; Chen, G.; Doyle, B.; Ikeda, Y. & Caplice, N.M. (2008). Myeloid lineage of high proliferative potential human smooth muscle outgrowth cells circulating in blood and vasculogenic smooth muscle-like cells in vivo. *Atherosclerosis*, Vol.198, No.1, (May 2008), pp. 29-38, ISSN 0021-9150.

Miano, J.M.; Cserjesi, P.; Ligon, K.L.; Periasamy, M. & Olson, E.N. (1994). Smooth muscle myosin heavy chain exclusively marks the smooth muscle lineage during mouse embryogenesis. *Circulation Research*, Vol.75, No.5, (November 1994), pp. 803-812, ISSN 0009-7330.

Miller, Y.I.; Chang, M.K.; Binder, C.J.; Shaw, P.X. & Witztum, J.L. (2003). Oxidized low density lipoprotein and innate immune receptors. *Current Opinion in Lipidology*, Vol.14, No.5, (October 2003), pp. 437-445, ISSN 0957-9672.

Mosse, P.R.; Campbell, G.R.; Wang, Z.L. & Campbell, J.H. (1985). Smooth muscle phenotypic expression in human carotid arteries. I. Comparison of cells from diffuse intimal thickenings adjacent to atheromatous plaques with those of the media. *Laboratory Investigation*, Vol.53, No.5, (November 1985), pp. 556-562, ISSN 0023-6837.

Muller, G. & Morawietz, H. (2009). Nitric oxide, NAD(P)H oxidase, and atherosclerosis. *Antioxidants and Redox Signaling*, Vol.11, No.7, (July 2009), pp. 1711-1731, ISSN 1523-0864.

Napoli, C.; Williams-Ignarro, S.; de Nigris, F.; Lerman, L.O.; D'Armiento, F.P.; Crimi, E.; Byrns, R.E.; Casamassimi, A.; Lanza, A.; Gombos, F.; Sica, V. & Ignarro, L.J. (2006). Physical training and metabolic supplementation reduce spontaneous atherosclerotic plaque rupture and prolong survival in hypercholesterolemic mice. *Proceedings of National Academy of Sciences of the United States of America*, Vol.103, No.27, (July 2006), pp. 10479-10484, ISSN 0027-8424.

Neureiter, D.; Zopf, S.; Dimmler, A.; Stintzing, S.; Hahn, E.G.; Kirchner, T.; Herold, C. & Ocker, M. (2005). Different capabilities of morphological pattern formation and its association with the expression of differentiation markers in a xenograft model of human pancreatic cancer cell lines. *Pancreatology*, Vol.5, No.4-5, pp. 387-397, ISSN 1424-3903.

Neuville, P.; Geinoz, A.; Benzonana, G.; Redard, M.; Gabbiani, F.; Ropraz, P. & Gabbiani, G. (1997). Cellular retinol-binding protein-1 is expressed by distinct subsets of rat arterial smooth muscle cells in vitro and in vivo. *The American Journal of Pathology*, Vol.150, No.2, (February 1997), pp. 509-521, ISSN 0002-9440.

Newby, A.C.; Libby, P. & van der Wal, A.C. (1999). Plaque instability--the real challenge for atherosclerosis research in the next decade?. *Cardiovascular Research*, Vol.41, No.2, (February 1999), pp. 321-322, ISSN 0008-6363.

Orlandi, A.; Di Lascio, A.; Francesconi, A.; Scioli, M.G.; Arcuri, G.; Ferlosio, A. & Spagnoli, L.G. (2008). Stem cell marker expression and proliferation and apoptosis of vascular smooth muscle cells. *Cell Cycle*, Vol.7, No.24, (December 2008), pp. 3889-3897, ISSN 1551-4005.

Orlandi, A. & Bennett, M. (2010). Progenitor cell-derived smooth muscle cells in vascular disease. *Biochemical Pharmacology*, Vol. 79, No.12, (June 2010), pp.1706-1713, ISSN 0006-2952.

Owens, G.K. (1995). Regulation of differentiation of vascular smooth muscle cells. *Physiological Reviews*, Vol.75, No.3, (July 1995), pp. 487-517, ISSN 0031-9333.

Owens, G.K.; Kumar, M.S. & Wamhoff, B.R. (2004). Molecular regulation of vascular smooth muscle cell differentiation in development and disease. *Physiological Reviews*, Vol.84, No.3, (July 2004), pp. 767-801, ISSN 0031-9333.

Packard, R.R. & Libby, P. (2008). Inflammation in atherosclerosis: from vascular biology to biomarker discovery and risk prediction. *Clinical Chemistry*, Vol.54, No.1, (January 2008), pp. 24-38, ISSN 0009-9147.

Partigulova, A.S. & Naumov, V.G. (2010). Inflammation and atherosclerosis: the role of Renin-Angiotensin system and its inhibition. *Kardiologiia*, Vol.50, No.10, pp. 50-55, ISSN 0022-9040.

Pasquinelli, G.; Tazzari, P.L.; Vaselli, C.; Foroni, L.; Buzzi, M.; Storci, G.; Alviano, F.; Ricci, F.; Bonafè, M.; Orrico, C.; Bagnara, G.P.; Stella, A. & Conte, R. (2007). Thoracic aortas from multiorgan donors are suitable for obtaining resident angiogenic mesenchymal stromal cells. *Stem Cells*, Vol.25, No.7, (July 2007), pp. 1627-1634, ISSN 1948-0210.

Pennathur, S. & Heinecke, J.W. (2007). Oxidative stress and endothelial dysfunction in vascular disease. *Current Diabetes Report*, Vol.7, No.4, (August 2007), pp. 257-264, ISSN 1534-4827.

Piechota, A.; Polańczyk, A. & Goraca, A. (2010). Role of endothelin-1 receptor blockers on hemodynamic parameters and oxidative stress. *Pharmacological Reports*, Vol.62, No.1, (January-February 2010), pp. 28-34, ISSN 1734-1140.

Rensen, S.S.; Doevendans, P.A. & van Eys, G.J. (2007). Regulation and characteristics of vascular smooth muscle cell phenotypic diversity. *Netherlands Heart Journal*, Vol.15, No.3, pp. 100-108, ISSN 1568-5888.

Roberts, N.; Jahangiri, M. & Xu, Q. (2005). Progenitor cells in vascular disease. *Journal of Cellular and Molecular Medicine*, Vol.9, No.3, (July-September 2005), pp. 583-591, ISSN 1582-4934.

Rodella, L.F.; Filippini, F.; Bonomini, F.; Bresciani, R.; Reiter, R.J. & Rezzani, R. (2010), a. Beneficial effects of melatonin on nicotine-induced vasculopathy. *Journal of Pineal Research*, Vol.48, No.2, (March 2010), pp. 126-132, ISSN 0742-3098 .

Rodella, L.F.; Favero, G.; Rossini, C.; Foglio, E.; Reiter, R.J. & Rezzani, R. (2010), b. Endothelin-1 as a potential marker of melatonin's therapeutic effects in smoking-induced vasculopathy. *Life Sciences*, Vol.87, No.17-18, (October 2010), pp. 558-564, ISSN 0024-3205.

Rodella, L.F.; Rossini, C.; Favero, G., Foglio, E., Loreto, C. & Rezzani, R. (2011). Nicotine-induced morphological changes in rat aorta: the protective role of melatonin. *Cells Tissues Organs*, (April 2011, Epub ahead of print), ISSN 1422-6405.

Ross, R. & Glomset, J.A. (1973). Atherosclerosis and the arterial smooth muscle cell: Proliferation of smooth muscle is a key event in the genesis of the lesions of atherosclerosis. *Science*, Vol.180, No.93, (June 1973), pp. 1332-1339, 0036-8075.

Ross, R. (1981-1982). Atherosclerosis: a question of endothelial integrity and growth control of smooth muscle. *Harvey Lectures*, Vol.77, pp. 161-182, ISSN 0073-0874.

Ross, R. (1999). Atherosclerosis is an inflammatory disease. *American Heart Journal*, Vol.138, No.5Pt 2, (November 1999), pp. S419-420, ISSN 0002-8703.

Rudijanto, A. (2007). The role of vascular smooth muscle cells on the pathogenesis of atherosclerosis. *Acta Medica Indonesiana*, Vol.39, No.2, (April-June 2007), pp. 86-93, ISSN 0125-9326.

Rzucidlo, E.M.; Martin, K.A. & Powell, R.J. (2007). Regulation of vascular smooth muscle cell differentiation. *Journal of Vascular Surgery*, Vol.45, No.SA, (June 2007), pp. A25-32, ISSN 0741-5214.

Schäfers, M.; Schober, O. & Hermann, S. (2010). Matrix-metalloproteinases as imaging targets for inflammatory activity in atherosclerotic plaques. *The Journal of Nuclear Medicine*, Vol.51, No.5, (May 2010), pp. 663-666, ISSN 0161-5505.

Schwartz, S.M.; Campbell, G.R. & Campbell, J.H. (1986). Replication of smooth muscle cells in vascular disease. *Circulation Research*, Vol.58, No.4, (April 1986), pp. 427-444, ISSN 0009-7330.

Schwartz, S.M.; deBlois, D. & O'Brien, E.R. (1995). The intima. Soil for atherosclerosis and restenosis. *Circulation Research*, Vol.77, No.3, (September 1995), pp. 445-465, ISSN 0009-7330.

Schwartz, S.M.; Virmani, R. & Rosenfeld, M.E. (2000). The good smooth muscle cells in atherosclerosis. *Current Atherosclerosis Reports*, Vol.2, No.5, (September 2000), pp. 422-429, ISSN 1523-3804.

Shah, P.K.; Falk, E.; Badimon, J.J.; Fernandez-Ortiz, A.; Mailhac, A.; Villareal-Levy, G.; Fallon, J.T.; Regnstrom, J. & Fuster, V. (1995). Human monocyte-derived macrophages induce collagen breakdown in fibrous caps of atherosclerotic plaques. Potential role of matrix-degrading metalloproteinases and implications for plaque rupture. *Circulation*, Vol.92, No.6, (September 1995), pp. 1565-1569, ISSN 0009-7322.

Shanahan, C.M.; Weissberg, P.L. & Metcalfe, J.C. (1993). Isolation of gene markers of differentiated and proliferating vascular smooth muscle cells. *Circulation Research*, Vol.73, No.1, (July 1993), pp. 193-204, ISSN 0009-7330.

Shanahan, C.M. & Weissberg, P.L. (1998). Smooth muscle cell heterogeneity: patterns of gene expression in vascular smooth muscle cells in vitro and in vivo. *Arteriosclerosis, Thrombosis and Vascular Biology*, Vol.18, No.3, (March 1998), pp. 333-338 ISSN 1079-5642.

Shanahan, C.M. & Weissberg, P.L. (1999). Smooth muscle cell phenotypes in atherosclerotic lesions. *Current Opinion in Lipidology*, Vol.10, No.6, (December 1999), pp. 507-513, ISSN 0957-9672.

Sies, H. (1991). Oxidative stress: from basic research to clinical application. *The American Journal of Medicine*, Vol.91, No.3C, (September 1991), pp. 31S-38S, ISSN 1548-2766.

Sima, A.V.; Stancu, C.S. & Simionescu, M. (2009). Vascular endothelium in atherosclerosis. *Cell and Tissue Research*, Vol.335, No.1, (January 2009), pp. 191-203, ISSN 0302-766X.

Simionescu, M. & Antohe, F. (2006). Functional ultrastructure of the vascular endothelium: changes in various pathologies. *Handbook of Experimental Pharmacology*, No.176Pt 1, pp. 41-69, ISSN 0171-2004.

Simper, D.; Stalboerger, P.G.; Panetta, C.J.; Wang, S. & Caplice, N.M. (2002). Smooth muscle progenitor cells in human blood. *Circulation*, Vol.106, No.10, (September 2002), pp. 1199-1204, ISSN 0009-7322.

Singh, U. & Jialal, I. (2006). Oxidative stress and atherosclerosis. *Pathophysiology*, Vol.13, No.3, (August 2006), pp. 129-142, ISSN 0928-4680.

Skålén, K.; Gustafsson, M.; Rydberg, E.K.; Hultén, L.M.; Wiklund, O.; Innerarity, T.L. & Borén, J. (2002). Subendothelial retention of atherogenic lipoproteins in early atherosclerosis. *Nature*, Vol.417, No.6890, (June 2002), pp.750-754, ISSN 0028-0836.

Skalska, A.B.; Pietrzycka, A. & Stepniewski, M. (2009). Correlation of endothelin 1 plasma levels with plasma antioxidant capacity in elderly patients treated for hypertension. *Clinical Biochemistry*, Vol.42, No.4-5, (March 2009), pp. 358-364, ISSN 0009-9120.

Slomp, J.; Gittenberger-de Groot, A.C.; Glukhova, M.A.; Conny van Munsteren. J.; Kockx, M.M.; Schwartz, S.M. & Koteliansky, V.E. (1997). Differentiation, dedifferentiation, and apoptosis of smooth muscle cells during the development of the human ductus arteriosus. *Arteriosclerosis, Thrombosis and Vascular Biology*, Vol.17, No.5, (May 1997), pp. 1003-1009, ISSN 1079-5642.

Sobue, K.; Hayashi, K. & Nishida, W. (1999). Expressional regulation of smooth muscle cell-specific genes in association with phenotypic modulation. *Molecular and Cellular Biochemistry*, Vol.190, No.1-2, (January 1999), pp. 105-118, ISSN 0300-8177.

Sprague, A.H. & Khalil, R.A. (2009). Inflammatory cytokines in vascular dysfunction and vascular disease. *Biochemical Pharmacology*, Vol.78, No.6, (September 2009), pp. 539-552, ISSN 0006-2952.

Steinberg, D. (2009). The LDL modification hypothesis of atherogenesis: an update. *Journal of Lipid Research*, Vol.50S, (April 2009), pp. 376-381, ISSN 0022-2275.

Stintzing, S.; Ocker, M.; Hartner, A.; Amann, K.; Barbera, L. & Neureiter, D. (2009). Differentiation patterning of vascular smooth muscle cells (VSMC) in atherosclerosis. *Virchows Archives*, Vol.455, No.2, (August 2009), pp. 171-185, ISSN 1432-2307.

Stocker, R. & Keaney, J.F. Jr. (2004). Role of oxidative modifications in atherosclerosis. *Physiological reviews*, Vol.84, No.4, (October 2004), pp.1381-1478, ISSN 0031-9333.

Tabas, I.; Williams, K.J. & Borén, J. (2007). Subendothelial lipoprotein retention as the initiating process in atherosclerosis: update and therapeutic implications. *Circulation*, Vol.116, No.16, (October 2007), pp.1832-1844, ISSN 0009-7322.

Tagliafico, E.; Brunelli, S.; Bergamaschi, A.; De Angelis, L.; Scardigli, R.; Galli, D.; Battini, R.; Bianco, P.; Ferrari, S.; Cossu, G. & Ferrari, S. (2004). TGFbeta/BMP activate the smooth muscle/bone differentiation programs in mesoangioblasts. *Journal of Cell Science*, Vol.117, No.Pt 19, (September 2004), pp. 4377-4388, ISSN 0021-9533.

Taniyama, Y. & Griendling, K.K. (2003). Reactive oxygen species in the vasculature: molecular and cellular mechanisms. *Hypertension*, Vol.42, No.6, (December 2003), pp.1075-1081, ISSN 0194-911X.

Teplyakov, A.I. (2004). Endothelin-1 involved in systemic cytokine network inflammatory response at atherosclerosis. *Journal of Cardiovascular Pharmacology*, Vol.44, No.S1, (November 2004), pp. S274-S275, ISSN 0160-2446.

Thom T.J. (1989). International mortality from heart disease: rates and trends. *International Journal of Epidemiology*, Vol.18, No.3(S1), pp.S20-S28, ISSN 1464-3685.

Thyberg, J. (2002). Caveolae and cholesterol distribution in vascular smooth muscle cells of different phenotypes. *The Journal of Histochemistry and Cytochemistry*, Vol.50, No.2, (February 2002), pp. 185-195, ISSN 0022-1554.

Tintut, Y.; Alfonso, Z.; Saini, T.; Radcliff, K.; Watson, K.; Boström, K. & Demer, L.L. (2003). Multilineage potential of cells from the artery wall. *Circulation*, Vol.108, No.20, (November 2003), pp. 2505-2510, ISSN 0009-7322.

Tîrziu, D.; Dobrian, A.; Tasca, C.; Simionescu, M. & Simionescu, N. (1995). Intimal thickenings of human aorta contain modified reassembled lipoproteins. *Atherosclerosis*, Vol.112, No.1, (January 1995), pp. 101-114, ISSN 0021-9150.

Topouzis, S. & Majesky, M.W. (1996). Smooth muscle lineage diversity in the chick embryo. Two types of aortic smooth muscle cell differ in growth and receptor-mediated transcriptional responses to transforming growth factor-beta. *Developmental Biology*, Vol.178, No.2, (September 1996), pp. 430-445, ISSN 0012-1606.

Torsney, E.; Mandal, K.; Halliday, A.; Jahangiri, M. & Xu, Q. (2007). Characterisation of progenitor cells in human atherosclerotic vessels. *Atherosclerosis*, Vol.191, No.2, (April 2007), pp. 259-264, ISSN 0021-9150.

Tousoulis, D.; Koutsogiannis, M.; Papageorgiou, N.; Siasos, G.; Antoniades, C.; Tsiamis, E. & Stefanadis, C. (2010). Endothelial dysfunction: potential clinical implications. *Minerva Medica*, Vol.101, No.4, (August 2010), pp. 271-284, ISSN 1827-1669.

Traub, O. & Berk, B.C. (1998). Laminar shear stress: mechanisms by which endothelial cells transduce an atheroprotective force. *Arteriosclerosis, Thrombosis and Vascular Biology*, Vol.18, No.5, (May 1998), pp. 677-685, ISSN 1079-5642.

Traupe, T.; Ortmann, J.; Münter, K. & Barton, M. (2003). Endothelial therapy of atherosclerosis and its risk factors. *Current Vascular Pharmacology*, Vol.1, No.2, (June 2003), pp. 111-121, ISSN 1570-1611.

van Oostrom, O.; Fledderus, J.O.; de Kleijn, D.; Pasterkamp, G. & Verhaar, M.C. (2009). Smooth muscle progenitor cells: friend or foe in vascular disease?. *Current Stem Cell Research & Therapy*, Vol.4, No.2, (May 2009), pp. 131-140, ISSN 1574-888X.

Vanhoutte P.M. (2009). Endothelial dysfunction: The first step toward coronary arterosclerosis. *Circulation Journal*, Vol.73, No.4, (April 2009), pp. 595-601, ISSN 1346-9843.

Vásquez-Vivar, J.; Kalyanaraman, B.; Martásek, P.; Hogg, N.; Masters, B.S.; Karoui, H.; Tordo, P. & Pritchard, K.A. Jr. (1998). Superoxide generation by endothelial nitric oxide synthase: the influence of cofactors. *Proceedings of the National Academy of Sciences of the United States of America*, Vol.95, No.16, (August 1998), pp. 9220-9225, ISSN 0027-8424.

Virdis, A.; Ghiadoni, L.; Giannarelli, C. & Taddei, S. (2010). Endothelial dysfunction and vascular disease in later life. *Maturitas*, Vol.67, No.1, (September 2010), pp. 20-24, ISSN 0378-5122.

Weissberg, P.L.; Clesham, G.J. & Bennett, M.R. (1996). Is vascular smooth muscle cell proliferation beneficial?. *Lancet*, Vol.347, No.8997, (February 1996), pp. 305-307, ISSN 0140-6736.

Williams, K.J. & Tabas, I. (2005). Lipoprotein retention--and clues for atheroma regression. *Arteriosclerosis, Thrombosis and Vascular Biology*, Vol.25, No.8, (August 2005), pp. 1536-1540, ISSN 1079-5642.

Willis, A.I.; Pierre-Paul, D.; Sumpio, B.E. & Gahtan, V. (2004). Vascular smooth muscle cell migration: current research and clinical implications. *Vascular and Endovascular Surgery*, Vol.38, No.1, (January-February 2004), pp. 11-23, ISSN 1538-5744.

Witztum, J.L. & Steinberg, D. (2001). The oxidative modification hypothesis of atherosclerosis: does it hold for humans?. *Trends in Cardiovascular Medicine*, Vol.11, No.3-4, (April-May 2001), pp. 93-102, ISSN 1050-1738.

Xu, Q. (2000). Biomechanical-stress-induced signaling and gene expression in the development of arteriosclerosis. *Trends in Cardiovascular Medicine*, Vol.10, No.1, (January 2000), pp. 35-41, ISSN 1050-1738.

Xu, Q. (2009). Disturbed flow-enhanced endothelial turnover in atherosclerosis. *Trends in Cardiovascular Medicine*, Vol.19, No.6, (August 2009), pp. 191-195, ISSN 1050-1738.

Yamada, N. (2001). Atherosclerosis and oxidative stress. *Japan Medical Association Journal*, Vol.44, No.12, pp. 529-534, ISSN 1346-8650.

Zachary, I.; Servos, S. & Herren, B. (1999). Identification of novel protein kinases in vascular cells. *Methods in Molecular Medicine*, Vol. 30, pp. 111-129, ISSN 1543-1894.

Zalewski, A.; Shi, Y. & Johnson, A.G. (2002). Diverse origin of intimal cells: smooth muscle cells, myofibroblasts, fibroblasts, and beyond?. *Circulation Research*, Vol.91, No.8, (October 2002), pp. 652-655, ISSN 0009-7330.

Zeng, L.; Zampetaki, A.; Margariti, A.; Pepe, A.E.; Alam, S.; Martin, D.; Xiao, Q.; Wang, W.; Jin, Z.G.; Cockerill, G.; Mori, K.; Li, Y.S.; Hu, Y.; Chien, S. & Xu, Q. Sustained activation of XBP1 splicing leads to endothelial apoptosis and atherosclerosis development in response to disturbed flow. (2009). *Proceedings of the National Academy of Sciences of the United States of America*,Vol.106, No.20, (May 2009), pp. 8326-8331, ISSN 0027-8424.

Zengin, E.; Chalajour, F.; Gehling, U.M.; Ito, W.D.; Treede, H.; Lauke, H.; Weil, J.; Reichenspurner, H.; Kilic, N. & Ergün, S. (2006). Vascular wall resident progenitor cells: a source for postnatal vasculogenesis. *Development*, Vol.133, No.8, (April 2006), pp. 1543-1551, ISSN 0950-1991.

Zhang, S.H.; Reddick, R.L.; Piedrahita, J.A. & Maeda, N. (1992). Spontaneous hypercholesterolemia and arterial lesions in mice lacking apolipoprotein E. *Science*, Vol.258, No.5081, (October 1992), pp. 468-471, ISSN 0036-8075.

Zhang, H.; Park, Y.; Wu, J.; Chen, X.; Lee, S.; Yang, J.; Dellsperger, K.C. & Zhang, C. (2009). Role of TNF-alpha in vascular dysfunction. *Clinical Science (London)*, Vol.116, No.3, (February 2009), pp. 219-230, ISSN 1470-8736.

Zoll, J.; Fontaine, V.; Gourdy, P.; Barateau, V.; Vilar, J.; Leroyer, A.; Lopes-Kam, I.; Mallat, Z.; Arnal, J.F.; Henry, P.; Tobelem, G. & Tedgui, A. (2008). Role of human smooth muscle cell progenitors in atherosclerotic plaque development and composition. *Cardiovascular Research*, Vol.77, No.3, (February 2008), pp. 471-480, ISSN 0008-6363.

6

Nutrigenomics and Atherosclerosis: The Postprandial and Long-Term Effects of Virgin Olive Oil Ingestion

Almudena Ortega, Lourdes M. Varela, Beatriz Bermudez,
Sergio Lopez, Francisco J.G. Muriana and Rocio Abia
Laboratory of Cellular and Molecular Nutrition, Instituto de la Grasa,
Consejo Superior de Investigaciones Científicas, Sevilla,
Spain

1. Introduction

Epidemiological studies over the past 50 years have revealed numerous risk factors for atherosclerosis. They can be grouped into factors with an important genetic component and environmental factors, particularly diet, which is one of the major, constant environmental factors to which our genes are expose through life. When a gene is activated, or expressed, functionally distinct proteins are produced which can initiate a host of cellular metabolic effects. Gene expression patterns produce a phenotype, which represents the physical characteristics of an organism (e.g., hair color), or the presence or absence of a disease. Nutrition scientists realize more and more that phenotypic treats (health status) are not necessarily produce by genes alone but also by the interaction of bioactive food components on the levels of DNA, RNA, protein and metabolites (Müller & Kersten, 2003). Nutritional genomics came into being at the beginning of the 1990s. There is some confusion about the delimitation of the concept, as often the terms of nutritional genomics, nutrigenetics, and nutrigenomics, are used as synonyms. Nutritional genomics refers to the joint study of nutrition and the genome including all the other omics derived from genomics: transcriptomics (mRNA), proteomics (proteins), and metabolomics (metabolites) (Fig. 1). The terms nutritional genomics would be equivalent to the wide-ranging term of gene-diet interaction. Within the wide framework of the concept of nutritional genomics, we can distinguish 2 subconcepts: nutrigenetics and nutrigenomics. Currently, there is a wide consensus on considering nutrigenetics as the discipline that studies the different phenotypic response to diet depending on the genotype of each individual. The term nutrigenomics is subject to a greater variability in its delimitation, but it seems that there is a certain consensus in considering nutrigenomics as the discipline which studies the molecular mechanisms explaining the different phenotypic responses to diet depending on the genotype, studying how the nutrients regulate gene expression, and how these changes are interrelated with proteomics and metabolomics (Corella & Ordovas, 2009). This interpretation of the nutrigenomics concept is the one that we shall use in this Chapter.

Atherosclerosis is a complex, multifactorial disease associated with accumulation of lipids in lesions along blood vessels, leading to the occlusion of blood flow, with oxidative and inflammatory components playing major roles in its cause. Environmental factors with particular emphasis on nutrition as well as genetic factors appear to be responsible for these aberrant oxidative and inflammatory components and the lipid abnormalities associated with the disease. Diet may contribute to the atherosclerotic process by affecting lipoprotein concentration, their composition and degree of oxidation. Although certain key risk factors affecting atherosclerosis have been identified, the full molecular characterization will remain a challenge in the next century to come. As a complex biological process, the cellular and molecular details of the growth, progression and regression of the vascular lesions of atherosclerosis call for application of the newly developing omics techniques of analysis. Profiling gene expression using microarrays has proven useful in identifying new genes that may contribute to features of the atherosclerosis lesion (transcriptomics). One of the interesting challenges of modern biology is to define the diet that best fits the needs of the human species. Understanding the details of gene-nutrient interactions and of how changes in a gene or in the amount or form of a nutrient influence atherosclerosis is essential to developing insight into how to support optimal health from a nutritional perspective. There has been much interest regarding the components that contribute to the beneficial health effects of the Mediterranean diet. Recent findings suggest that bioactive components found in extra-virgin olive oil (EVOO) (oleic acid and polyphenol compounds) are endowed with several biologic activities that may contribute to the lower incidence of atherosclerosis in the Mediterranean area. This review summarizes more recent studies, including omics technologies that have lead to the development of new hypothesis concerning the cellular response to virgin olive oil (VOO) ingestion and to identify the major cellular pathways responsive to them.

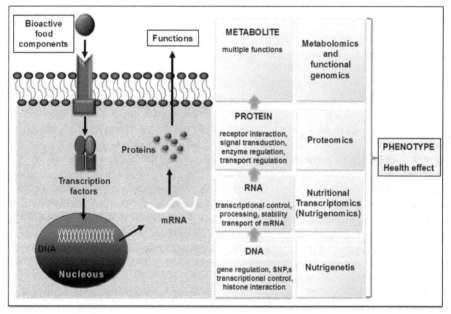

Fig. 1. Health effects of bioactive food components are related to specific interactions on a molecular level. (Adapted from Van Ommen, 2004; Müller & Kersten, 2003). SNP, single nucleotide polymorphism.

2. Olive oil and atherosclerosis

2.1 Olive oil classification according to International Olive Council

Olive oil is the main source of fat in the Mediterranean diet, and different categories of olive oils may be distinguished according to the International Olive Oil Council. Olive oil is obtained solely from the fruit of the olive tree (*Olea europaea*; family Oleaceae), and is not mixed with any other kind of oil. Olive oil extraction is the process of extracting the oil present in the olive drupes for food use. The oil is produced in the mesocarp cells, and is stored in a particular type of vacuole called a lipovacuole; every cell within an olive contains a tiny olive oil droplet. Olive oil extraction is defined as the process of separating the oil from the other fruit contents (vegetative extract liquid and solid material) and extracting the oil present in the drupes for food use. This separation is attained only by physical procedures under thermal conditions that do not alter the oil.

Several different types of oil can be oil extracted from the olive fruit and are classified as follows:

Virgin indicates that the oil was extracted by physical procedures only with no chemical treatment, and is in essence crude oil.

Refined indicates that the oil has been chemically treated to neutralise strong tastes (which are characterized as defects) and neutralise the acid content (free fatty acids). Refined oil is commonly regarded as a lower quality than virgin oil.

Pomace olive oil indicates oil that has been extracted from the pomace (ground flesh and pits left after pressing olives) using chemical solvents (typically hexane) and by heat.

Oil can be classified into different grades as follow:

Extra-virgin olive oil is the highest quality of olive oils and is produced by cold extraction of the olives; the oil has a free acidity of no more than 0.8 grams of oleic acid per 100 grams (0.8% acidity), and is often thought to have a superior taste. There can be no refined oil in extra-virgin olive oil.

Virgin olive oil has an acidity of less than 2%, and is often thought to have a good taste. There can be no refined oil in virgin olive oil.

Olive oil. Oils labelled as Olive oil are usually a blend of refined olive oil and one of the above two categories of virgin olive oil; typically, these blends contain less than or equal to 1.5% acidity. This grade of oil commonly lacks a strong flavour. Different blends are produced by adding more or less virgin oil to achieve different tastes.

Olive-pomace oil is a blend of refined pomace olive oil and possibly some virgin oil. This oil is safe to consume, but it may not be called olive oil.

Lampante oil is olive oil that is not used for consumption; lampante comes from olives that have strong physico-chemical and organoleptic defects and contain greater than 3,3% of acidity.

2.2 Olive oil composition

VOO is composed mainly of TGs (98-99 % of the total oil weight) and contains small quantities of free fatty acids (FFAs), and more than 230 chemical compounds such as aliphatic and triterpenic alcohols, sterols, hydrocarbons, volatile compounds and antioxidants. TGs are the major energy reserve for plants and animals. Chemically speaking, these are molecules derived from the natural esterification of three fatty acid molecules with a glycerol molecule. The glycerol molecule can simplistically be seen as an "E-shaped" molecule, with the fatty acids in turn resembling longish hydrocarbon chains, varying (in the case of olive oil) from about 14 to 24 carbon atoms in length (Fig. 2). The fatty acid composition of olive oil varies widely depending on the cultivar, maturity of the fruit, altitude, climate, and several other factors. A fatty acid has the general formula: CH3(CH2)nCOOH where n is typically an even number between 12 and 22. If no double bonds are present the molecules are called saturated fatty acids (SFAs). If a chain contains double bonds, it is called an unsaturated fatty acid. A single double bond makes monounsaturated fatty acids (MUFAs). More than one double bond makes polyunsaturated fatty acids (PUFAs). The major fatty acids in olive oil triglycerides are: oleic acid (C18:1), a monounsaturated omega-9 fatty acid. It makes up 55 to 83% of olive oil. Linoleic acid (C18:2), a polyunsaturated omega-6 fatty acid that makes up about 3.5 to 21% of olive oil. Palmitic acid (C16:0), a SFA that makes up 7.5 to 20% of olive oil. Stearic acid (C18:0), a SFA that makes up 0.5 to 5% of olive oil (Fig. 2). Linolenic acid (C18:3) (specifically alpha-Linolenic acid), a polyunsaturated omega-3 fatty acid that makes up 0 to 1.5% of olive oil. In the triglycerides the main fatty acids are represented by monounsaturates (oleic acid), with a slight amount of saturates (palmitic and stearic acids) and an adequate presence of polyunsaturates (linoleic and α-linolenic acid) (Bermudez et al., 2011). Most prevalent in olive oil is the oleic-oleic-oleic (OOO) triglyceride, followed, in order of incidence, by palmitic-oleic-oleic (POO), oleic-oleic-linoleic (OOL), palmitic-oleic-linoleic (POL), and stearic-oleic-oleic (SOO).

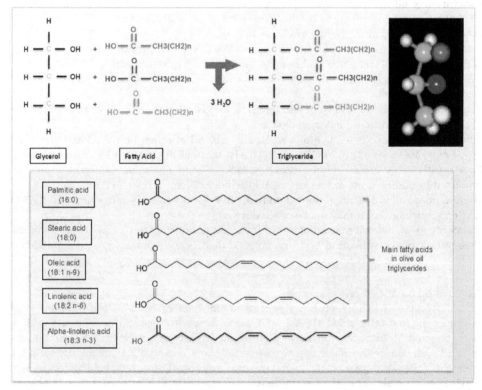

Fig. 2. Structure of triglycerides and main fatty acids in olive oil triglycerides.

The minor components of VOO are α-tocopherol, phenol compounds, carotenoids (β-carotene and lutein), squalene, pytosterols, and chlorophyll (in addition to a great number of aromatic substances). The factor that can influence the composition of VOO, especially in regard to its minor components, are the type of cultivar, the characteristics of the olive tree growing soil, climatic factors, fruit ripening stage, time of harvesting and degree of technology used in its production. The main antioxidants of VOO are phenols represented by lipophilic and hydrophilic phenols. Carotenes, on the contrary are contained in small concentrations. The lipophilic phenols, such as tocopherols and tocotrienols, can be found in other vegetable oils. In VOO more than 90% of total concentration of tocopherols is constituted by α-tocopherol. The VOO hydrophilic phenols constitute a group of secondary plant metabolites showing peculiar organoleptic and healthy properties. They are not generally present in other oils and fats (Servili et al., 2009). VOO contains four major classes of phenolic compounds: flavonoids, lignans, simple phenolics and secoiridois (Table 1). Although some cultivars contain flavonoids, the content in olive oil is low compared to other fruits and vegetables. Lignans are present at more significant

Phenolic alcohols (simple phenolics)	Phenolic acids and derivatives
(3,4-Dihydroxyphenil) ethanol (3,4 DHPEA) (HY)	Vanillic acid
(4-Hydroxyphenil) ethanol (p-HPEA) (TYR)	Syringic acid
(3,4-Dyhydroxyphenyl) ethanol-glucoside	p-Coumaric acid
Flavones	o-Coumaric acid
Apigenin	Gallic acid
Luteolin	Caffeic acid
Rutin	Protocatechuic acid
Lignans	p-Hydroxibenzoic acid
(+)-Acetoxypinoresinol	Ferulic acid
(+)-Pinoresinol	Cinnamic acid
(+)-Hydroxypinoresinol	4-(acetoxyithil)-1,2-Dihydroxybenzene
	Benzoic acid
	Hydroxy-isocromas
	Phenyl-6,7-dihydroxi-isochroman

Secoiridoids

Dialdehydic form of decarboxymethyl elenolic acid linked to 3,4-DHPEA (3,4 DHPEA-EDA)
Dialdehydic form of decarboxymethyl elenolic acid linked to p-HPEA (p-HPEA-EDA)
Oleuropein aglycon (3,4 DHPEA-EA)
Ligstroside aglycon
Oleuropein
p-HPEA-derivative
Dialdehydic form of oleuropein aglycon
Dialdehydic form of ligstroside aglycon

Table 1. Phenolic composition of a Virgin Olive Oil.

amounts. The levels of secoiridoids and simple phenolics, many of which are exclusive to VOO, are the major phenolics found in olive oil. The simple phenolics present in VOO are predominantly hydroxytyrosol (HT) (3,4-dihydroxyphenylethanol) and tyrosol (TYR) (4-hydroxyphenylethanol) whilst the secoiridoids are derived from the glusosides of oleuropein and ligstroside forms, they contain in their chemical structure an HT (oleuropein derivatives) or TYR (ligstroside derivatives) moiety linked to elenolic acid (Corona et al., 2009). After ingestion, olive oil polyphenols can be partially modified in the acidic environment of the stomach, aglycone secoiridoids are subject to hydrolysis leading to approximate 5-fold increase in the amount of free HT and 3-fold increase in free TYR. If the ingested secoiridoid is glucosylated it appears not to be subject to gastric hydrolysis, meaning that phenolics such as glucosides of oleuropein enter the small intestine unmodified, along with high amount of free HT and TYR and remaining secoiridoid aglycones. The major site for the absorption of olive oil polyphenols is the small intestine, HT and TYR are dose-dependently absorbed and they are metabolized primarily to O-glucuronidated conjugates. HT also undergoes O-methylation by the action of catechol-O-methyl-transferase, and both homovanillic acid and homovanillyl alcohol have been detected in human and animal plasma and urine after the oral administration of either VOO or pure HT and TYR. Studies have also demonstrated that secoiridoids, which appear not to be absorbed in the small intestine, undergo bacterial catabolism in the large intestine with oleuropein undergoing rapid degradation by the colonic microflora producing HT as the major end product (Corona, et al., 2006). The intense interest in VOO polyphenols and their metabolites can be attributed to the association of such substances with several biological activities; these include antioxidant activity as well as other important healthy properties that will be discussed later. For this reason, olive polyphenols are recognized as potential nutraceutical targets for food and pharmaceutical industries.

2.3 Atherosclerosis and virgin olive oil

Atherosclerosis underlies the leading cause of death in industrialised societies (Lloyd-Jones et al., 2010). The key-initiating step of early stages of atherosclerosis is the subendothelial accumulation of apolipoprotein B-containing lipoproteins. These lipoproteins are produced by the liver and the intestinal cells and consist of a core of neutral lipids, mainly cholesteryl esters and triglycerides (TGs), surrounded by a monolayer of phospholipids and proteins. Hepatic apoB-lipoproteins are secreted as very-low density lipoproteins (VLDL), and they are converted to atherogenic low-density lipoproteins (LDL) during the circulation; in contrast, the intestinal apoB-lipoproteins are secreted as chylomicrons. The VLDL and chylomicrons can be converted into atherogenic remnant lipoproteins by lipolysis. The VLDL, chylomicrons and their remnants, which are known as triglyceride-rich lipoproteins (TRLs), appear in the blood after a high-fat meal (postprandial state) and are considered to be highly atherogenic (Havel, 1994; Zilversmith, 1979). In fact, chylomicronemia causes atherosclerosis in mice (Weinstein et al., 2010) and decreasing the TRLs level reduces the progression of coronary artery disease to the same degree as decreasing the LDL-cholesterol level (Hodis et al., 1999). TRLs comprise a large variety of nascent and metabolically modified lipoprotein particles that vary in size and density, as well as lipid and apolipoprotein composition. Studies have indicated that the size and the specific structural arrangement of lipids and apolipoproteins are associated with atherogenicity. Morover, studies have consistently shown that there is an inverse relationship between the lipoprotein particle size and the ability to enter the arterial wall. Small TRLs and their remnants can enter the arterial wall and are independently associated with the presence, severity, and progression of atherosclerosis (Hodis, 1999). Short-term intake of the Mediterranean diet and the acute intake of an olive oil meal could favour the lower cardiovascular risk in Mediterranean countries by secreting a reduced number and higher-size TRLs particles compared with other fat sources (Perez-Martinez et al., 2011). Recent studies suggest that lipoproteins may also contribute to atherogenesis by affecting the mechanisms of the control of gene expression. Many lipoproteins-gene interactions have only been investigated under fasting conditions, Lopez et al., 2009 nicely reviews the emerging importance of gene-nutrient interactions at the postprandial state, which impacts ultimately on atherosclerosis risk.

A large body of knowledge exists from epidemiological, clinical, experimental animal models and in vitro studies that have indicated that olive oil can be regarded as functional food for its anti-atherogenic properties. Diets enriched with olive oil prevent the development and progression of atherosclerosis (Aguilera et al., 2002; Kanrantonis et al., 2006) and may also play an important role in atherosclerosis regression (Mangiapane et al., 1999; Tsalina et al., 2007, 2010). These and recent reports have suggested that the beneficial effects of olive oil on atherosclerosis may be influenced by the high oleic acid content and the minor fraction of the oil; potential benefitial microconstituents include tocopherols, phenolic compounds, phytosterols, triterpenoids and unusual glycolipids that exert an antagonistic effect on PAF (1-O-hexadecyl-2-acetyl-sn-glycero-3-phosphocholine). There are several mechanisms by which olive oil affects the development of atherosclerosis. Theses mechanisms have been nicely reviewed by Carluccio et al., 2007, and include the following: 1) regulation of cholesterol levels as olive oil decreases LDL-cholesterol and increases HDL-cholesterol; 2) decreased susceptibility of human LDL to oxidation, because of the lower susceptibility of its MUFAs content and to the ability of its polyphenol fraction to scavenge free radicals and reduce oxidative stress; 3) both, oleic acid and olive oil antioxidant polyphenols inhibit endothelial activation and monocyte recruitment during early atherogenesis; 4) decreased macrophage production of inflammatory cytokines, eicosanoid inflammatory mediators derived from arachidonic acids and increased nitric oxide (NO) production, which improves vascular stability; 5) decreased macrophages matrix-metalloproteinases (MMPs) production, which improves plaque stability; 6) oleic acid and olive oil polyphenols are associated with a reduced risk of hypertension; 7) oleic acid and olive oil polyphenols also affect blood coagulation and fibrinolytic factors, thereby reducing the risk of acute thrombotic cardiovascular events; and 8) a decreased rate of oxidation of DNA (Machowetz et al., 2007); human atherosclerosis is associated with DNA damage in both circulating cells and cells that comprise the vessel wall.

EVOO is therefore becoming more important due to its beneficial effects on human health. EVOO has proven effective in controlling atherosclerotic lesions, mainly within the framework of a Mediterranean-type diet (low cholesterol). An animal model that reproduces the processes taking place in the development of human atherosclerosis has been crucial to obtaining these conclusions, and this has been provided by the apoE-deficient mouse. Using this model, it has been proved that EVOO possesses beneficial antiatherogenic effects, and its enrichment with polyphenols (Rosenblat et al., 2008) and with long chain n-3 PUFAs (Eilertsen et al., 2011) further improves these effects, leading to the attenuation of atherosclerosis development. Feeding these mice with various olive oils rich in different minor components or with these components in isolation has made it possible to assess the contribution of those molecules to the beneficial effect of this food, these effects have been review by Guillen et al., 2009 and include the following: 1) increase of small, dense HDL enriched with apo A-IV tightly bound to paraoxonase; these apolipoprotein A-IV-enriched particles were very effective in inactivating the peroxides present in the low-density lipoproteins (LDL) which are thought to initiate atherosclerosis; 2) minor components decrease plasma triglycerides and LDL-colesterol and very low density lipoprotein cholesterol (VLDL-colesterol), as well as 3) parameters of oxidative stress, such as isoprostane (8-iso-prostaglandin F2a); 4) EVOO acts against oxidative stress, which occurs primarily through a direct antioxidant effect as well as through an indirect mechanism that involves greater expression and activity of certain enzymes with antioxidant activities such as catalase and glutathione peroxidase-1 (Oliveras-Lopez et al., 2008). Among the antioxidants from EVOO, phenolic compounds have received the most attention. Oleuropein derivatives, especially HT, have been shown to have protective effects against markers associated with the atherogenic process (González-Santiago et al., 2006; Zrelli et al., 2011), some studies (Acin et al., 2006), however, have shown opposite results with HT administration in the atherosclerotic process. Given the anti-atherogenic properties of EVOO evident in animal models fed a Western diet, clinical trials are needed to establish whether these oils are a safe and effective means of treating atherosclerosis.

3. Nutrigenomics of olive oil

3.1 Gene-diet interactions after acute ingestion of olive oil

In addition to the mechanisms described above, olive oil components can exert an anti-atherogenic affect by acting at the genomic level. Nearly all evidence for the impact of olive oil on gene expression is derived from research using animal or human cells in culture. Carefully designed human clinical studies to establish a cause-and-effect relationship between olive oil affecting gene expression and the atherosclerotic process are scare and will be review here. Recent in vivo studies have shown that sustained consumption of VOO influence peripheral blood mononuclear cells (PBMNCs) gene expression (nutritional transcriptomics) (Table 2). PBMNCs are often used to asses changes in gene expression in vivo because the leucocytes recruitment from the circulation to the vessel wall for subsequent migration into the sub-endothelial layer is a critical step in atherosclerotic plaque formation; additionally, PBMNCs can be easily obtained from volunteers through simple blood draws. Previous studies have shown that in healthy individuals, a 3-week consumption of VOO as a principal fat source in a diet low in natural antioxidants (Khymenets et al., 2009) up-regulated the expression of genes associated with DNA repair proteins such as, the excision repair cross complementation group (ERCC-5) and the X-ray repair complementing defective repair Chinese hamster cells 5 (XRCC-5). VOO consumption also up-regulated aldehyde dehydrogenase 1 family, member A1 (ALDH1A1) and LIAS (lipoic acid synthetase) gene expression. ALDH1A1 is a gene encoding protein which protect cells from the oxidative stress induced by lipid peroxidation; the LIAS protein plays an important role in α-(+)-lipolitic acid (LA) synthesis. LA is an important antioxidant that has been shown to inhibit atherosclerosis in mouse models of human atherosclerosis due to its anti-inflammatory, antihyperglyceridemic and weight-reducing effects. Morover, apoptosis-related genes such as, BIRC-1 (baculoviral IAP repeat-containing protein 1) and TNSF-10 (tumor necrosis factor (ligand) superfamily, member 10), were also upregulated. BIRC-1 inhibits apoptosis while TNSF-10 promotes macrophages and lymphocytes apoptosis. VOO ingestion also modified OGT gene expression (O-linked N-acetylglucosamine (GlcNAc) transferase). Nuclear and cytoplasmic protein glycosylation is a widespread and reversible posttranslational modification in eukaryotic cells; intracellular glycosylation via the addition of N-acetylglucosamine to serine and threonine is catalysed by OGT. Thus, OGT plays a significant role in modulating protein stability, protein-proteins interactions, transactivation processes, and the enzyme activity of target proteins; moreover OGT plays a critical role in regulating cell function and survival in the cardiovascular system. VOO consumption also profoundly impacted the expression of the USP-48 (ubiquitin specific peptidase-48) gene. USP-48 is a member of the ubiquitin proteasome system that removes damaged, oxidized and /or misfolded proteins; it also plays a role in inflammation, proliferation and apoptosis. PPARBP (peroxisome proliferator-activated receptor-binding protein), which is an essential transcriptional mediator of adipogenesis, lipid metabolism, insulin sensitivity and glucose homeostasis via peroxisome proliferator-activated receptor-γ (PPAR-γ) regulation, and ADAM-17 (a disintegrin and metalloproteinase domain 17), a membrane –anchored metalloprotease, were also upregulated. ADAM-17 is a candidate gene of atherosclerosis susceptibility in mice models of atherosclerosis (Holdt et al., 2008), it mediates the release of several cell-signaling and cell adhesion molecules such as vascular endothelial (VE)-cadherin, vascular cell adhesion molecule-1   (VCAM-1), intercellular adhesion molecule-1 (ICAM-1) or L-selectin affecting endothelial permeability and leukocyte transmigration. According with this study, Reiss et al. 2011, have recently show that unsaturated FFA increase ADAM-mediated substrate cleavage, with corresponding functional consequences on cell proliferation, cell migration, and endothelial permeability, events of high significance in atherogenesis.

LLorent-Cortes et al. 2010, have also concluded that a Mediterranean-type diet in a high-risk cardiovascular population impacts the expression of genes involved in inflammation, vascular foam cell formation and vascular remodelling in human monocytes. Inflammation plays a role in the onset and development of atherosclerosis. In this study, VOO ingestion prevented an increase in cyclo-oxygenase-2 (COX-2) expression and decreased monocyte chemotactic protein-1 (MCP-1) gene expression compared with a traditional Mediterranean diet (TMD) with nuts or a low fat diet. COX-2 is a pro-inflammatory enzyme that increases prostanoid levels (thromboxane A2; TXA2 and prostaglandine E2; PGE2); bioactive molecules present in VOO such as 1-hydroxityrosol and phenyl-6,7-dihydroxi-isochroman which is an ortho-diphenol present in EVOO, down-regulate COX-2 synthesis by preventing nuclear factor-kappaB (NF-kB) activation in macrophages and monocytes (Maiuri et al., 2005; Trefiletti et al., 2011). MCP-1 is a potent regulator of leucocyte trafficking, and animal studies have shown that a VOO diet can reduce neutrophil accumulation and decreases the MCP-1 blood levels (Leite et al., 2005); again, these data support the hypothesis that VOO is anti-inflammatory. Morover, the dietary intervention with VOO specifically prevented low density lipoprotein receptor-related protein-1 (LRP-1) overexpression in the high cardiovascular risk population. LRP-1 plays a major role in macrophage-foam cell formation and migration; additionally, LRP-1 is also a key receptor for the prothrombotic transformation of the vascular wall. Morover, VOO dietary intervention prevented an increase in the expression of genes involved in intracellular lipid accumulation in macrophages and monocytes (e.g., CD36 antigen; CD36) and in the process of thrombosis (e.g., tissue factor pathway inhibitory, FFPI) compared to a TMD enriched with nuts (high in PUFAs).

Reference	Subjects	Study design	Intervention	Gene Expression	Function
Khyments et al., 2009	Healthy men (6) and women (4)		Virgin olive oil in a diet low in antioxidants (1 wk washout, 3 wk 25ml VOO)	XRCC5, ERCC5 ALDH1A1, LIAS OGT, BIRC1, TNFSF-10 PPARBP, USP48, ADAM17.	DNA repair Oxidative stress Protein stability Apoptosis PPAR-γ regulation Tissue remodelling Endothelial permeability
Llorente-Cortes et al., 2010	Asymptomatic high cardiovascular-risk subjects (type 2 diabetes, hypertension, hypercholesterolemia, low HDL-cholesterol) (23 men, 26 women)	Randomized, controlled	Virgin olive oil or nuts in the context of a traditional Mediterranean diet (3 mo).	COX-2, MCP-1, TFPI, LRP1, CD36.	Inflammation Thrombosis Lipid accumulation
Konstantinidou et al., 2010	Healthy men and women (90)	Randomized, parallel, controlled	Virgin olive oil or washed virgin olive oil (without polyphenols) in the context of a traditional Mediterranean diet.	IFNγ, ARHGAP15, IL7R ADRB2 POLK	Inflammation Oxidative stress DNA repair

Table 2. Changes in gene expression of atherosclerotic-related genes after acute ingestion of virgin olive oil in human studies.

The last two nutritional interventions, suggest that the benefits associated with a TMD and VOO consumption can reduce cardiovascular risk via nutrigenomic effects; however, these studies could not distinguish between the effects elicited by minor components of VOO and those promoted by the fat content of the oil. A recent study by Konstantinidou et al, 2010 indicated that olive oil polyphenols play a significant role in the down-regulation of pro-atherogenic genes in human PBMNCs after 3 months of a dietary intervention with a TMD+VOO and TMD+WOO (washed virgin olive oil which has the same characteristics as VOO except for a lower polyphenol content). The dietary intervention decreased the expression of genes related to inflammation (e.g., interferon-γ, IFN-γ; Rho GTPase activating protein-15, ARHGAP-15; and Interleukin 7 receptor, IL7R) oxidative stress (e.g., adrenergic β-2 receptor surface, ADRB2) and DNA damage (e.g., polymerase DNA directed k, POLK). Changes in the expression of all of these genes, except POLK, were particularly observed when VOO, rich in polyphenols, was present in the TMD. The decrease in gene expression associated with inflammatory that was observed in this study agrees with previous studies that have reported a decrease in systemic inflammatory markers and oxidative stress due to the ingestion of polyphenols from olive oil and olive leaf extract (Poudyal et al., 2010; Puel et al., 2008). IFN-γ is considered to be a key inflammatory mediator and the release of this cytokine is regulated by polyphenols from red wine and dietary tea polyphenols (Deng et al., 2010; Magrone et al., 2008). ARHGAP-15 encodes for a Rho GTPase-activating protein that regulates the activity of GTPases. To date, little is known about the physiological role of ARHGAP-15, however, recent studies by Costa et al., 2011 have shown that this protein is associated with the selective regulation of multiple neutrophil functions. The protein encoded by the IL7R gene is a receptor for IL-7, which is associated with inflammation; interestingly, olive oil consumption has been shown to reduce the IL-7 serum concentration in patients with the metabolic syndrome (Esposito et al., 2004). POLK is a DNA repair gene that copies undamaged DNA templates. Previous studies have indicated that down-regulation of POLK is not associated with polyphenol content of VOO. Thus, the protective effect of VOO associated with DNA repair is related to the fat content (MUFA) and other minor oil components. ADRB2 has previously been associated with body composition (Bea et al., 2010), overexpression of the receptor that enhances reactive oxygen species (ROS) signalling (Di Lisa et al., 2011), and ADRB2 inhibition, which reduces macrophage cytokine production. Down-regulation of the ADRB2 gene, particularly in the TDM+VOO intervention group, along with an improvement in the oxidative status of the volunteers, may indicate that olive oil polyphenols protect against oxidative stress. Collectively, these studies support the hypothesis that olive oil polyphenol consumption in the context of a TMD may protect against cardiovascular disease by modulating the expression of atherosclerosis-related genes.

3.2 Influence of olive oil on gene-diet interaction at the postprandial state

Humans that reside in industrialised societies spend most of the daytime in a non-fasting state that is influence by meal consumption patterns and the amounts of food ingested. Postprandial lipaemia is characterised by an increase in TGs, specifically in the form of TRLs. Over 25 years ago, Zilversmit, 1979 proposed that atherogenesis was a postprandial phenomenon because high concentrations of lipoproteins and their remnants following food ingestion could deposit on the arterial wall and accumulate in atheromatous plaques. In postprandial studies, subjects usually receive a fat-loading test meal with a variable composition according to the nutrient to be tested. In these studies, both, the amount and the type of fat ingested influence postprandial lipaemia. Although, controversial results have been obtained for comparing an olive oil fat meal with other dietary fats, some studies have shown that VOO intake decreases the postprandial TGs concentration and results in a faster TRLs clearance from the blood in normolipidemic subjetcs (Abia et al., 2001). The amount of fat ingested influences the results as small doses of olive oil (25 ml) did not promote postprandial lipaemia, whereas larger doses (40 and 50 ml) of any type of olive oil promoted lipaemia (Fitó et al., 2002; Covas et al., 2006). Olive oil is considered to be an optimal fat for the modulation of extrinsic cardiovascular risk factors in the postprandial state. The influence of olive oil on postprandial insulin release and action, endothelial function, blood pressure, inflammatory processes and hemostasis has been recently review by Bearmudez et al., 2011.

3.2.1 Postprandial effect of olive oil in PBMNCs

Early in vivo postprandial human studies have shown that VOO activates PBMCs immediately after ingestion and may induce changes in gene expression (Bellido et al., 2004). Postprandial studies have shown that high-fat meals can induce β cell dysfunction and insulin resistance in healthy individuals, as well as in subjects with type 2 diabetes or the metabolic syndrome. However, postprandial olive oil (MUFAs) can buffer β cell hyperactivity and insulin intolerance compared to butter (SFAs) in subjects with high fasting triglyceride concentrations (Lopez et al., 2011). Moreover, changes in expression of insulin sensitivity related genes occur in human PBMNCs after an oral fat load of VOO (Konstantinidou et al., 2009) (Table 3). In this study, the expression of genes such as OGT, arachidonate 5-lipoxygenase-activating protein (ALOX5AP), LIAS, PPARBP, ADBR2 and ADAM-17 were up-regulated at 6 h after VOO ingestion. LIAS and PPARBP regulate insulin sensitivity by activating and co-activating PPARγ, respectively. PPARγ is a nuclear hormone receptor that plays a crucial role in adipogenesis and insulin sensitisation. The authors hypothesised that the up-regulation of both of these genes may be one feed back mechanism that counteracts the postprandial oxidative stress that plays a role in the development of insulin resistance. The ADRB2 gene encodes for a major lipolytic receptor in human fat cells that modulates insulin secretion and protects against oxidative stress. Because insulin signaling activates the OGT gene, the authors attributed the increase in OGT expression with the several feedback mechanisms that serve to attenuate sustained insulin signalling. CD36 is an integral membrane glycoprotein expressed on the surface of cells active in fatty acid metabolism (adipocytes, muscle cells, platelets, monocytes, heart and intestine cells). This protein plays diverse functions, including uptake of long-chain fatty acids and oxidized low-density lipoproteins. CD36 deficiency underlies insulin resistance, defective fatty acid metabolism and hypertriglyceridemia in spontaneously hypertensive rats (SHRs), furthermore, lipid-induced insulin resistant has been associated with atherogenesis through mechanisms mediated by the expression of scavenger receptor CD36 (Kashyap et al., 2009). CD36 gene expression was modulated during the postprandial period after VOO ingestion (Konstantinidou et al., 2009), however the authors did not find a relationship between in CD36 gene expression and insulin levels in the subjects. Rather, they found an association with a postprandial increase in plasma fatty acids and the satiety response after VOO ingestion. ADAM-17 is considered to be an attractive target for controlling insulin resistance. It also regulates tumor necrosis factor (TNF-α), major negative regulator of the

Reference	Subjects	Study design	Intervention	Gene Expression	Function
Jimenez-Gomez et al., 2009	Healthy men (20)	Randomized, crossover Postprandial	Three diet intervention period of 4 wks [SFA (butter), MUFA (VOO) and PUFA (walnut)] followed by fat-load rich in either SFA, MUFA, or PUFA (60% fat)	TNF-α, IL-6	Inflammation
Konstantinidou et al., 2009	Healthy men (11)	Postprandial	Virgin olive oil (1 wk washout, followed by 50mL fat-load).	LIAS, PPARBP, ADRB2, ADAM17 OGT, ALOX5AP CD36	Insulin-sensitivity Scavenger receptor, satiety
Konstantinidou et al., 2009	Healthy men (6)	Postprandial	Virgin olive oil (1 wk washout, followed by 50mL fat-load).	IL-10, IFN-Y DCLRE1C, POLK OGT, ADAM17 USP48, ABCA7	Inflammation DNA repair Oxidative stress Tissue remodelling Apolipoprotein-dependent formation of HDL
Camargo et al., 2010	20 patiens (9 men, 11 women) suffering metabolic syndrome	Double-blinded, randomized, crossover postprandial	Virgin olive oil-based breakfast with high and low content of phenolic compounds. (1 wk washout period, followed by 40 mL fat-load)	CCL3, CXCL1, CXCL2, CXCL3, CXCR4 PTGS2 ILB1, IL6 SGK1, NFKBIA DUSP1, DUSP2, TRIB1	Leucocyte infiltration Prostaglandin biosynthesis Inflammation NF-kB activation Migration Proliferation, chemotaxis.

Table 3. Changes in gene expression of atherosclerotic-related genes after the ingestion of virgin olive oil in human studies during the postprandial period.

insulin receptor pathway, at posttranscriptional level. PPARBP may also increase insulin sensitivity by down-regulating the expression of TNF-α. The consumption of an olive oil-enriched breakfast decreases postprandial expression of TNF-α mRNA compared with a breakfast rich in butter and walnuts (Jimenez-Gomez et al., 2009). Correspondingly, acute consumption of EVOO decreased the circulating levels of soluble TNF-α in young healthy individuals (Papageorgiou et al., 2011). TNF-α activates a cytokine production cascade and thereby has a crucial role in the inflammatory process that is associated with atherogenesis; thus, dietary modification of TNF-α may prevent atherosclerosis.

In human interventional studies, an acute intake of olive oil increased the HDL cholesterol level, decreased inflammation, decreased lipid oxidation and decreased DNA oxidative damage. Studies by Konstantinidow et al. 2009, showed that there was a postprandial increase in the expression of PBMNCs genes related to DNA-repair (DNA-cross-link repair 1C, DCLRE1C and POLK) and inflammation (interleukin-10, IL-10; IFN-γ) 6h after ingestion of 50 mL of VOO. IL-10 is an anti-inflammatory cytokine that inhibits the production of interleukin-6 (IL-6), which is considered to be the most important inflammatory mediator. Il-6 release from rat adipocytes is regulated by the dietary fatty acid composition, and lower values of IL-6 are released with an olive oil diet (Garcia-Escobar et al., 2010); however, the postprandial change in plasma IL-6 concentrations does not seem to be altered by VOO ingestion (Teng et al., 2011; Manning et al., 2008). Postprandial VOO down-regulated IFN-γ gene expression. IFN-γ is a key pro-atherogenic cytokine that induces expression of adhesion molecules in endothelium and recruit leucocytes (Zhang et al., 2011), induces the expression of genes that have been implicated in atherosclerosis, promotes uptake of modified LDL (N. Li et al., 2010), and regulates macrophage foam cell formation and plaque stability, which are essential steps that mediate the pathogenesis of atherosclerosis. ATP-binding cassette, subfamily A, member 7 (ABCA7) is a protein that mediates the biogenesis of HDL with cellular lipids and helical apolipoproteins. In agreement with this, an increase in ABCA7 gene expression was observed in the postprandial studies after VOO ingestion.

The authors also observed up-regulation of several oxidative stress related genes and genes that may regulate NF-kB activation such as USP48 and a-kinase anchor protein-13 (AKAP-13). NF-kB regulates numerous processes in the cardiovascular system, including inflammation, cell survival, differentiation, proliferation and apoptosis. In vascular cells, NF-kB activation is mediated by diverse extracellular signals including Ang II, oxLDL, TRLs, advanced glycation end-products, and inflammatory cytokines. NF-kB activation by circulating cytokines has been linked to atherosclerosis and thrombosis and a number of NF-kB-regulated pro-inflammatory proteins are relevant for the initiation and progression of atherosclerosis. The induction of NF-κB signalling, results in transcriptional regulation of pro-inflammatory genes, including cytokines, chemokines, adhesion molecules, antioxidants, transcription factors, growth factors, and apoptosis and angiogenesis regulators (van der Heiden et al., 2010). The data showed so far, suggest that olive oil ingestion may protective during the postprandial by altering gene expression changes. However, the authors could not distinguish whether the protective effect was caused by the minor components of olive oil or to the fat content.

To adress this problem, Camargo et al., 2010 performed postprandial studies with two VOO based breakfast, with a high and low phenolic compounds content, administered to patients suffering form metabolic syndrome. The phenol fraction of VOO repressed the expression of several PBMNCs genes that are involved in inflammation processes mediated by cytokine-cytokine receptor interactions, arachidonic acid metabolism, mitogen-activated protein kinases (MAPKs) and transcription factor NF-kB/AP-1, such as the SGK1 (serum/glucocorticoid-regulated kinase-1) and the NFKBIA (nuclear factor of kappa light chain gene enhancer in B cells inhibitor, alpha) genes. SGK1 encodes a serum/glucocorticoid-regulated kinase that enhances nuclear NF-kB activity by phosphorylating the inhibitory kinase IKKα. The NFKBIA gene, encodes the IkBα protein,which is a member of an inhibitory IkB protein family that sequesters NF-kB into the cytoplasm. As NF-kB binds to the IKBα promoter to activate its transcription, a decrease in NFKBIA expression should be associated with a decrease in NF-kB activation. The hypothesis that olive oil polyphenols decreases NF-kB activation is supported by in vivo studies, which showed that VOO ingestion reduces inflammatory response of PMBSCs mediated by transcription factor NF-kB when compared to, butter and walnut-enriched diets during the postprandial state (Bellido et al., 2004). The study also showed the VOO consumption decreased the expression of PTGS2 (prostagladin-endoperoxide synthase-2), interleukin 1- β (IL-1β) and IL-6. The PTGS2 gene encodes for COX-2, which is an inducible isozyme that mediates prostaglandin biosynthesis from the substrate arachidonic acid. Pro-inflammatory cytokines, prostaglandins and NO, which are produced by monocytes and activated macrophages, play critical roles in inflammatory diseases such as atherosclerosis. VOO and hydrolysed olive vegetation water (Bitler et al., 2005) exhibit anti-inflammatory activities in the human monocytic leukemia cell line (THP-1). Previous studies have shown that, HT down-regulates iNOS and COX-2 gene expression in THP-1 cells (Zhang et al., 2009) and in murine macrophages by preventing NF-kB, STAT-1alpha (signal transducer and activator of transcription-1) and IRF-1 (interferon regulatory factor-1) activation (Maiuri et al., 2005). In vitro studies by Graham et al., 2011 have recently shown that TRLs, isolated from healthy volunteers after ingestion of VOO and pomace olive oil, enriched in minor components, produces a decrease in IL-6 and IL-1B secretion along with a down-regulation of COX-2 mRNA in macrophages. IL-6 is a pro-inflammatory cytokines that may contribute to the development of atherosclerosis by promoting insulin resistance, dyslipidaemia and endothelial dysfunction (Wilson, 2008). IL-6 synthesis is stimulated by IL-1β, which is another pro-inflammatory cytokine that regulates endothelial cell proliferation and the expression of adhesion molecules on the arterial wall (Andreotti et al., 2002). Studies, with a high-fat diet induced insulin-resistant animal model, showed that the ingestion of green tea polyphenols decreased IL-1β and IL-6β mRNA expression in cardiac muscle (Qin et al., 2010).

Circulating monocytes are components of innate immunity, and many pro-inflammatory cytokines and adhesion molecules facilitate monocyte adhesion and migration to the vascular endothelial wall. Monocyte migration is a key event in the pathogenesis of atherosclerosis. Therefore, modulating PMBCs activity and creating a less deleterious inflammatory profile may decrease leucocytes recruitment from the circulation to the vessel wall, important process in the initiation of atherosclerosis. According to this, Camargo et al., 2010 observed a decreased expression of chemokine, cc motif, ligand-3 (CCL3), chemokine, cxc motif, ligan-1 (CXCL1), chemokine, cxc motif, ligan-2 (CXCL2), chemokine, cxc motif, ligan-3 (CXCL3) and chemokine, cxc motif, receptor-4 (CXCR4) after acute-intake of phenol-rich olive oil. The CCL3 gene, which encodes for macrophage inflammatory protein-1 (MIP-1) has been implicated in inducing leucocyte-endothelial cell interactions and leucocyte recruitment in vivo (Gregory et al., 2006). CXCL1, CXCL2 and CXCL3, regulate leucocytes cell trafficking. CXCR4 have been shown to mediate bone mesenchymal stem cells migration through the endothelium in response to ox-LDL (M. Li et al., 2010). Dual-specificity phosphatase-1 (DUSP-1), dual-specificity phosphatase-2 (DUSP-2) and tribbes homology-1 (TRIB-1), gene expression were decreased by phenol-rich olive oil. DUSP-1 is actively involved in atherosclerosis and a chronic deficiency of DUSP-1 in ApoE(-/-) mice leads to decreased atherosclerosis via mechanisms involving impaired macrophage migration and defective extracellular signal-regulated kinase signalling (Shen et al., 2010). TRBIR1 is also involved in MAPK signalling and is up-regulated in vascular smooth muscle cells (SMCs) of human atherosclerotic plaques; TRBIR1 expression levels are key for modulating the extent of vascular SMCs proliferation and chemotaxis (Sung et al., 2007). Extracellular matrix degradation occurs in several pathological conditions such as atherosclerosis. Among the circulating cells, activated monocytes may directly contribute to atherosclerosis by expressing MMPs. In particular, monocytes express matrix metalloproteinase-9 (MMP-9), which is a member of the MMPs family that acts on the extracellular matrix, facilitates the migration of recruited monocytes to the sub-endothelial layer and acts on precursors of inflammatory cytokines, thereby amplifying the inflammatory response. In vitro studies showed that oleuropein aglycone, which a typical olive oil polyphenol, prevented an increase in MMP-9 expression and secretion in THP-1 cells (Dell´Agli et al., 2010); these data provide further evidence regarding the mechanisms by which olive oil reduces inflammation during atherosclerosis.

3.2.2 Postprandial effect of olive oil on the endothelium

Low-grade inflammation is often associated with endothelial dysfunction, which is associated with the development of atherosclerosis. Moreover, remnant like-lipoproteins have been associated with endothelial dysfunction and coronary artery disease in subjects with metabolic syndrome (Nakamura et al., 2005). A large number of genes are regulated after endothelial cells are exposed to TRLs with the net effect reflecting receptor and non-receptor mediated pathways that are activated or inhibited depending on the fatty acid type, lipid and apolipoprotein composition of TRLs and the presence or absence of lipoprotein lipase (Williams et al., 2004). TRLs have been shown to induce pro- and anti-inflammatory responses in the endothelium, and TRL composition plays a key role in determining these responses. TRLs that were isolated after a meal enriched in SFAs induced E-selectin, VCAM-1 and lectin-like oxidised-LDL receptor-1 (LOX-1) gene expression to a higher extent compared to TRLs that were isolated after a meal enriched in MUFAs and PUFAs (Williams et al., 2004); similarly, chylomicrons separated after ingestion of safflower oil, which is rich in polyunsaturated linoleic acid, induced a higher expression level of adhesion molecules compared with chylomicrons that were separated after ingestion of olive oil, rich in monounsaturated oleic acid (Jagla & Schrezenmeir, 2001). The effects of lipoproteins on vasoactive substances may also play a role in endothelial dysfunction. The endothelium-derived relaxing factor NO has gained wide attention because the current data suggests that it may protect against hypertension and atherosclerosis. In general, high-fat meals have often been associated with a loss of postprandial vascular reactivity compared to low fat meals. However several studies have shown that differences in food composition and the fatty acid content of meals may contribute to the observed effects on vascular reactivity via postprandial lipoproteins modifications. Thus, meals that contain MUFAs and eicosapentaenoic/docosahexaenoic acids (EPA/DHA) can attenuate the endothelial function impairment likely by reducing the most atherogenic postprandial lipoprotein subclass containing apolipoproteins B and C (Hilpert et al., 2007). Olive oil polyphenols can also inhibit endothelial adhesion molecule expression through NF-kB inhibition (Carluccio et al., 2003). In endothelial cell models, oleic acid (Carluccio et al., 1999) and phenolic extracts from EVOO, strongly reduced the gene expression of the vascular wall cell adhesion molecules (ICAM-1, VCAM-1), being HT, oleuropein and oleuropein aglycone the main polyphenols responsible for these effects (Dell´Agli et al., 2006; Carluccio et al., 2003)

3.2.3 Postprandial effect of olive oil in smooth muscle cells

SMCs are essential for proper vasculature function. SMCs contract and relax to alter the luminal diameter, which enables the blood vessels to maintain an appropriate blood pressure. However, vascular SMCs can also proliferate and migrate and synthesise large amounts of extracellular matrix (ECM) components. Thus, SMCs plays an important role in atherogenesis. TRLs induce the SMCs proliferation and migration via MAPKs activation, G protein–coupled receptor (GPCR)–dependent or independent protein kinase C (PKC) activation, epidermal growth factor receptor (EGF) transactivation and heparing-binding EGF-like growth factor shedding. TRLs can exert their effects on SMCs by acting at the genomic level (Lopez et al., 1999). TRL up-regulates the expression of genes involved in proliferation (e.g., cycin D1, CCND1; cyclin E, CCNE1; proliferating cell nuclear antigen, PCNA), inflammation (e.g., interleukin-8, IL-8; IL-1B; COX-2; suppressor of cytokine signaling 5, SOCS-5), signal transduction (e.g., mitogen-activated protein kinase 1, MAP3K-1; mitogen-activated protein kinase phosphatase-3, MKP-3; dual-specificity tyrosine phosphorylation-regulated kinase 1A, DYRK1A), oxidative stress (e.g., stress-activated protein kinase-3, SAPK-3 and stress-activated protein kinase-2A, SAPK-2A) and cytoskeleton function and motility (e.g., vimentin, VIM; keratin 19, KRT-19; fibrillin, FBN; tubulin beta, TUBB) (Bermudez et al., 2008). Furthermore, increasing evidence has shown that the pathophysiological contribution of TRLs to atherosclerosis development of plaque stability depends on the fatty acid composition of TRLs. The same study showed that TRLs obtained after the ingestion of olive oil produced a less deleterious pro-atherogenic profile compared to TRLs obtained after ingestion of butter (SFAs) or a mix of vegetable and fish oils (PUFAs). Since the olive oil contained no minor components, the effects were mainly attributed to oleic acid. However, oleic acid is not the sole component of olive oil that confers health benefits. In that sense, oleanolic acid, which is a natural triterpenoid that is present in pommace olive oil, induces prostaglandine I2 (PGI2) production through a mechanism that involves COX-2 mRNA upregulation via MAPKs signalling pathways (Martinez-Gonzalez et al., 2008).

4. Conclusions

Nutrigenomic analyses directly asseses the influence of bioactive food compounds on gene expression. An increasing amount of data indicate that the fatty acids and polyphenols present in EVOO modulate the expression of key atherosclerotic-related genes, in vascular (macrophages, endothelial and smooth muscle cells) and peripheral blood mononuclear cells, towards a less-atherogenic gene profile. These compounds exert an effect after acute ingestion of the oil and during the postprandial state, and may provide protection during several stages of atherosclerosis. These data presented here, suggest that the traditional Mediterranean diet (rich in VOO) is optimal for both healthy and high-risk cardiovascular populations for the prevention of atherosclerosis plaque progression. The current literature suggests that EVOO, with its adequate PUFAs content, being poor in SFAs, high in MUFAs, and rich in antioxidants, is the best dietary fat for the prevention of atherosclerotic disease and ischemic cardiopathy. The ultimate goal in the prevention and treatment of coronary atherosclerosis is to reduce the risk of new heart attacks and reduce the mortality associated with cardiovascular failure. Thus, identification of an optimal diet may aid in the prevention of disease development and decrease the risk of associated cardiovascular events.

5. Abbreviations

ABCA-7 = ATP-binding cassette, subfamily A, member-7
ADAM-17 = A disintegrin and metalloproteinase domain-17
ADRB2 = Adrenergic β-2 receptor surface
ARHGAP-15 = Rho GTPase activating protein-15
BIRC-1 = Baculoviral IAP repeat-containing protein-1
CCL3 = Chemokine, cc motif, ligand-3
CD36 = CD36 antigen
COX-2 = Cyclo-oxygenase-2
CXCL1 = Chemokine, cxc motif, ligan-1
CXCL2 = Chemokine, cxc motif, ligan-2
CXCL3 = Chemokine, cxc motif, ligan-3
CXCR4 = Chemokine, cxc motif, receptor-4
DUSP-1 = Dual-specificity phosphatase-1
DUSP-2 = Dual-specificity phosphatase-2
EVOO = Extra-virgin olive oil
FFA = Free fatty acids
HDL = High density lipoprotein
HT = Hydroxytyrosol
IFN-γ = Interferon-γ
ICAM-1 = Intercellular adhesion molecule-1
IL-1β = Interleukin 1-β
IL-6 = Interleukin-6
IL7R = Interleukin 7 receptor
IL-10 = Interleukin 10
LA = α-(+)-Lipolitic acid
LDL = Low-density lipoproteins
LIAS = Lipoic acid synthetase
LRP-1 = Lipoprotein receptor-related protein-1
MCP-1 = Monocyte chemotactic protein-1
MMPs = Matrix-metalloproteinases
MMP-9 = Matrix metalloproteinase-9
MUFAs = Monounsaturated fatty acids
NF-κB = Nuclear factor-kappaB
NFKBIA = Nuclear factor of kappa light chain gene enhancer in B cells inhibitor, alpha
NO = Nitric oxide
OGT = O-linked N-acetylglucosamine (GlcNAc) transferase

PBMNCs = Peripheral blood mononuclear cells
POLK = Polymerase DNA directed k
PPARBP = Peroxisome proliferator-activated receptor-binding protein
PPAR-γ = Peroxisome proliferator-activated receptor-γ
PTGS2 = Prostagladine-endoperoxide synthase-2
PUFAs = Polyunsaturated fatty acids
SFAs = Saturated fatty acids
SGK-1 = Serum/glucocorticoid-regulated kinase-1
SMCs = Smooth muscle cells
TGs = Triglycerides
TMD = Traditional Mediterranean diet
TNF-α = Tumor necrosis factor
TNSF-10 = Tumor necrosis factor (ligand) superfamily, member 10
TRIB-1 = Tribbes homology-1
TRLs = Triglyceride-rich lipoproteins
TYR = Tyrosol
USP-48 = Ubiquitin specific peptidase- 48
VCAM-1=Vascular cell adhesion molecule-1
VLDL = Very-low density lipoproteins
VOO = Virgin olive oil

6. Acknowledgements

This work has been supported by grant (AGL2008-02811) from the Spanish Ministry of Innovation and Science and Marie Curie grant PERG07-GA-2010-268413.
AO, LMV, BB, SL contributed equally to this work.

7. References

Abia, R; Pacheco, YM; Perona, JS; Montero, E; Muriana, FJ. & Ruiz-Gutiérrez, V. (2001). The metabolic availability of dietary triacylglycerols from two high oleic oils during the postprandial period does not depend on the amount of oleic acid ingested by healthy men. *Journal of Nutrition*, Vol.131, No.1, pp. 59-65.

Acín, S; Navarro, MA; Arbonés-Mainar, JM; Guillén, N; Sarría, AJ; Carnicer, R; Surra, JC; Orman, I; Segovia, JC; Torre, R; Covas, MI; Fernández-Bolaños, J; Ruiz-Gutiérrez, V. & Osada J. Hydroxytyrosol administration enhances atherosclerotic lesion development in apo E deficient mice. *Journal of Biochemistry*, Vol.140, No.3, pp. 383-391.

Aguilera, CM; Ramirez-Tortosa, MC; Mesa, MD; Ramirez-Tortosa, CL. & Gil, A. (2002). Sunflower, virgin-olive and fish oils differentially affect the progression of aortic lesions in rabbits with experimental atherosclerosis. *Atherosclerosis*, Vol.162, no.2, pp. 335-344.

Andreotti, F; Porto, I; Crea, F. & Maseri, A. (2002). Inflammatory gene polymorphisms and ischaemic heart disease: review of population association studies. *Heart*, Vol.87, pp. 107–112.

Bea, JW; Lohman, TG; Cussler, EC; Going, SB. & Thompson, PA. (2010). Lifestyle modifies the relationship between body composition and adrenergic receptor genetic polymorphisms, ADRB2, ADRB3 and ADRA2B: a secondary analysis of a randomized controlled trial of physical activity among postmenopausal women. *Behavior Genetics*, Vol.40, No.5, pp. 649-659.

Bellido, C; López-Miranda, J; Blanco-Colio, LM; Pérez-Martínez, P, Muriana, FJ; Martín-Ventura, JL, Marín, C; Gómez, P; Fuentes, F; Egido, J. & Pérez-Jiménez, F. (2004). Butter and walnuts, but not olive oil, elicit postprandial activation of nuclear transcription factor kappaB in peripheral blood mononuclear cells from healthy men. *American Journal of Clinical Nutrition*, Vol.80, No.6, pp. 1487-1491.

Bermudez, B; Lopez, S; Ortega, A; Varela, LM; Pacheco, YM; Abia, R. & Muriana FJ. (2011). Oleic acid in olive oil: from a metabolic framework toward a clinical perspective. *Current Pharmacology Design*, Vol.17, No.8, pp. 831-843.

Bermúdez, B; López, S; Pacheco, YM; Villar, J; Muriana, FJ; Hoheisel, JD, Bauer, A. & Abia, R. (2008). Influence of postprandial triglyceride-rich lipoproteins on lipid-mediated gene expression in smooth muscle cells of the human coronary artery. *Cardiovascular Research*, Vol.79, No.2, pp. 294-303.

Bitler, CM; Viale, TM; Damaj, B. & Crea, R. (2005). Hydrolyzed olive vegetation water in mice has anti-inflammatory activity. *Journal of Nutrition*, Vol.135, No.6, pp. 1475-1479.

Camargo, A; Ruano, J; Fernandez, JM; Parnell, LD; Jimenez, A; Santos-Gonzalez, M; Marin, C; Perez-Martinez, P; Uceda, M; Lopez-Miranda, J. & Perez-Jimenez, F. (2010). Gene expression changes in mononuclear cells in patients with metabolic syndrome after acute intake of phenol-rich virgin olive oil. *BMC Genomics*, Vol.11, No.253, pp. 1-11.

Carluccio, MA; Massaro, M; Bonfrate, C; Siculella, L, Maffia, M; Nicolardi, G; Distante, A; Storelli, C. & De Caterina, R. (1999). Oleic acid inhibits endothelial activation : A direct vascular antiatherogenic mechanism of a nutritional component in the mediterranean diet. *Arteriosclerosis Thrombosis and Vascular Biology*, Vol.19, No.2, pp. 220-228.

Carluccio, MA; Massaro, M; Scoditti, E. & De Caterina, R. (2007). Vasculoprotective potential of olive oil components. *Molecular Nutrition Food Research*, Vol.51, No.10, pp. 1225-1234.

Carluccio, MA; Siculella, L; Ancora, MA; Massaro, M; Scoditti, E; Storelli, C; Visioli, F; Distante, A. & De Caterina, R. (2003). Olive oil and red wine antioxidant polyphenols inhibit endothelial activation: antiatherogenic properties of Mediterranean diet phytochemicals. *Arteriosclerosis Thrombosis and Vascular Biology*, Vol.23, No.4, pp. 622-629.

Corella, D. & Ordovas, JM. (2009). Nutrigenomics in cardiovascular medicine. *Circulation: Cardiovascular Genetics*, Vol.2, No.6, pp. 637-651.

Corona, G; Tzounis, X; Assunta Dessì, M; Deiana, M; Debnam, ES; Visioli, F. & Spencer, JP. (2006). The fate of olive oil polyphenols in the gastrointestinal tract: implications of gastric and colonic microflora-dependent biotransformation. *Free Radical Research*, Vol.40, No.6, pp. 647-658.

Corona, G; Spencer, JP. & Dessì MA. (2009) Extra virgin olive oil phenolics: absorption, metabolism, and biological activities in the GI tract.Toxicology and Industrial Health, Vol. 25, No.(4-5), pp. 285-293.

Costa, C; Germena, G; Martin-Conte, EL; Molinaris, I; Bosco, E; Marengo, S; Azzolino, O; Altruda, F, Ranieri, VM. & Hirsch, E. (2011). The RacGAP ArhGAP15 is a master negative regulator of neutrophil functions. Blood, (ahead of publication)

Covas, MI; de la Torre, K; Farré-Albaladejo, M, Kaikkonen, J; Fitó, M; López-Sabater, C; Pujadas-Bastardes, MA; Joglar, J; Weinbrenner, T; Lamuela-Raventós, RM. & de la Torre, R. (2006). Postprandial LDL phenolic content and LDL oxidation are modulated by olive oil phenolic compounds in humans. Free Radical Biology and Medicine, Vol.40, No.4, pp. 608-616.

Dell'Agli, M; Fagnani, R; Mitro, N; Scurati, S; Masciadri, M; Mussoni, L; Galli, GV; Bosisio, E; Crestani, M; De Fabiani, E, Tremoli, E. & Caruso D. (2006). Minor components of olive oil modulate proatherogenic adhesion molecules involved in endothelial activation. Journal of Agricultural and Food Chemistry, Vol.54, No.9, pp. 3259-3264.

Dell'Agli, M; Fagnani, R; Galli, GV; Maschi, O; Gilardi, F; Bellosta, S; Crestani, M; Bosisio, E; De Fabiani, E. & Caruso, D. (2010). Olive oil phenols modulate the expression of metalloproteinase 9 in THP-1 cells by acting on nuclear factor-kappaB signaling. Journal of Agricultural and Food Chemistry, Vol.58, No.4, pp. 2246-2252.

Deng, Q; Xu, J; Yu, B; He, J; Zhang, K; Ding, X. & Chen, D. (2010). Effect of dietary tea polyphenols on growth performance and cell-mediated immune response of post-weaning piglets under oxidative stress. Archives of Animal Nutrition, Vol.64, No.1, pp. 12-21.

Di Lisa, F; Kaludercic, N. & Paolocci, N. (2011). β_2-Adrenoceptors, NADPH oxidase, ROS and p38 MAPK: another 'radical' road to heart failure?. British Journal of Pharmacology, Vol.162, No.5, pp, 1009-1011.

Eilertsen, KE; Mæhre, HK; Cludts, K; Olsen, JO. & Hoylaerts, MF. (2011). Dietary enrichment of apolipoprotein E-deficient mice with extra virgin olive oil in combination with seal oil inhibits atherogenesis. Lipids in Health and Disease, Vol.3, No.10, 41-49.

Esposito, K; Marfella, R; Ciotola, M; Di Palo, C; Giugliano, F; Giugliano, G; D'Armiento, M; D'Andrea, F. & Giugliano, D. (2004). Effect of a mediterranean-style diet on endothelial dysfunction and markers of vascular inflammation in the metabolic syndrome: a randomized trial. JAMA, Vol.292, No.12, pp. 1440-1446.

Fitó, M; Gimeno, E; Covas, MI; Miró, E; López-Sabater, Mdel C; Farré M. & Marrugat J. (2002). Postprandial and short-term effects of dietary virgin olive oil on oxidant/antioxidant status. Lipids, Vol.37, No.3, pp. 245-251.

García-Escobar, E; Rodríguez-Pacheco, F; García-Serrano, S; Gómez-Zumaquero, JM; Haro-Mora, JJ; Soriguer, F. & Rojo-Martínez, G. (2010). Nutritional regulation of interleukin-6 release from adipocytes. International Journal of Obesity (London), Vol.34, No.8, pp. 1328-1332.

González-Santiago, M; Martín-Bautista, E; Carrero, JJ; Fonollá, J; Baró, L; Bartolomé, MV; Gil-Loyzaga, P. & López-Huertas E. (2006). One-month administration of hydroxytyrosol, a phenolic antioxidant present in olive oil, to hyperlipemic rabbits improves blood lipid profile, antioxidant status and reduces atherosclerosis development. *Atherosclerosis*, Vol.188, No.1, pp. 35-42.

Graham, VS; Lawson, C; Wheeler-Jones, CP; Perona, JS; Ruiz-Gutierrez, V. & Botham, KM. (2011). Triacylglycerol-rich lipoproteins derived from healthy donors fed different olive oils modulate cytokine secretion and cyclooxygenase-2 expression in macrophages: the potential role of oleanolic acid. *European Journal of Nutrition*, (ahead of publication).

Gregory, JL; Morand, EF; McKeown, SJ; Ralph, JA; Hall, P; Yang, YH; McColl, SR. & Hickey, MJ. (2006). Macrophage migration inhibitory factor induces macrophage recruitment via CC chemokine ligand 2. *Journal of Immunology*, Vol.177, No.11, pp. 8072-8079.

Guillén, N; Acín, S; Navarro, MA; Surra, JC; Arnal, C; Lou-Bonafonte, JM; Muniesa, P; Martínez-Gracia, MV. & Osada, J. (2009). Knowledge of the biological actions of extra virgin olive oil gained from mice lacking apolipoprotein E. *Revista Española de Cardiologia*, Vol.62, No.3, pp.294-304.

Havel, RJ. (1994). Postprandial hyperlipidemia and remnant lipoproteins. *Current Opinion of Lipidology*, Vol. 5, No.2, pp. 102–119.

Hilpert, KF; West, SG; Kris-Etherton, PM; Hecker, KD; Simpson, NM. & Alaupovic, P. (2007). Postprandial effect of n-3 polyunsaturated fatty acids on apolipoprotein B-containing lipoproteins and vascular reactivity in type 2 diabetes. *American Journal of Clinical Nutrition*, Vol.85, No.2, pp. 369-376.

Hodis, HN; Mack, WJ; Krauss, RM. & Alaupovic, P. (1999). Pathophysiology of triglyceride-rich lipoproteins in atherothrombosis: clinical aspects. *Clinical Cardiology*, Vol.22, No.6 Suppl, pp. 15-20.

Hodis, HN. (1999). Triglyceride-rich lipoprotein remnant particles and risk of atherosclerosis. *Circulation*. Vol. 99, No. 22, pp. 2852-2854.

Holdt, LM; Thiery, J; Breslow, JL. & Teupser, D. (2008). Increased ADAM17 mRNA expression and activity is associated with atherosclerosis resistance in LDL-receptor deficient mice. *Arteriosclerosis Thrombosis and Vascular Biology*, Vol.28, No.6, pp. 1097-1103.

Jagla, A. & Schrezenmeir, J. (2001). Postprandial triglycerides and endothelial function. *Experimental and Clinical Endocrinology and Diabetes*, Vol.109, No.4, pp. S533-547.

Jiménez-Gómez, Y; López-Miranda, J; Blanco-Colio, LM; Marín, C; Pérez-Martínez, P; Ruano, J; Paniagua, JA; Rodríguez, F; Egido, J. & Pérez-Jiménez, F. (2009). Olive oil and walnut breakfasts reduce the postprandial inflammatory response in mononuclear cells compared with a butter breakfast in healthy men. *Atherosclerosis*, Vol.204, No.2, pp. e70-76.

Karantonis, HC; Antonopoulou, S; Perrea, DN; Sokolis, DP; Theocharis, SE; Kavantzas N; Lliopoulos, DG. &Demopoulos, CA. (2006). In vivo antiatherogenic properties of olive oil and its constituent lipid classes in hyperlipidemic rabbits. *Nutrition, Metabolism and Cardiovascular Disease*, Vol.16, No.3, pp 174-185.

Kashyap, SR; Loachimescu, AG; Gornik, HL; Gopan, T; Davidson, MB; Makdissi, A; Major, J; Febbraio, M. & Silverstein, RL. (2009). Lipid-induced insulin resistance is associated with increased monocyte expression of scavenger receptor CD36 and internalization of oxidized LDL. *Obesity (Silver Spring)*, Vol.17, No.12, pp. 2142-8.

Khymenets, O; Fitó, M; Covas, MI; Farré, M; Pujadas, MA, Muñoz, D; Konstantinidou, V. & de la Torre, R. (2009). Mononuclear cell transcriptome response after sustained virgin olive oil consumption in humans: an exploratory nutrigenomics study. *OMICS*, Vol.13, No.1, pp. 7-19.

Konstantinidou, V; Covas, MI; Muñoz-Aguayo, D; Khymenets, O; de la Torre, R; Saez, G; Tormos Mdel, C; Toledo, E; Marti, A; Ruiz-Gutiérrez, V; Ruiz Mendez, MV. & Fito, M. (2010). In vivo nutrigenomic effects of virgin olive oil polyphenols within the frame of the Mediterranean diet: a randomized controlled trial. *FASEB Journal*, Vol.24, No.7, pp. 2546-2557.

Konstantinidou, V; Khymenets, O; Covas, MI; de la Torre, R; Muñoz-Aguayo, D; Anglada, R; Farré, M. & Fito, M. (2009). Time course of changes in the expression of insulin sensitivity-related genes after an acute load of virgin olive oil. *OMICS*. Vol.13, No.5, pp. 431-438.

Leite, MS; Pacheco, P; Gomes, RN; Guedes, AT; Castro-Faria-Neto, HC; Bozza, PT. & Koatz, VL. (2005). Mechanisms of increased survival after lipopolysaccharide-induced endotoxic shock in mice consuming olive oil-enriched diet. *Shock*, Vol.23, No.2, pp. 173-178.

Lopez, S; Bermudez, B; Ortega, A; Varela, LM; Pacheco, YM; Villar, J; Abia, R. & Muriana, FJ. (2011). Effects of meals rich in either monounsaturated or saturated fat on lipid concentrations and on insulin secretion and action in subjects with high fasting triglyceride concentrations. *American Journal of Clinical Nutrition*, Vol.93, No.3, pp. 494-499.

Lopez, S; Ortega, A; Varela, LM; Bermudez, B; Muriana, FJ. & Abia, R. (2009). Recent advances in lipoprotein and atherosclerosis: a nutrigenomics approach. *Grasas y Aceites*, Vol.60, No.1, pp.33-40.

Li, M; Yu, J; Li, Y; Li, D; Yan, D; Qu, Z. & Ruan, Q. (2010). CXCR4 positive bone mesenchymal stem cells migrate to human endothelial cell stimulated by ox-LDL via SDF-1alpha/CXCR4 signaling axis. *Experimental Molecular Pathology*, Vol.88, No.2, pp. 250-255.

Li, N; McLaren, JE; Michael, DR; Clement, M; Fielding, CA. & Ramji, DP. (2010). ERK is integral to the IFN-γ-mediated activation of STAT1, the expression of key genes implicated in atherosclerosis, and the uptake of modified lipoproteins by human macrophages. *Journal of Immunology*, Vol.185, No.5, pp. 3041-3048.

Llorente-Cortés, V; Estruch, R; Mena, MP; Ros, E; González, MA; Fitó, M; Lamuela-Raventós, RM. & Badimon, L. (2010). Effect of Mediterranean diet on the expression of pro-atherogenic genes in a population at high cardiovascular risk. *Atherosclerosis*, Vol.208, No.2, pp. 442-450.

Lloyd-Jones, D; Adams, RJ; Brown, TM; Carnethon, M; Dai, S; De Simone, G; Ferguson, TB; Ford, E; Furie, K; Gillespie, C; Go, A; Greenlund, K; Haase, N; Hailpern, S; Ho, PM; Howard, V; Kissela, B; Kittner, S; Lackland, D; Lisabeth, L; Marelli, A; McDermott, MM; Meigs, J; Mozaffarian, D; Mussolino, M; Nichol, G; Roger, VL; Rosamond, W; Sacco, R; Sorlie, P; Stafford, R; Thom, T; Wasserthiel-Smoller, S; Wong, ND. & Wylie-Rosett, J. (2010). Executive summary: heart disease and stroke statistics-2010 update: a report from the American Heart Association. American Heart Association

Statistics Committee and Stroke Statistics Subcommittee. *Circulation*, Vol.121, No.7, pp 948-954.

Machowetz, A; Poulsen, HE; Gruendel, S; Weimann, A; Fitó, M; Marrugat, J; de la Torre, R; Salonen, JT; Nyyssönen, K; Mursu, J; Nascetti, S; Gaddi, A; Kiesewetter, H; Bäumler, H; Selmi, H; Kaikkonen, J; Zunft, HJ; Covas, MI. & Koebnick, C. (2007). Effect of olive oils on biomarkers of oxidative DNA stress in Northern and Southern Europeans. *FASEB Journal*, Vol.21, No.1, pp. 45-52.

Magrone, T; Candore, G; Caruso, C; Jirillo, E. & Covelli, V. (2008). Polyphenols from red wine modulate immune responsiveness: biological and clinical significance. *Current Pharmaceutical Design*, Vol.14, No.26, pp. 2733-2748.

Mangiapane, EH; McAteer, MA; Benson, GM; White, DA. & Salter, AM. (1999). Modulation of the regression of atherosclerosis in the hamster by dietary lipids: comparison of coconut oil and olive oil. *British Journal of Nutrition*, Vol.82, No.5, pp. 401-419.

Maiuri, MC; De Stefano, D; Di Meglio, P; Irace, C; Savarese, M; Sacchi, R; Cinelli, MP. & Carnuccio, R. (2005). Hydroxytyrosol, a phenolic compound from virgin olive oil, prevents macrophage activation. *Naunyn-Schmiedebergs Archives of Pharmacology*, Vol. 371, No.6, pp. 457-465.

Manning, PJ; Sutherland, WH; McGrath, MM; de Jong, SA; Walker, RJ. & Williams, MJ. (2008). Postprandial cytokine concentrations and meal composition in obese and lean women. *Obesity (Silver Spring)*, Vol.16, No.9, pp. 2046-2052.

Martínez-González, J; Rodríguez-Rodríguez, R; González-Díez, M, Rodríguez, C, Herrera, MD, Ruiz-Gutierrez, V. & Badimon, L. (2008). Oleanolic acid induces prostacyclin release in human vascular smooth muscle cells through a cyclooxygenase-2-dependent mechanism. *Journal of Nutrition*, Vol.138, No.3, pp. 443-448.

Müller, M. & Kersten S. (2003). Nutrigenomics: goals and strategies. *Nature Reviews. Genetics*, Vol.4, No.4, pp. 315-22.

Nakamura, T; Takano, H; Umetani, K; Kawabata, K; Obata, JE; Kitta, Y; Kodama, Y; Mende, A; Ichigi, Y; Fujioka, D; Saito, Y. & Kugiyama, K. (2005). Remnant lipoproteinemia is a risk factor for endothelial vasomotor dysfunction and coronary artery disease in metabolic syndrome. *Atherosclerosis*, Vol. 181, No.2, pp. 321-327.

Oliveras-López, MJ; Berná, G; Carneiro, EM; López-García de la Serrana, H; Martín, F. & López, MC. (2008). An extra-virgin olive oil rich in polyphenolic compounds has antioxidant effects in OF1 mice. Journal of Nutrition, Vol.138, No.6, pp. 1074-1078.

Papageorgiou, N; Tousoulis, D; Psaltopoulou, T; Giolis, A; Antoniades, C; Tsiamis, E; Miliou, A; Toutouzas, K; Siasos, G. & Stefanadis C. (2011). Divergent anti-inflammatory effects of different oil acute consumption on healthy individuals. *European Journal Clinical Nutrition*, Vol.65, No.4, pp. 514-519.

Perez-Martinez, P; Ordovas, JM; Garcia-Rios, A; Delgado-Lista, J; Delgado-Casado, N; Cruz-Teno, C; Camargo, A; Yubero-Serrano, EM; Rodriguez, F; Perez-Jimenez, F. & Lopez-Miranda J. (2011). Consumption of diets with different type of fat influences triacylglycerols-rich lipoproteins particle number and size during the postprandial state. *Nutrition, Metabolism & Cardiovascular Diseases*, Vol.21, pp. 39-45.

Poudyal, H; Campbell, F. & Brown, L. (2010). Olive leaf extract attenuates cardiac, hepatic, and metabolic changes in high carbohydrate-, high fat-fed rats. *Journal of Nutrition*, Vol.140, No.5, pp. 946-53.

Puel, C; Mardon, J; Agalias, A; Davicco, MJ; Lebecque, P; Mazur, A; Horcajada, MN; Skaltsounis, AL. & Coxam, V. (2008). Major phenolic compounds in olive oil modulate bone loss in an ovariectomy/inflammation experimental model. *Journal of Agricultural and Food Chemistry*, Vol.56, No.20, pp. 9417-9422.

Qin, B; Polansky, MM; Harry, D. & Anderson, RA. (2010). Green tea polyphenols improve cardiac muscle mRNA and protein levels of signal pathways related to insulin and lipid metabolism and inflammation in insulin-resistant rats. *Molecular Nutrition and Food Research*, Vol.54, Suppl 1, pp. S14-23.

Reiss, K; Cornelsen, I; Husmann, M; Gimpl, G. & Bhakdi S. (2011). Unsaturated fatty acids drive ADAM-dependent cell adhesion, proliferation and migration by modulating membrane fluidity. *Journal Biological Chemistry*, (ahead of print).

Rosenblat, M; Volkova, N; Coleman, R; Almagor, Y. and Aviram, M. (2008). Antiatherogenicity of extra virgin olive oil and its enrichment with green tea polyphenols in the atherosclerotic apolipoprotein-E-deficient mice: enhanced macrophage cholesterol efflux. *Journal of Nutritional Biochemistry*, Vol.19, No.8, pp. 514-523.

Servili, M; Esposto, S; Fabiani, R; Urbani, S; Taticchi, A; Mariucci, F; Selvaggini, R. & Montedoro GF. (2009). Phenolic compounds in olive oil: antioxidant, health and organoleptic activities according to their chemical structure. *Inflammopharmacology*, Vol.17, No.2, 76-84.

Shen, J; Chandrasekharan, UM; Ashraf, MZ; Long, E; Morton, RE; Liu, Y; Smith, JD. & DiCorleto, PE. (2010). Lack of mitogen-activated protein kinase phosphatase-1 protects ApoE-null mice against atherosclerosis. *Circulation Research*, Vol.106, No.5, pp. 902-910.

Sung, HY; Guan, H; Czibula, A; King, AR; Eder, K; Heath, E; Suvarna, SK; Dower, SK; Wilson, AG; Francis, SE; Crossman, DC. & Kiss-Toth, E. (2007). Human tribbles-1 controls proliferation and chemotaxis of smooth muscle cells via MAPK signaling pathways. *Journal of Biological Chemistry*, Vol.282, No.25, pp. 18379-18387.

Teng, KT; Nagapan, G; Cheng, HM. & Nesaretnam, K. (2011). Palm olein and olive oil cause a higher increase in postprandial lipemia compared with lard but had no effect on plasma glucose, insulin and adipocytokines. *Lipids*, Vol.46, No.4, pp. 381-388.

Trefiletti, G; Rita Togna, A; Latina, V; Marra, C; Guiso, M. & Togna, GI. (2011). 1-Phenyl-6,7-dihydroxy-isochroman suppresses lipopolysaccharide-induced pro-inflammatory mediator production in human monocytes. *British Journal of Nutrition*, Vol.106, No.1, pp. 33-36.

Tsantila, N; Karantonis, HC; Perrea, DN; Theocharis, SE; Iliopoulos, DG; Antonopoulou, S. & Demopoulos CA. (2007). Antithrombotic and antiatherosclerotic properties of olive oil and olive pomace polar extracts in rabbits. *Mediators of Inflammation*, Vol.2007, No. 36204, pp.1-11.

Tsantila, N; Karantonis, HC; Perrea, DN; Theocharis, SE; Iliopoulos, DG; Iatrou, C; Antonopoulou, S. & Demopoulos, CA. (2010) Atherosclerosis regression study in rabbits upon olive pomace polar lipid extract administration. *Nutrition, Metabolism and Cardiovascular Disease*, Vol. 20, No. 10, pp. 740-747.

Van der Heiden, K; Cuhlmann, S; Luong, Le A; Zakkar, M. & Evans, PC. (2010). Role of nuclear factor kB in cardiovascular health and disease. *Clinical Sciences (London)*, Vol.118, No.10, pp. 593-605.

Van Ommen, B. (2004). Nutrigenomics: exploiting systems biology in the nutrition and health arenas. *Nutrition*, Vol.20, No.1, pp. 4-8.

Weinstein, MM; Yin, L; Tu, Y; Wang, X; Wu, X; Castellani, LW; Walzem, RL; Lusis, AJ; Fong, LG; Beigneux, AP. & Young, SG. (2010). Chylomicronemia elicits atherosclerosis in mice--brief report. *Arteriosclerosis Thrombosis and Vascular Biology*, Vol.30, No.1, pp. 20-23.

Williams, CM; Maitin, V. & Jackson, KG. (2004). Triacylglycerol-rich lipoprotein-gene interactions in endothelial cells. *Biochemical Society Transations*, Vol.32, No.6, pp. 994-998.

Wilson, PW. (2008). Evidence of systemic inflammation and estimation of coronary artery disease risk: a population perspective. *American Journal of Medicine*, Vol.121, No.10 Supple1, pp. S15-S20.

Zhang, J; Alcaide, P; Liu, L; Sun, J; He, A; Luscinskas, FW. & Shi, GP. (2011). Regulation of endothelial cell adhesion molecule expression by mast cells, macrophages, and neutrophils. *PLoS One*, Vol.6, No.1, pp. e14525.

Zhang, X; Cao, J. & Zhong, L. (2009). Hydroxytyrosol inhibits pro-inflammatory cytokines, iNOS, and COX-2 expression in human monocytic cells. *Naunyn-Schmiedebergs Archives of Pharmacology*, Vol.379, No.6, pp. 581-586.

Zilversmit, DB. (1979). Atherogenesis: a postprandial phenomenon. *Circulation*, Vol. 60, No.3, pp, 473–485.

Zrelli, H; Matsuoka, M; Kitazaki, S; Zarrouk, M. & Miyazaki, H. (2011). Hydroxytyrosol reduces intracellular reactive oxygen species levels in vascular endothelial cells by upregulating catalase expression through the AMPK-FOXO3a pathway. *European Journal of Pharmacology*. Vol.660, No.(2-3), pp. 275-282.

7

Emerging Epigenetic Therapy for Vascular Proliferative Diseases

Kasturi Ranganna[1], Frank M. Yatsu[2] and Omana P. Mathew[1]
[1]Texas Southern University, Department of Pharmaceutical Sciences,
[2]University of Texas Health Science Center at Houston, Texas, Department of Neurology
USA

1. Introduction

Atherosclerosis and restenosis, complex pathologies of blood vessels, are multifactorial diseases triggered by the inflammatory response to injury of endothelium. Remodeling of the injured vessel, proliferation and migration of vascular smooth muscle cells (VSMC) and elaboration and accumulation of extracellular matrix proteins are main traits of these diseases (Dzau et al., 2002; Libby, 2002; Pons et al., 2009; Ranganna et al., 2006; Ross, 1995;). Despite the substantial progress in understanding the etiology and the clinical management of atherosclerosis and restenosis, they are still life threatening diseases. Precise reasons are not still fully transparent. Different cell types; distinct cellular pathways and processes; and multiple genes within each participating cell types that are vulnerable to both genetic and environmental risk factors participate in the pathogenesis of atherosclerosis and restenosis.

Recently, it is recognized that besides the genetic control epigenetic mechanisms regulate development and maintenance of organisms or their interaction with surrounding environment through the coordination of a set of reversible modifications that turn parts of the genome 'off' and 'on' at strategic times and at specific sites causing changes in gene expression with no changes in DNA sequences (Ekstrom, 2009; Pons et al., 2009; Ranganna et al., 2006; Turunen, 2009). The two well-known epigenetic mechanisms, DNA methylation and histone modifications change the chromatin structure and dynamics that alter gene functions by influencing gene expressions. Dysregulation of epigenetic processes has been linked to human diseases, which influences many aspects of cell biology including cell growth, cell cycle control, proliferation, differentiation, and cell death. Reversing the dysregulation of epigenetic mechanisms may offer effective treatment strategy for many diseases including cardiovascular disease due to atherosclerosis and restenosis. This review presents the current advancement in the epigenetics of VSMC proliferation and potential use of histone epigenetic modifiers in the intervention of atherosclerosis and restenosis.

2. Overview of pathogenesis of atherosclerosis

Atherosclerosis, a disease of medium to large arterial vessels, accounts for over 55% of all deaths in western countries. It is typically asymptomatic for decades but ultimately result in life-threatening pathological outcomes like myocardial infarction and stroke, both with tissue infarction because of intra-arterial thrombosis provoked by atherosclerosis.

Atherosclerosis is a complex progressive disease in which intimal thickening of the arterial wall promotes luminal stenosis by vascular remodeling, accumulation of cellular and extracellular substances and VSMC proliferation and migration. Integrity of arterial wall is crucial for the regulation of vascular tone, control inflammation, thrombosis, and angiogenesis, enhance regional blood flow, and inhibit cancer metastasis. Arterial wall is composed of three tunics that surround a central lumen through which blood flows. The innermost layer is the tunica intima composed of endothelial cells that form a smooth lining that minimizes interaction with circulating cellular and non-cellular components as blood moves through the vessel. The middle layer, tunic media, is composed of vascular smooth muscle cells (VSMC) and layers of flexible proteins, which enables the lumen to contract and dilate to regulate blood flow in the body. The outer layer, tunica adventitia is a protective layer of connective tissue that anchors the blood vessel to surrounding structures.

Under normal conditions, a delicate balance between proliferation and apoptosis of local vascular cell types maintains the thickness of arterial vessel wall. A number of regulatory factors produced by the endothelial cells are responsible for the homeostatic balance by controlling vessel tone, coagulation state, leukocyte trafficking, and cellular proliferative response. Any damage to the vessel wall by mechanical, biochemical, or immunological insults triggers endothelial dysfunction or denudation of endothelial layer overwhelming the normal homeostatic balance, thus, upsets the normal vascular tone setting the stage for the activation of proinflammatory and immune response. Escalating evidence indicates that inflammatory or atherogenic stimuli promote ROS generation in endothelial milieu causing oxidative stress (Freeman & Crapo, 1982; Kehrer, 1993; Kunsch & Medford, 1999; Madamanchi et al., 2005). Inflammatory response fueled by the oxidative stress is also linked to oxidation of lipoproteins. LDL molecules that enter the subendothelial space are oxidized to form oxidized LDL (OxLDL) by different mechanisms including enzymatic and nonenzymatic pathways, which are taken up by macrophages via scavenger receptors to become foam cells. Besides stimulating proinflammatory and proatherogenic effects, OxLDL also appears to elicit highly immunogenic response resulting in the generation of autoantibodies that appears to be of pathogenic significance (Hansson, 2009; Klingenberg, R., & Hansson, G.K. 2009; Steinberg & Witztum, 2010; Witztum, 1997). Moreover, elevated levels of ROS appear to function as second-messenger molecules transmitting the extracellular signals to nucleus via redox-sensitive signaling pathways to turn on the expression of atherogenic gene products such as adhesion molecules and inflammatory cytokines. Expression of these gene products elicit changes in the vessel wall promoting inflammation, infiltration of monocytes and T cells, proliferation, migration and activation of VSMC and matrix alteration (Freeman & Crapo, 1982; Hansson, 2007; Kehrer, 1993; Klingenberg & Hansson, 2009; Kunsch & Medford, 1999; Madamanchi et al., 2005; Steinberg & Witztum, 2010; Witztum, 1997). These processes involve synthesis and release of a host of regulatory molecules, both by cellular components in the blood and vascular cells of the arterial wall triggering autocrine, paracrine, and endocrine type of interactions between cells and the molecules they produce. Outcome of these complex interactions leads to migration of VSMCs from their normal residence in the arterial media to the intima where they change their phenotype from a contractile to a proliferative type (Libby, 2002; March et al., 1999; Ross, 1995). This phenotypic change, in conjunction with excessive production and accumulation of extracellular matrix proteins, is the main contributor to vascular remodeling.

2.1 Vascular remodeling in atherosclerosis and restenosis

Atherosclerosis and restenosis both are multifactorial vascular occlusive processes but exhibit certain similarities and differences in the origin and progression of their development (Dzau et al., 2002; Pons et al., 2009). Inflammatory response of activated endothelial cells to injury or insults elicits both these processes. Activation of endothelial cells leads to a cascade of events, which promotes vascular remodeling by changing the size, structure and composition of vessel wall. Moreover, both processes involve proliferation, migration and activation of VSMC and modulation of extracellular matrix by elaborating and accumulating extracellular matrix proteins. Although they share some of the risk factors such as hypertension and diabetes, there is a consensus that atherosclerosis develops in response to elevated low-density lipoproteins (LDL) and cigarette smoke. On the other hand, VSMC proliferation is the primary pathophysiological mechanism in restenosis, which is largely due to transcending wound healing response to clinical procedures such as balloon angioplasty, stent placement and vein graft surgery [Dzau et al., 2002; Pons et al., 2009]. While restenosis appears to be insensitive to circulating lipids, accumulation of oxidized LDL is the characteristic feature of atherosclerosis. Additionally, while development and progression of atherosclerosis is a gradual process, the restenotic process is a relatively a rapid process caused by surgical revascularization procedures such as angioplasty and stent placement. Despite substantial progress in understanding the etiology and the clinical management of atherosclerosis and restenosis, they are still life-threatening diseases. Possible reasons are multiple factors, different cellular pathways and processes, and multiple genes are contributory to these complex vascular disease processes.

2.2 VSMC proliferation

VSMC are highly specialized cells, which play vital roles in the regulation of blood pressure, blood flow and in many pathological states. In mature individuals, the typical function of arterial VSMC is contraction and maintenance of vascular tone. As such, VSMC in adult artery exhibit contractile or differentiated phenotype displaying quiescent proliferation state, decreased synthetic activity and expression of proteins unique to contractile phenotype like contractile proteins, ion channels and signaling proteins. However, VSMC retain their remarkable plasticity to undergo reversible phenotypic change in response to alterations in the local environment like during development, physiological conditions like pregnancy or in response to vascular injury. This remarkable flexible persona of VSMC makes them vulnerable to phenotypic modification from contractile to proliferative, synthetic, or de-differentiated phenotype in conjunction with vessel remodeling by altering cell number and composition of vessel wall (Pons et al., 2009; Ross, 1993).

VSMC proliferation is also the primary pathophysiological mechanism in different clinical pathologies such as postangioplasty restenosis, in-stent restenosis, vein bypass graft failure and transplant vasculopathy (Dzau et al., 2002; Holmes, 2003). The clinical procedures performed to clear the occluded vessel fortuitously become precursors for restenosis in 30-40% of the patients, mainly due to proliferation and activation of VSMC. While entry into cell cycle followed by proliferation of VSMC contributes to the formation of neointima, activation of VSMC induces expression of proinflammatory cytokines, adhesion molecules, chemoattractants, proteolytic enzymes and other molecules not usually present in normal, quiescent, contractile VSMC of the medial layer (Kleemann et al., 2008; Li et al., 1993; O'Brien et al., 1996; Zeffer et al., 2004). Expression of these molecules amplifies the inflammatory response, and in turn, increases further proliferation of VSMC and elaboration of vessel remodeling.

2.3 Antiproliferative therapeutics to target VSMC proliferation

The current therapies used for atherosclerosis aim to minimize the risk factors that promote atherosclerosis, such as reducing elevated levels of cholesterol or enhancing the blood flow by surgical intervention of an already occluded vessel. Ironically, the surgical procedures performed to clear the occluded vessel become a precursor for restenosis, mainly due to VSMC proliferation, in significant number of patients (Dzau et al., 2002; Ferns et al., 1991). Because proliferation of VSMC is the hallmark of atherosclerosis and clinical conditions such as arterial stenosis, transplant vasculopathy, and bypass graft failure, the suitable therapeutic approach is to develop strategies that inhibit or block VSMC proliferation. Based on the current understanding of the molecular basis of vascular proliferative diseases, there is an abundance of potential therapeutic possibilities. Accordingly, a number of agents are tested for antiproliferative activity including heparins, cytostatic agents, inhibitors of angiotensin converting enzyme, and antagonists to growth factors (Dzau et al., 2002; Ferns et al., 1991; Gershlick, 2002; Stephen et al., 2005; Toshiro et al., 2005). Although some of these agents have shown promise in animal models, they failed to elicit any protection in human clinical studies (Gershlick, 2002). Species differences, potential toxicity, and lack of potency are possible culprits. Furthermore, the probability of successfully treating a multifactorial disease by targeting a single factor is unlikely. Additionally, all vascular cell types secrete growth factors and cytokines that activate signaling pathways that are redundant and thus prevent the success of targeting one or two factors.

2.4 Cell cycle as the therapeutic target

Based on the current knowledge of cell cycle mechanisms, it appears that targeting specific parts of the cell cycle is a better strategy to inhibit or block the development of vascular proliferative diseases such as arterial restenosis; in-stent-stenosis and vein bypass graft failure. Moreover, cell cycle is the final common pathway where all the growth regulatory signals converge, and thus, makes a rational target of antiproliferative therapeutics to inhibit vascular proliferative diseases. Some of the experimental studies indeed reveal that inhibition of cell cycle progression emerges as an important therapeutic target for prevention of vascular proliferative diseases (Dzau et al., 2002; Ranganna et al., 2006; Von der Leyen & Dzau, 2001). Different approaches such as pharmacological agents, irradiation, and gene therapy have been used for arresting VSMC proliferation. These approaches inhibit proliferation by cytostatic or cytotoxic mechanism. However, cytostatic mechanism of cell cycle arrest is desired over cytotoxic mechanism to avoid unintended damage to the vessel wall due to cytotoxic treatment. Three different approaches have been tried for arresting VSMC proliferation by targeting cell cycle, which include: 1) brachytherapy, 2) gene therapy, and 3) pharmacotherapy.

2.4.1. Brachytherapy

Endovascular radiotherapy is a promising method for effective antiproliferative treatment of restenosis (Teirstein & King, 2003; Waksman, 2000). Radiotherapy directed at restenosis has two objectives, one to treat restenosis by killing the cells that re-occluded and to prevent further restenosis by inhibiting tissue growth. Brachytherapy with either beta or gamma radiation sources are used to diminish restenosis in patients with post-angioplasty restenosis or with in-stent restenosis. The rationale for using radiation for treating restenosis is that uncontrolled proliferation of VSMC is similar to neoplastic cells that can be targeted for radiation therapy just as transformed cells in cancer tissue. Brachytherapy-induced DNA damage of VSMC can result in arrest of VSMC at the G1 checkpoint or induction of apoptosis through p53 induced p21Cip1 upregulation. A key feature of brachytherapy is that the irradiation only affects a precise localized area around the radiation sources. Exposure to radiation of healthy tissues further away from the sources is therefore, reduced. In addition, brachytherapy is associated with a low risk of serious adverse side effects. More than a dozen randomized trials established its safety and efficacy. However, it exhibits two radiotherapy-related problems, arterial narrowing adjacent to the edge of the target site and unexpected late coronary thrombo-occlusive events (Raizner, 2000).

2.4.2 Gene therapy

Gene therapy techniques provide a unique opportunity to genetically engineer vessels and grafts to become impervious to atherosclerosis and neointimal formation that contributes to arterial restenosis, in-stent restenosis and vein graft failure (Dzau et al., 2002; Khanna, 2008; Kishore & Losordo, 2007; Gaffney et al., 2007; Melo et al., 2005; Von der Leyen & Dzau, 2001). Gene therapy approach has potential not only against monogenic diseases, but also against complex diseases where multiple genes are involved in the disease pathogenesis like in cardiovascular diseases and cancer. One of the key challenges of the gene therapy is appropriate vector for the delivery of functional gene or a concoction of genes in multigenic diseases as in cardiovascular diseases. Besides the choice of vector, other parameters such as, appropriate gene targets and efficient methods of vector delivery for a specific target have to be optimized. Vectors can be either viral or non-viral. The ideal vector is the one, which is nonpathogenic, less immunogenic, more efficient, and enhanced tissue specificity.

Delivery of therapeutic genes to the cardiovascular tissues is challenging. To facilitate local gene delivery to lesions in the vasculature catheter-based vector delivery has been tried using a variety of balloon catheters in animal models and human trials (Khanna, 2008; Kishore & Losordo, 2007; Gaffney et al., 2007; Melo et al., 2005). Stents are ideal gear for localized gene delivery to the vascular wall because of their widespread use, safety and permanent scaffold structure. Stents can be coated with genetically engineered cells or plasmid or adenoviral vectors carrying therapeutic genes (Khanna, 2008; Kishore & Losordo, 2007; Gaffney et al., 2007; Melo et al., 2005). Experimental studies have demonstrated usefulness of gene therapy in treating atherosclerosis and restenosis in various animal models and in some clinical trials. It can be used to transfer exogenous genes to express functional gene products to overcome defective or downregulated endogenous gene expressions through vector-based delivery system. It also can be used to knockdown or suppress the expression of gene products that contribute to pathogenesis of disease by one of the several methods of gene silencing. These include antisense oligonucleotides (ODNs), short segments of RNA with enzymatic activity (ribozymes) and small interfering RNAs [siRNA] (Dzau et al., 2002; J.M. Li et al., 2010; Banno, et al., 2006).

A number of studies have shown that gene therapies can be targeted for reducing cholesterol levels, inflammation and thrombosis (Feldman & Isner, 1995); for upregulating apo-A1 and downregulating chemoattractant protein-1 (MCP1)receptor expression (Tangirala, 1999); transferring pleiotropic atheroprotective nitric oxide synthase [NOS]

(Qian, 1999); targeting vascular redox biology through heme oxygenase-1, superoxide dismutase, catalase and glutathione peroxidase antioxidant gene therapy to attenuate oxidative stress (Van Assche, 2011); and lipid-lowering gene therapy to reduce plasma LDL levels (Grossman et al., 1995). Furthermore, neointimal hyperplasia that contributes to pathogenesis of arterial stenosis, in-stent stenosis and vein graft failure is also a good target for gene therapy. A number of potential therapeutic genes, which are key to the development of neointimal hyperplasia, have been identified. The ones that are promising for gene therapy include tissue inhibitors of matrix metalloproteinases (Akowuah et al., 2005; Gaffney et al., 2007; Khanna, 2008); NOS (Cooney, 2006; Dzau et al., 2002; Khanna, 2008; Kishore & Losordo, 2007; Gaffney et al., 2007; Melo et al., 2005; Von der Leyen & Dzau, 2001) and p53 (Gaffney et al., 2007). Importantly, delivery of antiproliferative genes such as those coding for p21Cip1, p27Kip1, and iNOS are used to inhibit stenosis and neointimal hyperplasia (Dzau et al., 2002; Von der Leyen & Dzau, 2001]. Conversely, silencing the genes that contribute to proliferation via antisense ODNs (Dzau et al., 2002; Khanna, 2008; Kishore & Losordo, 2007; Gaffney et al., 2007; Melo et al., 2005) or siRNA approach is also effective in preventing in-stent and graft neointimal hyperplasia (Banno, et al., 2006; F. Li et al., 2005; J.M. Li et al., 2010; Matsumae et al., 2008). Antisense ODNs–based inhibition of cell proliferation-related genes such as PCNA, c-myc, c-myb or different cyclin-dependent kinases (cdks) have been successfully carried out in experimental models of vascular lesion formation (Braun-Dullaeus et al., 1998; Dzau et al., 2002; Morishita et al., 1993; Simons et al., 1994).

RNA interference (RNAi) technology is becoming popular approach to alter gene expressions to interrogate their role in pathogenesis of disease, which has utility in the inhibition of VSMC proliferation and neointimal hyperplasia (Banno, et al., 2006; F. Li et al., 2005; J.M. Li et al., 2010; Matsumae et al., 2008). To determine whether Angiotensin II (ANG II)-induced neointimal thickening is mediated via cytoplasmic phospholipase A2 (cPLA2) - and phospholipase D2 (PLD2)-activated Akt, injured carotid arteries were exposed to a retrovirus containing cPLA$_2$ siRNA or PLD2 siRNA to test whether their knockdown will result in the reduction of ANG II-induced neointimal thickening (F. Li et al., 2005). SiRNA-mediated downregulation of cPLA2 and PLD2 resulted in the reduction of ANG II-induced neointimal thickening. The involvement of CCN1, an extracellular matrix-associated protein, in the development of neointimal hyperplasia is confirmed by siRNA-mediated knockdown approach (Matsumae et al., 2008). The atheroprotective role of midkine (MK), a heparin-binding growth factor, is corroborated by the use of MK-siRNA (Banno, et al., 2006). NADPH oxidase has a critical role in the development of neointimal hyperplasia and restenosis due to its contribution to oxidative stress, which is blocked by siRNA specific to NOX2 gene *Cybb*, an important component of NADPH oxidase (J.M. Li, et al., 2010).

Several experimental gene transfer and gene silencing strategies are evaluated as potential treatments for cardiovascular disease, which resulted in Phase I, and Phase I to Phase III clinical studies for inducible iNOS (Tzeng, 1996; Von der Leyen & Dzau, 2001) and transcription factor E2F, respectively (Dzau et al., 2002; McCarthy, 2001; Mann et al., 1999). E2F, a transcription factor that leads to upregulation of up to 12 cell-cycle genes is an ideal target for cell-cycle blockade. A double-stranded E2F decoy ODN that bears the consensus E2F-binding site (*cis*-elements) was designed as an agent for prevention of vein graft disease. In rabbits, treatment of vein grafts with E2F decoy ODN resulted in inhibition of neointimal hyperplasia and graft atherosclerosis for up to 6 months. This led to phase I

PREVENT trial for human vascular bypass grafts, which resulted in about 75% reduction in VSMC proliferation and fewer graft occlusions. Similar gene manipulation approach was used for coronary bypass grafts in PREVENT II trial. Although the phase 1 trial (PREVENT Trial) showed promising results, later studies were less positive including the phase III, multicentre, randomized double-blinded, placebo-controlled trial of 3014 patients undergoing primary coronary artery bypass graft surgery with at least two planned saphenous grafts (Alexander et al., 2005; Conte et al., 2005, 2006). Although appears to be promising, the use of gene therapy in the treatment of vascular proliferative diseases is still in infancy. Various feasibility and efficacy issues as well as design and delivery of the genes have to be addressed taking into account the complexity of the pathological processes leading to atherosclerosis and restenosis.

2.4.3 Pharmacotherapy

A number of pharmacological agents have been used to target injury-induced VSMC proliferation that contributes to neointimal growth in balloon-injured arteries. Among these rapamycin or sirolimus, a cytostatic agent, arrests VSMC proliferation and migration *in vitro* and reduces neointimal growth in animal models of balloon-injury (Dzau et al., 2002; Guerin et al., 2005). Its action appears to be mediated through the inhibition of mammalian target of rapamycin (mTOR). One of the downstream events induced by the inhibition of mTOR is induction of p27Kip1, an inhibitor of cyclin-dependent kinases (cdk), causes cells to arrest in G1 phase of the cell cycle. In doing so, it inhibits cell proliferation. Paclitaxel, a derivative of Taxol, is another promising agent for proliferation arrest, which by collapsing the mitotic spindle formation causes mitotic arrest (Jordan et al., 1993). It prevents neointima formation in animal models, and its clinical effect in the blockade of restenosis is investigated in several human trials (the ELUTES, TAXUS and ASPECT trials) via local delivery through stents coated with paclitaxel (Finn et al., 2007; Wilson et al., 2007).

2.4.4 Immunotherapy

Over the past several years, accumulating data have identified involvement of several antigens in the initiation of immune response during atherosclerosis. These include exogenous infectious microbial pathogens like, cytomegalovirus and chlamydia pneumonia and endogenous proteins such as oxLDL, heat shock proteins (HSPs) and β_2-glycoprotein-1b (Habets et al., 2010). Among these, the epitopes recognized on oxLDL are important because of the role of oxLDL in the pathogenesis of atherosclerosis ((Hansson, 1997; 2007; Steinberg & Witztum, 2010; Witztum, 1997). In addition to its proinflammatory and proatherogenic effects, and participation in the formation of foam cells, oxLDL is also immunogenic due to the presence of several neoepitopes. A number of neoepitopes generated during the oxidation of LDL are highly immunogenic and cause the generation of autoantibodies, which are detected in atherosclerotic lesions. Since the different epitopes of oxLDL induce atherogenic immune response, it may be possible to inhibit proatherogenic effects of oxLDL by modulating the immune response towards oxLDL through the immunization against oxLDL. Several antigens have been identified and investigated for immunization against atherosclerosis in animal models. Immunization against oxLDL show reduction in atherosclerosis in several animal models (Habets et al., 2010). This discovery of atheroprotective immunity has resulted in the emergence of immunotherapy approach against atherosclerosis. Indeed, several animal studies indicate that immunization against oxLDL offers protection against atherosclerosis, which appears to operate both through cellular and humoral immunity (Zhou, 2001). The increased titers of T cell-dependent IgG antibodies to oxLDL (Habets et al., 2010; Zhou, 2001) and natural IgM antibodies to phosphocholine (Binder et al., 2004) are also in agreement with the atheroprotection. Furthermore, two recent studies report promising immunotherapeutic approach for the prevention of atherosclerosis. In one study, LDL-receptor deficient mice were vaccinated with oxLDL-pulsed mature dendritic cells to determine the effect on atherosclerosis (Habets et al., 2010). In the second immunotherapy study, tolerogenic apo-B100-loaded dendritic cells in combination with immunosuppressive cytokine interleukin-10 were injected intravenously to hypercholesterolemic mice. This immunotherapy significantly prevented atherosclerosis by reducing autoimmune response against LDL (Hermansson et al., 2011) Although, these studies are encouraging and promising from a clinical perspective to translate these promising outcomes to the clinics, antigens that can be easily manufactured under good manufacturing practice conditions and that have a reproducible quality are necessary. However, several clinical studies are currently underway to evaluate the therapeutic implications of immunotherapy.

3. Epigenetics and vascular proliferative diseases

Advancement in technological innovations during the past 25 years has resulted in far-reaching in-depth comprehension of the biology and the etiology of vascular diseases, and thus influencing the perception of the pathophysiology of vascular proliferative diseases like atherosclerosis and restenosis. In spite of the substantial understanding of the etiology and the clinical management of these vascular proliferative diseases, they are still life threatening diseases and reasons are not fully evident. Based on the recent finding of the role of epigenetics in human diseases, it is proper to expect that epigenetic mechanisms enforces an additional layer of gene regulation that alters chromatin structure, and dynamics in the pathogenesis of vascular proliferative diseases (Ekstrom, 2009; Pons et al., 2009; Ranganna et al., 2006; Turunen, 2009). Epigenetic mechanisms are essential for the functioning of genomes to regulate normal development and maintenance of organisms, and to facilitate their interaction with surrounding environment. Compilation of the past 10 to 20 years of studies has resulted in the identification of three highly interrelated epigenetic mechanisms that alter the chromatin structure and accessibility. These include, DNA methylation, histone posttranslational modifications and non-coding RNA (ncRNA) expression based mechanisms, each of these mechanisms is essential for regulation of gene expression. Therefore, it is anticipated that the genetic and environmental factors that are relevant to the development of vascular proliferative diseases by their effect on inflammation, VSMC proliferation and vessel remodeling, is regulated by epigenetic mechanisms through the modification of chromatin structure, dynamics and accessibility (Ekstrom, 2009; Pons et al., 2009; Ranganna et al., 2006; Turunen, 2009). Although there is an outbreak of interest and enthusiasm in linking altered epigenetic mechanisms to human pathologies particularly cancers, it is relatively unexplored area regarding cardiovascular diseases. Moreover, deregulation of epigenetic processes are linked to changes in many aspects of cell biology including cell growth, cell cycle control, and cell death by altering the expression and in turn functions of target genes without changing their primary gene structure. Because VSMC proliferation is the hallmark of vascular proliferative diseases, understanding the epigenetics of VSMC proliferation and in particular their susceptibility to perturbation by the epigenetic modifiers may offer novel insights into disease pathogenesis and epigenetic therapeutic approaches. Therefore, it is appropriate to review the current knowledge of epigenetics in the regulation of VSMC proliferation.

3.1 VSMC epigenetics

Curiosity in epigenetics has surged during past decade even though the principle question it aims to address has been there for decades. That is, how a multicellular organism maintain drastically different gene expression profile in different cell types of the organism, while all the different cell types of the organism have exactly the same DNA. This is where epigenetics come into picture. Epigenetics refers to the inheritance of gene function/activity/expression that may be stable over long periods, last through several cell divisions or inherit through several generations, all without any change in their primary DNA (Ng & Gurdon, 2008; Probst, 2009). The three interrelated epigenetic mechanisms, which involve: methylation of DNA at CpG dinucleotides at specific position in the DNA molecule suppress expression of nearby genes (Esteller, 2008); posttranslational modifications of histones alters chromatin structure and changes promoter accessibility (Kouzarides, 2007); and small RNA molecules generated from non-coding RNAs (ncRNAs) inhibit gene expression (Mattick et al., 2009). All these mechanisms involved in epigenetic regulation contribute to epigenome. This review focuses on the role of posttranslational modifications of histones in the regulation of VSMC proliferation, and on the epigenetic regulators of histone modifications as potential candidates for drug targeting in the treatment and management of vascular proliferative disease.

3.2 Chromatin structure

Chromatin is a nucleoprotein complex consisting of repeating units of nucleosomal core particles. It offers a dynamic platform for all DNA-mediated processes within the nucleus. The nucleosomal core particles are the basic units of chromatin consisting of 147 base pair (bp) of DNA that wraps almost twice around two copies of each of the four core histone proteins, H3, H4, H2A and H2B. Each nucleosome is separated by 10-16 bp long linkers DNA, which gives an appearance of a bead on a string structure that constitutes the chromatin fiber of ~10 nm in diameter. The linker DNA assists further compaction of chromatin structure into higher-order chromatin structure, which is essential for packaging of remarkable lengths of DNA into the cell nucleus. Furthermore, this compact chromatin structure limits accessibility of DNA to DNA-mediated processes like transcription, DNA replication, and DNA repair (Kouzarides, 2007). Evidence accumulated during the past 15 years reveals that three interrelated epigenetic mechanisms alter the highly compacted chromatin structure and facilitate accessibility of DNA for gene transcription. The interrelated epigenetic mechanisms that include DNA methylation, histone modification and ncRNA expression contribute to the epigenome making the epigenome dynamic rather than static like genome and thus, being predisposed to and influenced by environmental factors and extracellular stimuli. Deregulation of epigenetic mechanisms is observed in many different cancers and other human diseases. Thus, understanding of how epigenetic mechanisms contribute to gene regulation will provide insight into the disease process.

3.3 Histone modifications

Histones are highly conserved basic proteins that undergo an amazing number and types of posttranslational modifications, which contributes to the active or inactive chromatin (Ekstrom, 2009; Kouzarides, 2007; Pons et al., 2009; Ranganna et al., 2006; Turunen, 2009). Each of the four core histones are composed of a conserved globular domain that forms the nucleosome core, and a highly dynamic amino-terminal tail of 20-35 residues rich in basic amino acids. Additionally, H2A histone has an extended tail of about 35 residues at the carboxy-terminal end. Both amino- and carboxy-terminal tails protrude from nucleosome into the nucleoplasm. Histones tails are the targets of an array of site-specific posttranslational modifications including lysine acetylation/deacetylation, lysine and arginine methylation, serine and threonine phosphorylation, lysine ubiquitylation and sumoylation, and glutamic acid ADPribosylation (Fischle et al., 2003; Ito, 2007; Jenuwein & Allis, 2001; Turner, 2003).

Histone modifications are dynamic and reversible, and their 'off' and 'on" modification states are influenced by different physiological and environmental factors like developmental state, stress condition and environmental cues. Many of histone modifications are associated with transcriptionally active euchromatin regions, while other histone modifications are localized to transcriptionally inactive heterochromatin regions. Even though issues such as how the process of modification is regulated, and how many modifications are required for their biological effect are still elusive, recognition of specific histone modifications by various effector proteins is suggested to mediate specific biological processes like gene activation or gene suppression by altering the chromatin structure and gene accessibility. Generally, conformationally relaxed and decondensed chromatin structure that is associated with histone acetylation and DNA hypomethylation is the feature of transcriptionally active chromatin. On the other hand, compact and condensed chromatin structure that is associated with deacetylation of histones and hypermethylation of DNA is transcriptionally silent. Condensed chromatin structure is essential during cell cycle, mitosis and meiosis, whereas decondensed chromatin structure is required for gene expression, replication, repair and recombination. The combinatorial pattern of the histone modifications indicates the state of the chromatin structure, and thus, regulates the accessibility of the DNA to the transcription-regulatory complexes, through it controls gene expression. The collection of various covalent histone modifications serve as epigenetic marks for the recruitment of different proteins or protein complexes to regulate disparate chromatin functions such as gene expression, gene suppression, mitosis, repair, replication and chromosome segregation (Taverna et al., 2007). Furthermore, there is also crosstalk between different histone modifications like acetylation, methylation and phosphorylation at independent sites forming a "histone code" that is translated to a specific biological event through the mediation of various effector proteins. For example, phosphorylation of serine 10 of histone H3 facilitates acetylation of lysine 14 and methylation of lysine 4, which create an open or relaxed chromatin conformation associated with an active gene. Serine 10-phosphorylation also facilitates the acetylation of lysine 9, thus preventing the repressive lysine 9-methylation associated with an inactive gene (Jenuwein & Allis., 2001; Lund & van Lohuizen, 2004; Mathew et al., 2010; Schreiber & Bernstein, 2002; Turner, 2003).

3.4 Chromatin modifying enzymes

Consistent with the variety of posttranslational modifications of histones, a disparate family of enzymes, which are referred as histone modification writers, catalyzes addition of specific functional groups to histones. These modifications of histones alter the chromatin structure and function by two distinct manner: First, by directly altering the charges of histone proteins, certain posttranslational modifications cause localized relaxation of chromatin structure and second, by serving as recognition and binding sites for various classes of effector proteins that participate in chromatin remodeling, certain histone modifications indirectly alter the chromatin structure. However, most histone modification are reversible and diverse families of proteins, which include histone acetyltransferases (HATs) /histone deacetylases (HDACs), histone methyltransferases (HMTs)/demethylases, histone kinases/phosphatases, and ubiquitin ligases, catalyze addition and removal of the modifications from histones. One of the highlights of epigenetics is that it offers new therapeutic targets for diseases including cardiovascular diseases. The epigenetic regulators, HATs/HDACs and HMTs/demethylases, which exhibit counterbalancing activities are essential for the regulation of gene expression, which are required for the basic cellular processes such as cell proliferation and differentiation. This essential role of epigenetic regulators in basic cellular processes identifies potential therapeutic targets for diseases including cardiovascular diseases. Moreover, identification of those HATs and HDACs that plays a role in the transcriptional regulation of genes, products of which contributes to the processes of neointima formation like inflammation, VSMC proliferation, and matrix formation is also important in designing potential epigenetic therapy to target vascular proliferative diseases. Thus, pharmacological inhibition of enzyme activities involved in epigenetic DNA and histone modifications designed to induce or silence the transcription of disease-relevant genes offers an amenable therapeutic intervention for atherosclerosis and restenosis. In addition to modifying the effects of diseased genes, it is possible to change the effects of environmental risk factors by targeting epigenetic mechanisms. Here we will focus on HATs/HDACs, the principal epigenetic regulators that control histone acetylation, a major epigenetic modification for transcriptional control of gene expression. Because HATs/HDACs are essential for the regulation of gene expression, in all probability, they play crucial role in the development of multigene and multifactorial diseases such as atherosclerosis and restenosis.

4. Histone acetyltransferases (HATs) and histone deacetylases (HDACs)

One of the best- and most-studied posttranslational histone modifications is lysine acetylation catalyzed by HATs, the modification that is generally associated with gene activation (Ekstrom, 2009; Kouzarides, 2007; Pons et al., 2009; Ranganna et al., 2006; Turunen, 2009). Hyperacetylation of histones causes decondensation of chromatin allowing a more relaxed or open and active chromatin structure, which allows accessibility of DNA to basal transcription initiation machinery (Kouzarides, 2007; Roth, 2001). In contrast, gene repression is mediated by HDACs, and other co-repressors, which cause deacetylation of hyperacetylated histones and offset the activity of HATs resulting in a closed conformation of chromatin structure. Thus, the acetylation status of the chromatin associated with particular genes is dictated by the balance between the activities of HATs and HDACs. These enzymes are shown to regulate expression of genes associated with various cellular processes like inflammation, proliferation and matrix modulation (Cao et al., 2005; Pons et al., 2009; Sahar et al., 2007; Vinh et al., 2008; Waltregny et al., 2005; Xu et al., 2007; Yan et al., 2009). HATs and HDACs are also recruited to gene promoters by multiprotein transcriptional complexes, where they regulate transcription through chromatin modification without directly binding the DNA.

A number of different HATs are identified and organized as families based on the presence of highly conserved structural motifs, which include PCAF/Gcn5, p300/CBP, MYST, SRC, and TAF$_{II}$250 families. While they all differ in their HAT domains and substrate specificity, they all require the assembly of multiprotein complexes for acetylation of nucleosomes (Marmorstein, 2001). Likewise a number of HDACs are identified and are classified into three different classes based on cellular localization, substrates and binding site features (Lindemann et al., 2004; Santini et al., 2007). Class I and class II include zinc-dependent HDACs, and class III includes NAD-dependent HDACs, which are also called as sirtuins. Class I HDACs are widely expressed and include HDACs 1-3 and 8 that are exclusively localized to nucleus. They are known to modulate cell proliferation and survival. Class II HDACs are HDACs 4-7, 9, and 10, which shuttle between the nucleus and cytoplasm in response to certain cellular signals. They may be involved in cell differentiation (Pons et al., 2009; Santini et al., 2007). Class II HDACs are further divided into Class IIa and Class IIb , which include HDACs 4, 5 ,7, and 9, and, HDACs 6 and 10, respectively. While Class IIa members have an extended N-terminal regulatory domain, Class IIb exhibit an extra catalytic domain (Lindemann et al., 2004; Pons et al., 2009; Santini et al., 2007). Class III HDACs are sirtuins (SIRT), which include NAD$^+$-dependent enzymes (SIRT 1-7) potentially involved in apoptosis (Pons et al., 2009).

HATs and HDACs are also recruited to gene promoters by multiprotein transcriptional complexes. There they regulate transcription through chromatin modification without directly binding the DNA (Johnstone & Licht, 2003; Pons et al., 2009). Moreover, HATs and HDACs are also involved in the acetylation status of lysine residues of transcription factors such as p53, E2F1, GATA1, RelA, YY1 and hormone receptors. Acetylation status of these transcription factors affects their DNA binding and transcriptional activity (Glozak et al., 2005; Johnstone & Licht., 2003; Marks, 2001; Pons et al., 2009). Besides histones and transcription factors, several other non-histone proteins like α-tubulin, nuclear import protein importin-α7, and signal transduction protein β-catenin are also modified by HATs and HDACs, but their effects on gene expression is not dependent on chromatin remodeling (Johnstone & Licht., 2003; Marks, 2001).

4.1 Epigenetic therapy targeting VSMC proliferation

Because HATs/HDACs are involved in dynamic reversible epigenetic processes that contribute to modulation of gene expression profiles specific to cellular processes like cell proliferation, they probably play important role in cardiovascular pathologies such as atherosclerosis and restenosis. Moreover, epigenetic deregulation affects several aspects of cell biology, including cell growth, cell cycle control, differentiation, DNA repair, and cell death. This elevates the strong possibility that reversing deregulated epigenetic mechanisms may be an effective treatment strategy for proliferative diseases. Incidentally, the property of HDACs, suppression of gene expression by epigenetic mechanism, has been exploited in the field of cancer to reactivate transcriptionally silent tumor suppressor gene to arrest proliferation of cancer cells and growth (Pons et al., 2009; Ranganna, et al., 2005, 2007; Sharma et al., 2010). Moreover, HDAC inhibitors (HDACi) are emerging as a new class of anticancer agents that are under clinical trials for different cancer treatment. Some of the early clinical studies have demonstrated that certain HDACi exhibit promising activity against several neoplasms (Bhalla, 2005). Naturally, it has stimulated great interest to determine how HATs/HDACs regulate transcriptome of different processes that are linked to the development of atherosclerosis and restenosis like inflammation, VSMC proliferation and matrix modification and to assess therapeutic potential of HDACi in these vascular proliferative diseases (Ekstrom, 2009; Pons et al., 2009; Ranganna et al., 2006; Turunen, 2009). The following sections will focus on the role of HATs and HDACs in the transcriptional regulation of genes in the context of their contribution to VSMC proliferation and its disorders as well as on the potential applicability of HDACi in vascular disease management.

4.1.1 Histone deacetylase inhibitors (HDACi)

In the past few years, great effort has been focused on seeking and designing most effective HDACi because of their potential roles in reversing the silenced genes in tumor cells by modulating transcriptional processes. The balance between the acetylated/deacetylated states of histones, which is mediated by the counterbalancing activities of HATs and HDACs, contributes to the transcriptional states of chromatin structure. The structural modification of histones by acetylation/deacetylation of their N-terminal tails is crucial in modulating gene expression, because it affects the accessibility of DNA for the transcription-regulatory protein complexes. HATs preferentially acetylate specific lysine residues of histones, which relaxes the DNA conformation, thus allowing its access to transcription machinery to turn on gene expression. On the contrary, HDACs restore the positive charge on lysine residues by removing acetyl groups, which promotes condensed chromatin structure. This promotes silencing of gene expression by blocking the access of transcription machinery to DNA. Inappropriate silencing of critical genes such as tumor suppressor genes can result in cancer based on the recent understanding of the cancer cell cycle (Kristeleit et al., 2004). This provides a rationale for using inhibition of HDAC activity to release transcriptional repression. As result, a flurry of HDACi has been recognized for their ability to inhibit HDACs activity.

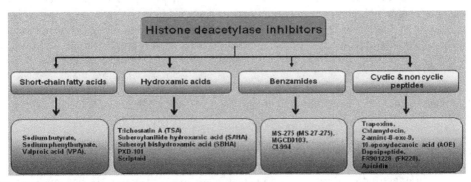

Fig. 1. Structural class of histone deacetylase inhibitors

Structurally diverse classes of naturally occurring and synthetic compounds have been recognized for their ability to bind to the catalytic pocket of HDACs and chelate the zinc ion at its base, thereby inhibiting HDAC activity (Marks et al., 2000). A wide range of structures inhibits activity of class I/II HDAC enzymes with a few exceptions [Figure 1]. The HDACi are classified into structural classes including 1) short-chain fatty acids (carboxylates), 2) hydroxamic acids, 3) benzamides, and 4) cyclic and non-cyclic peptides. The various HDACi studied so far have been shown to inhibit class I (HDACs 1, 2, 3, and 8) and II (HDACs 4, 5, 6, 9, and 10) HDACs. Their activities have been tested in cell lines and preclinical murine models, and appropriate drugs that are selected for clinical trials, demonstrated good tolerance and clinical activity against different human neoplasms (Santini et al., 2007). However, Class III HDACs (SIRT 1, 2, 3, 4, 5, 6, and 7), also known as sirtuins, require NAD rather than zinc as a co-factor for their activity, and are not inhibited by the HDACi. Instead, they are inhibited by Nicotinamide (Luo et al., 2001).

4.1.2 HDACi effects on cellular processes

HDACi exhibit multiple cellular effects, which are linked to chromatin-mediated altered transcriptional activity. In general, most HDACi exhibit inhibition of cell proliferation, stimulation of cell differentiation and/or induction of cell death by selectively modulating gene expression (Bhalla, 2005; Mathew et al., 2010; Ranganna, 2005). HDACi arrest cells at the G1 or G2/M, and promote cell differentiation mainly by stimulating cyclin-dependent kinase inhibitor (cdkI) p21Cip1 expression (Bhalla, 2005; Mathew et al., 2010; Ranganna et al., 2005). HDACi also cause cell cycle blockade through the modulation of mechanisms that involve repression of cyclin D and cyclin A and upregulation of other cdkI like p27Kip1, p16INK4A and p15INK4B, which blocks pRb/E2F pathway, thus preventing the cell cycle progression (Mathew et al., 2010; Bhalla, 2005) [Figure 2]. Now with the array technologies, it is recognized that HDACi selectively modulate about 2% to 10% of all genes, with as many genes upregulated as are downregulated genes in different cell types (Bhalla, 2005; Ranganna et al., 2003). One of the genes that are universally upregulated is the cdkI p21Cip1, in a p53-independent manner, which is necessary for HDACi-induced G1 arrest. Induction of GADD45α and β and upregulation of transforming growth factor beta, which inhibits c-*myc* expression may also contribute to the cell cycle arrest in G1 or G2 (Bhalla, 2005.). HDACi treatment is also shown to transcriptionally downregulate the expression of CTP synthetase and thymidylate synthetase, which are required for DNA synthesis, thus, causing inhibition of S phase progression [Figure 3].

HDACi also stimulate differentiation of several cancer cells by inhibiting cell proliferation (Bhalla, 2005). Again, upregulation of p21Cip1 appears to be essential for differentiation because cells lacking p21Cip1 fail to respond to HDACi treatment (Bhalla, 2005). Furthermore, acute promyelocytic leukemic cells and primary leukemia blasts, expressed differentiated phenotype in response to a combination of ATRA, a retinoid-based chemotherapeutic drug and HDACi (Bhalla, 2005). HDACi stimulated gelsolin, an actin-binding protein required for morphological and cytostructural changes associated with differentiation (Bhalla, 2005).

It is interesting that HDACi induce growth arrest and cell differentiation in some cell, and in others, they cause apoptosis (Bhalla, 2005; Johnstone & Licht, 2003). HDACi-induced apoptosis triggers both the intrinsic and extrinsic pathways of apoptosis. Several types of HDACi, particularly hydroxamic acid analogs are shown to induce mitochondrial permeability transition, which releases prodeath molecules such as cytochrome c, Smac and Omi into cytosol (Bhalla, 2005). This triggers activation of Apaf-1, which leads to the processing and activation of caspases-9 and-3 (Bhalla, 2005). HDACi appear to promote apoptotic cell death not only by upregulating several proteins that participate in apoptotic cell death including Bak, Bax, Bim, DR4, DR5, and TRAIL, but also by attenuating the levels of a number of antiapoptotic proteins such as Bcl-xL, Bcl-2, XIAP, and survivin (Bhalla, 2005).

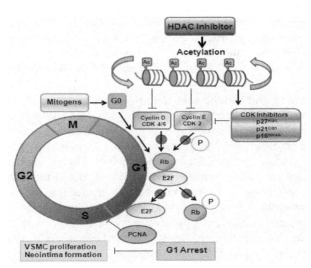

Fig. 2. Display of cell cycle targets of HDAC inhibition.

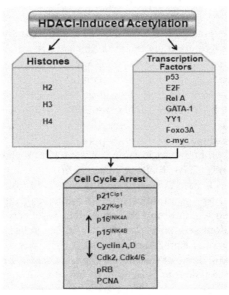

Fig. 3. Cell cycle regulatory proteins that are altered by the HDACi-induced acetylation of histones and transcription factors.

Besides affecting cell proliferation, differentiation and apoptosis, HDACi also alter the function of some of the non-histone transcription factors like p53, RelA, GATA1 and FoxO3A because HDACi enhance their acetylation, which may affect their DNA binding and transcriptional activity (Marks et al, 2001; Lindemann et al., 2004). Similarly, stimulating acetylation status of other non-histone protein such as nuclear import protein importin-α7, signaling protein β-catenin, DNA repair enzyme Ku70, and the cytoskeletal protein β-tubulin, HDACi alter their activity (Bhalla, 2005). Taken together, by inducing acetylation of histones and non-histones, HDACi alter the levels of proteins that control cell cycle progression, differentiation and apoptosis appropriately by transcriptional and post-transcriptional mechanisms, which implicate their potential use in disease treatment.

4.2 VSMC proliferation and histone acetylation

Although the common mechanism of pathogenesis shared by the atherosclerosis and cancer are linked to abnormal cell proliferation, very limited information is available with reference to anti-atherogenic potential of HDACi. Because HDACi not only alter gene expressions, but also cause inhibition of cell proliferation and induction of differentiation and/or apoptosis, a number of studies are initiated in the past few years to test the effects of HDACi as potential antiatherogenic agents. Even though both in vitro and in vivo studies have been done with the intention of targeting VSMC proliferation for the intervention and management of vascular proliferative diseases, most of the information that is available currently is from in vitro cell culture studies. There is limited in vivo data supporting the protective role of HDACi but needs further evaluation in models of VSMC injury.

4.2.1 VSMC proliferation

In general, HDACi exhibit almost same effects in VSMC as they do in cancer cells. They arrest cell proliferation, induce differentiation and/or apoptosis, and modulate expression of cell cycle regulators. Several studies have shown that trichostatin A (TSA), a well-known HDACi, arrests VSMC proliferation via upregulation of p21Cip1 and subsequent reduction of the phosphorylation of Rb protein at the G1-S phase (Okamoto et al., 2006; Pons et al., 2009), the effects consistently observed in cancer cell (Bhalla, 2005). In contrast, in one of the studies TSA unexpectedly exhibited paradoxical pro-atherogenic effect on VSMCs via the reduction of thioredoxin 1 instead of antiatherogenic properties (Song et al., 2010).

Besides TSA, butyrate, a well-known dietary HDACi, which has been used in different human cancer and other disease treatments, appears to exhibit potential antiatherogenic effect by arresting VSMC proliferation and appropriately altering both negative and positive cell cycle regulators (Davie, 2003; Mathew et al., 2010; Ranganna et al, 2005). Butyrate belongs to the class of short-chain fatty acids and is a derived from the intestinal microbial fermentation of dietary fiber. A number of epidemiological, animal and interventional studies suggest an inverse relationship between dietary fiber and chronic diseases such as bowel disorders and colorectal cancer, cancer of other tissues, cardiovascular disease, diabetes, obesity and hypertension (Anderson, 2003; Dashwood et al., 2006; Kim, 2000; Ranganna et al., 2005, 2006). Some of the studies suggest that the protective effect of dietary fibers in chronic diseases is linked to bioactivity of butyrate (Anderson, 2003; Dashwood et al., 2006; Kim, 2000; Ranganna et al., 2005, 2006). Butyrate elicits many cytoprotective, chemopreventive and chemotherapeutic activities mainly through inhibition of cell proliferation, stimulation of cell differentiation and/or induction of cell death by selectively modulating certain gene expressions, but the mechanistic basis for these actions are far from clear. Butyrate has been known to alter chromatin structure and organization via hyperacetylation of histone amino-terminal tails, modulate gene expression and play a protective role in the prevention of cancer and inflammatory diseases of colon for a long time (Ranganna et al., 2005, 2006). However, its importance in the prevention of cancer of other tissues and different diseases has been recognized during the past ten years (Anderson, 2003; Dashwood et al., 2006; Kim, 2000; Ranganna et al., 2005, 2006). On the other hand, no similar studies are performed to indicate the protective role of butyrate in cardiovascular diseases due to atherosclerosis and restenosis.

During last few years, significant interest is focused on potential utility of butyrate and its stable derivatives in the intervention of vascular proliferative diseases, besides their therapeutic applications in other diseases including cancers. Butyrate and its more stable in vivo analogue tributyrin, arrested proliferation and inhibited DNA synthesis of smooth muscle cells in a cAMP-independent manner. Butyrate also abolished serum-induced c-fos, c-myc, and Ki-Ras expression that are important for early G1 events initiated by serum growth factors, but stimulated the expression of PS4 and thromospondin (Feng et al., 1996). Moreover, studies performed in our own lab further supports the efficacy of butyrate and its stable derivatives in vascular proliferative diseases. Treatment of VSMC with butyrate inhibited serum and PDGF-induced proliferation and abolished expression of proliferation markers such as c-myc and proliferating cell nuclear antigen [PCNA] (Ranganna et al., 1995, 2000). Furthermore, our analysis of profiles of VSMC transcriptome by array technology disclosed that butyrate-arrested VSMC proliferation is a multigene and multipathway-mediated process. Our array data identified differential expression of several genes in butyrate arrested VSMC proliferation, which are mainly belonging to four different functional classes: cell proliferation and differentiation; stress response; vascular function; and genes normally present in neuronal cells (Ranganna, et al., 2003). Extension of this study reveals that an upper level regulatory mechanism mediated through epigenetic modification of chromatin structure controls the expression of both positive and negative cell cycle regulatory genes linked to VSMC proliferation arrest by butyrate (Mathew et al., 2010). To establish the mechanistic link between chromatin remodeling and antiproliferation action of butyrate, influence of butyrate on posttranslational modifications of histone H3 and its consequence on G1-specific cell cycle regulators were investigated [Figure 2]. Outcomes of the study indicate interplay between different site-specific posttranslational modifications of histone H3 in butyrate treated VSMCs that seem to alter chromatin structure and organization that supports downregulation of cdk2, cdk4/6, and PCNA, and upregulation of cdkI, p21Cip1 and p15INK4B. This causes inhibition of Rb phosphorylation resulting in arrest of VSMC proliferation [Figure 2 and Figure 3]. The effects of HDACi on cell cycle-related gene expressions appear to be highly selective, leading to transcriptional activation of certain genes such as the cdkIs but repression of others like cdks to efficiently block cell proliferation.

4.2.2 Histone acetylation

Hypernuclear acetylation (HNA) also plays a role in proliferation (Kawahara et al., 2003). Presence of increased histone acetylation is observed in VSMC of atherosclerotic lesions unlike in normal arteries. Thrombin, a humoral factor that is known to activate and stimulate VSMC proliferation, strongly induced HNA in cultures of VSMC. MAP kinase pathway and CBP are implicated in thrombin-induced HNA suggesting that coactivators cooperating with signaling-dependent transcription activators play a role in atherosclerosis through HNA (Kawahara et al., 1999).

5. Conclusions and perspectives

Over the past few years, it has become abundantly evident that several interdependent epigenetic changes collaborate with genetic changes in the development of human diseases including cardiovascular diseases such as atherosclerosis and restenosis. Since the genetic foundations of diseases are generally immutable, but their epigenetic and chromatin changes are reversible, they are suitable for epigenetic therapy with epigenetic and chromatin modifiers. Therefore, thorough understanding on the roles of epigenetic processes in the etiology of atherosclerosis and restenosis is essential to launch an epigenetic therapy designed to target the epigenetic processes. Although a number of different therapeutic approaches have been investigated in the treatment of atherosclerosis and restenosis such as brachytherapy, pharmacotherapy, gene therapy, and immunotherapy, the therapeutic efficacy of these treatment modalities for atherosclerosis and restenosis is not adequate for a number of patients. Possible reasons are multiple factors, genes, pathways are involved in the disease pathogenesis, and targeting one or two genes or pathways are not sufficient to treat complex vascular pathologies. In these scenarios, epigenetic therapy, which is reversible, appears to be appropriate because HDACi exhibit multiple cellular effects that play major roles in vascular pathogenesis. HDACi exhibit antiproliferative, antioxidant and antiinflammatory effects and cause inhibition of cell proliferation and stimulation of differentiation or apoptosis by modulating expression of multiple genes (Natarajan, 2011; Ranganna, et al.,2005; 2006; 2007). For example, HDACi inhibit cell proliferation by appropriately altering both positive and negative regulators of cell cycle. While cell cycle inhibitors such as p21Cip1, p27kip1, p16INK4a and p15INK4b are upregulated, expressions of cyclin D, cyclin A, cdk2, cdk4/6, PCNA and pRb that promote cell cycle progression are downregulated (Figure 2 and Figure 3). With one single HDACi, multiple genes are altered that control cell cycle progression unlike gene therapy, where a cocktail of genes is required to bring about inhibition of cell proliferation. Furthermore, stents are ideal platform for the localized delivery of HDACi to the vascular wall because of their widespread use and safety in the treatment of restenosis. It is recognized that many of the processes that play critical role in atherosclerosis and restenosis such as VSMC proliferation, migration, inflammation, cellular redox state and matrix protein synthesis (Natarajan, 2011) are regulated by epigenetic mechanisms. As such, they present an exciting opportunity for therapeutic intervention, particularly to refractory or recurrent vascular pathologies such as restenosis and in-stent restenosis and vein graft failure. A number of natural and synthetic HDACi are already in the pipeline for the treatment of cancer either stand alone, or in combination with other anticancer drugs and several clinical trials are in progress. Exploring these particulars will speed the necessary epigenetic treatment strategies for the management of atherosclerosis and restenosis.

6. Acknowledgements

The work from our laboratory described in this review is supported by G12RR0345 and C06RR012537-01 grants from National Institutes of Health/National Center for Research Resources.

7. References

Akowuah, E.F., Gray, C., Lawrie, A., Sheridan, P.J., Su, C.H., Bettinger, T., et al. (2005). Ultrasound-mediated delivery of TIMP-3 plasmid DNA into saphenous vein leads to increased lumen size in a porcine inteposition graft model. *Gene Therapy* 12, No. 14, (July 2005), pp. 1154-1157, ISSN 0969-7128

Anderson, J.W. (2003). Whole grains protect against atherosclerotic cardiovascular disease. *Proceedings of Nutrition Society*, Vol. 62, No. 1, (February 2003), pp. 135-142, ISSN 0029-6651

Banno, H., Takei, Y., Muramatsu, T., Komori, K., & Kadomatsu, K. (2006). Controlled release of small interfering RNA targeting midkine attenuates intimal hyperplasia in vein grafts. *Journal of Vascular Surgery*, Vol. 44, No. 3 (September 2006), pp. 633-641, ISSN 0741-5214

Bhalla, K.N. (2005). Epigenetic and chromatin modifiers as targeted therapy of hematologic malignancies. *Journal of Clinical Oncology*, Vol. 23, No. 17, (June 2005), pp. 3971-3993, ISSN 0732-183X

Binder, C.J., Hartvigsen, K., Chang, M. K., Miller, M., Broide, D., Palinski, W. et al. (2004). IL-5 links adaptive and natural immunity specific for epitopes of oxidized LDL and protects from atherosclerosis. *Journal of Clinical Investigsation*, Vol.114, No. 3, (August 2004), pp. 427-37 ISSN 0021-9738

Braun-Dullaeus, R.C., Mann, M.J., & Dzau, V.J. (1998). Cell cycle progression: New therapeutic target for vascular proliferative disease. *Circulation*, Vol. 98, No. 1, (July 1998), pp. 82-89, ISSN 0009-7322

Cao, D., Wang, Z., Zhang, C.L., Oh, J., Xing, W., Li, S., et al. (2005). Modulation of smooth muscle gene expression by association of histone acetyltransferases and deacetylases with myocardin. *Molecular and Cellular Biology*, Vol. 25, No. 1, (January 2005), pp. 364 -376, ISSN 0270-7306

Cooney, R., Hynes, S.O., Sharif, F., Howard, L., & O'Brien, T. (2006). Effect of gene delivery of NOS isoforms on intimal hyperplasia and endothelial regeneration after balloon injury. *Gene Therapy*, Vol. 14, No 5, (March 2007), pp. 396-404, ISSN 0969-7128

Dashwood, R.H., Myzak, M.C., & Ho, E. (2006). Dietary HDAC inhibitors: time to rethink weak ligands in cancer chemoprevention? *Carcinogenesis*, Vol. 27, No. 2, (February 2006), pp. 344-349, ISSN 0143-3334

Davie, J.R. (2003). Inhibition of histone deacetylase activity by butyrate. *Journal of Nutrition*, Vol. 133, No. 7 Suppl, (July 2003), pp. 2485S-2493S, ISSN 0022-3166

Doran, A.C., Meller, N., & McNamara, C.A. (2008). Role of smooth muscle cells in the initiation and early progression of atherosclerosis. *Arteriosclerosis Thrombosis and Vascular Biology*, Vol. 28, No. 5, (May 2008), pp. 812- 819, ISSN 1079-5642

Dzau, V.J., Braun-Dullaeus, R.C., & Sedding, D.G. (2002). Vascular proliferation and atherosclerosis: new perspectives and therapeutic strategies. *Nature Medicine*, Vol. 8, No. 11, (November 2002), pp. 1249-56, ISSN 1078-8956

Ekström, T.J. (2009). Epigenetic control of gene expression. *Biochemical Biophysical Acta*, Vol. 1790, No. 9, (September 2009), pp. 845-846, ISSN 0006-3002

Esteller, M. (2008). Epigenetics in cancer. *New England Journal of Medicine, Vol.* 358, No.11, (March 2008), pp. 1148-1159, ISSN 0096-6762

Fasciano, S., Patel, R.C., Handy, I. & Patel, C.V. (2005). Regulation of vascular smooth muscle proliferation by heparin. Inhibition of cyclin-dependent kinase 2 activity by p27kip1. *Journal of Biological Chemistry*, Vol. 280, No.16, (April 2005), pp. 15682-15689, ISSN 0021-9258

Feldman, L.J., & Isner, J.M. (1995). Gene therapy for vulnerable plaque. *Journal of the American College of Cardiology*, Vol. 26, No. 3, (September 1995), pp. 826-833, ISSN 0735-1097

Feng, P., Ge, L., Akyhani, N., & Liau, G. (1996). Sodium butyrate is a potent modulator of smooth muscle cell proliferation and gene expression. *Cell Proliferation*, Vol. 29, No. 5, (May 1996), pp. 231-241, ISSN 0960-7722

Ferns, G.A., Raines. E.W., Sprugel, K.H., Motani, A.S., Reidy, M.A., & Ross, R. (1991). Inhibition of neointimal smooth muscle accumulation after angioplasty by an antibody to PDGF. *Science*, Vol. 253, No. 5024, (September 1991), pp. 1129-1132, ISSN 0036-8075

Finn, A.V., Nakazawa, G., Joner, M., Kolodgie, F.D., Mont, E.K., Gold, H.K., et al. (2007). Vascular responses to drug eluting stents. Importance of delayed healing. *Arteriosclerosis Thrombosis and Vascular Biology*, Vol. 27, No. 7, (July, 2007), pp. 1500-1510, ISSN 1079-5642

Fischle, W., Wang, Y., & Allis, C.D. (2003). Histone and chromatin cross-talk. *Current Opinions in Cell Biology*, Vol. 15, No. 2, (April 2003), pp. 172-183, ISSN 0955-0674

Freeman, B.A., & Crapo, J.D. (1982). Biology of disease: free radicals and tissue injury. *Laboratory Investigation*, Vol. 47, No. 5, (November 1982), pp. 412-426, ISSN 0023-6837

Gaffney, M.M., Hynes, S.O., Barry, F., & O'Brien, T. (2007). Cardiovascular gene therapy: status and therapeutic potential. *British Journal of Pharmacology*, Vol. 152, No. 2, (September 2007), pp. 175-188, ISSN 1476-5381

Gershlick, A.H. (2002). Treating atherosclerosis: Local drug delivery from laboratory studies to clinical trials. *Atherosclerosis*, Vol. 160, No. 2, (February 2002), pp. 259-271, ISSN 0021-9150

Grossman, M., Rader, D.J., Muller, D.W., Kolansky, D.M., Kozarsky, K., Clark, B.J., et al. (1995). A pilot study of ex vivo gene therapy for homozygous familial hypercholesterolemia. *Nature Medicine*, Vol. 1, No. 11, (November 1995), pp. 1148-1154, ISSN 1078-8956

Guerin, P., Sauzeau, V., Rolli-Derkinderen, M., Al Habbash, O., Scalbert, E., Crochet, D., et al. (2005). Stent implantation activates Rho A in human arteries: Inhibitory effect of rapamycin. *Journal of Vascular Research*, Vol. 42, No. 1, (January-February 2005), pp. 21-28, ISSN 1018-1172

Habets, K.L., van Puijvelde, G.H., van Duivenvoorde, L. M., van Wanrooij, E. J., de Vos, P. Tervaert, J. W. et al. (2010). Vaccination using oxidized low-density lipoprotein-pulsed dendritic cells reduces atherosclerosis in LDL receptor-deficient mice. *Cardiovascular Research*, Vol. 85, No. 3, (February 2010), pp. 622-630, ISSN 0008-6363

Holmes, Jr. D.R. (2003). State of the art in coronary intervention. *American Journal of Cardiology*, Vol. 91, No. 3A, (February 2003), pp. 50A-53A, ISSN 1423-0135

Ito T. (2007). Role of histone modifications in chromatin dynamics. *Journal of Biochemistry*, Vol. 141, No. 5, (May 2007), pp. 609-614, ISSN 0021-924X

Jenuwein, T., & Allis, C.D. (2001). Translating the histone code. *Science*, Vol.293, No.5532, (August 2001), pp. 1074-1080, ISSN 0036-8075

Jordan, M.A., Toso, R.J., Thrower, D., & Wilson, L. (1993). Mechanism of mitotic block and inhibition of cell proliferation by taxol at low concentrations. *Proceedings of National Academy of Sciences, USA*, Vol. 90, No. 20, (October 1993), pp. 9552-9556, ISSN 0027-8424

Kawahara, K., Kawabata, H., Aratani, S., & Nakajima, T. (2003). Hypernuclear acetylation (HNA) in proliferation, differentiation and apoptosis. *Ageing Research Review*, Vol. 2, No. 3, (July 2003), pp. 287-297, ISSN 1568-1637

Kawahara, K., Watanabe, S., Ohshima, T., Soejima, Y., Oish, T., Aratani, S., et al. (1999). Hypernuclear acetylation in atherosclerotic lesions and activated vascular smooth muscle cells. *Biochemical and Biophysical Research Communications*, Vol. 266, No. 2, (December 1999), pp 417–424, ISSN 0006-291X

Kehrer, J. P. (1993). Free radicals as mediators of tissue injury and disease. *Critical Reviews in Toxicology*, Vol. 23, No. 1, (January 1993), pp. 21-48, ISSN 1040-8444

Khanna, A. (2008). Strategies and vectors for gene therapy: Its prospective therapeutic attributes against restenosis. *Journal of Clinical and Diagnostic Research*, Vol. 2, No. 3, (June 2008), pp. 871-878, ISSN 0973-709X

Kim, Y.I. (2000). AGA technical review: impact of dietary fiber on colon cancer occurrence. *Gastroenterology*, Vol. 118, No. 6, (June 2000), pp. 1235 -1257, ISSN 0016-5085

Kishore, R., & Losordo, D.W. (2007). Gene therapy for restenosis: biological solution to a biological problem. *Journal of Molecular and Cellular Cardiology*, Vol. 42, No. 3, (March 2007), pp. 461-468, ISSN 0022-2828

Kleeman, R., Zadelaar, S., & Kooistra, T. (2008). Cytokines and atherosclerosis: a comprehensive review of studies in mice. *Cardiovascular Research*, Vol. 79, No. 3, (August 2008), pp. 360-376, ISSN 0008-6363

Klingenberg, R., & Hansson, G.K. (2009). Treating inflammation in atherosclerotic cardiovascular disease: emerging therapies. *European Heart Journal*, Vol. 30, No.23, (December 2009), pp. 2838–2844, ISSN 0195-668x

Kouzarides, T. (2007). Chromatin modifications and their function. *Cell, Vol.* 128, No. 4, (February 2007), pp. 693–705, ISSN 0092-8674

Kristeleit, R., Stimson, L., Workman, P., & Aherne, W. (2004). Histone modification enzymes: novel targets for cancer drugs. *Expert Opinion Emerging Drugs*, Vol. 9, No. 1, (May 2004), pp. 135–154, ISSN 1472-8214

Kunsch, C., &, Medford, R.M. (1999). Oxidative stress as a regulator of gene expression in the vasculature. *Circulation Research*, Vol. 85, No. 8, (October 1999), pp. 753-766, ISSN 0009-7330

Li, F., Zhang, C., Schaefer, S., Estes, A., & Malik, K.U. (2005). ANG II-induced neointimal growth is mediated via cPLA2- and PLD2-activated Akt in balloon-injured rat carotid artery. *American Journal of Physiology, Heart and Circulatory Physiology*, Vol. 289, No. 6, (December 2005), pp. H2592–H2601, ISSN 0363-6135

Li, J.M., Newburger, P.E., Gounis, M.J., Dargon, P., Zhang, X., & Messina, L.M. (2010). Local arterial nanoparticle delivery of siRNA for NOX2 knockdown to prevent restenosis in an atherosclerotic rat model. *Gene Therapy*, Vol. 17, No. 10 (October 2010), 1279-1287, ISSN 0969-7128

Libby, P. (2002). Inflammation in atherosclerosis. *Nature*, Vol. 420, No. 6917, (December 2002), pp. 868-874, ISSN 0028-0836

Lindemann, R.K., Gabrielli, B., & Johnstone, R.W. (2004). Histone-deacetylase inhibitors for the treatment of cancer. *Cell Cycle*, Vol. 3, No. 6, (June 2004), pp. 779-788, ISSN 1538-4101

Lund, A.H., & van Lohuizen, M. (2004). Epigenetics and cancer. *Genes and Development*, Vol. 18, No. 19, (October 2004), pp. 2315-2335, ISSN 0890-9369

Luo, J., Nikolaev, A.Y., Imai, S., Chen, D., Su, F., Shiloh, A., et al (2001). Negative control of p53 by Sir2alpha promotes cell survival under stress. *Cell*, Vol. 107, No. 2, (October 2001), pp. 137-148, ISSN 0092-8674

Madamanchi, N.R., Vendrov, A., & Runge, M.S. (2005). Oxidative stress and vascular disease. *Arteriosclerosis Thrombosis and Vascular Biology*, Vol. 25, No. 1, (January 2005), pp. 29-38, ISSN 1079-5642

Mann, M.J., Whittemore, A.D., Donaldson, M.C., Belkin, M., Conte, M.S., Polak, J.F., et al. (1999). Ex-vivo gene therapy of human vascular bypass grafts with E2F decoy: the PREVENT single-centre, randomized, controlled trial. *Lancet*, Vol. 354, No. 9189, (October 1999), pp.1493-1498, ISSN 0099-5355

March, F., Sauty, A., Iarossi, A.S., Sukhova, G.K., Neote, K., Libby, P., etal. (1999). Differential expression of three T lymphocyte-activating CXC chemokines by human atheroma-associated cells. *Journal of Clinical Investigation*, Vol. 104, No. 8, (October 1999), pp. 1041-1050, ISSN 0021-9738

Marks, P.A., Richon, V.A., & Rifkind, R.A. (2000). Histone deacetylase inhibitors: Inducers of differentiation or apoptosis of transformed cells. *Journal of National Cancer Institute*, Vol. 92, No. 15, (August 2000), pp. 1210-1216, ISSN 0027-8874

Marmorstein, R. (2001). Structure of histone acetyltransferases. *Journal of Molecular Biology*, Vol. 311, No. 3, (August 2001), pp. 433-444, ISSN 0022-2836

Mathew, O.P., Ranganna, K., & Yatsu, F.M. (2010). Butyrate, an HDAC inhibitor, stimulates interplay between different posttranslational modifications of histone H3 and differently alters G1-specific cell cycle proteins in vascular smooth muscle cells. *Biomedicine & Pharmacotherapy*, Vol. 64, No. 10, (December 2010), pp. 733–740, ISSN 0753-3322

Matsumae, H., Yoshida, Y., Ono, K., Togi, K., Inoue, K., Furukawa, Y., et al. (2008). CCN1 knockdown suppresses neointimal hyperplasia in a rat artery balloon injury model. *Arteriosclerosis Thrombosis and Vascular Biology*, Vol. 28, No. 6 (June 2008), pp. 1077-1083, ISSN 1079-5642

Mattick, J.S., Amaral, P.P., Dinger, M.E., Mercer, T.R., & Mehler, M.F. (2009). RNA regulation of epigenetic processes. *Bioessays*, Vol. 31, No. 1, (January 2009), pp. 51-59, ISSN 1521-1878

McCarthy, M. (2001). Molecular decoy may keep bypass grafts open. *Lancet*, Vol. 358, No. 9294, (November 2001), pp. 1703, ISSN 0099-5355

McManus, K.J., & Hendzel, M.J. (2006). The relationship between histone H3 phosphorylation and acetylation throughout the mammalian cell cycle. *Biochemistry and Cell Biology*, Vol. 84, No. 4, (August 2006), pp. 640-657, ISSN 0829-8211

Melo, L.G., Pachori, A.S., Gnecchi, M., & Dzau, V.J. (2005). Genetic therapies for cardiovascular diseases. *Trends in Molecular Medicine*, Vol.11, No.5, (May 2005), pp. 240-250, ISSN 1471-4914

Morishita, R., Gibbons, G.H., Ellison, K.E., Nakajima, M., Zhang, L., Kaneda, Y., et al. (1993). Single intraluminal delivery of antisense cdc2 kinase and proliferating- cell nuclear antigen oligonucleotides results in chronic inhibition of neointimal hyperplasia. *Proceedings National Academy of Sciences, USA*, Vol. 90, No. 18, (September 1993), pp.8474-8478 ISSN 0027-8424

Natarajan, R. (2011). Drugs targeting epigenetic histone acetylation in vascular smooth muscle cells for restenosis and atherosclerosis. *Arteriosclerosis Thrombosis and Vascular Biology*, Vol. 31, No. 4, (April 2011), pp. 725-727 ISSN 1079-5642

Ng, R.K., & Gurdon, J.B. (2008). Epigenetic inheritance of cell differentiation status. *Cell Cycle*, Vol. 7, No. 9 (May 2008), pp. 1173-77, ISSN 1538-4101

O'Brien, K.D., McDonald, T.O., Chait, A., Allen, M.D., & Alpers, C.E. (1996). Neovascular expression of E-Selectin, intercellular adhesion molecule-1, and vascular cell adhesion molecule-1 in human atherosclerosis and their relation to intimal leukocyte content. *Circulation*, Vol. 93, No. 4, (February 1996), pp. 672-682, ISSN 0009-7322

Okamoto, H., Fujioka, Y., Takahashi, A., Takahashi, T., Taniguchi, T., Ishikawa, Y., etal. (2006). Trichostatin A, an inhibitor of histone deacetylase, inhibits smooth muscle cell proliferation via induction of p21 (WAF1). *Journal of Atherosclerosis and Thrombosis*, Vol. 13, No. 4, (August 2006), pp. 183-191, ISSN 1079-5642

Pons, D., de Vries, F.R., van den Elsen, P.J., Heijmans, B.T., Quax, P.H., & Jukema, J.W. (2009). Epigenetic histone acetylation modifiers in vascular remodeling: new targets for therapy in cardiovascular disease. *European Heart Journal*, Vol. 30, No. 3, (February 2009), pp. 266-277, ISSN 0195-668X

Probst, A.V., Dunleavy, E., & Almouzni, G. (2009). Epigenetic inheritance during the cell cycle. *Nature Reviews, Molecular and Cell Bioliology*. Vol. 10, No. 3, (March 2009), pp. 192-206, ISSN 1471-0072

Qian, H., Neplioueva, V., Shetty, G.A., Channon, K. M., George, S. E. (1999). Nitric oxide synthase gene therapy rapidly reduces adhesion molecule expression and inflammatory cell infiltration in carotid artery of cholesterol-fed rabbits. *Circulation*, Vol. 99, No. 23, (June 1999), pp. 2979-2982, ISSN 0009-7322

Raizner, A.E., Oesterle, S.N., Waksman, R., Serruys, P.W., Colombo, A., Lim, Y.L., et al. (2000). Inhibition of restenosis with b-emitting radiotherapy. Report of the proliferation reduction with vascular energy trial (PREVENT). *Circulation*, Vol. 102, No. 9, (August 2000), pp. 951-958, ISSN 0009-7522

Ranganna, K., Yatsu, F.M., & Hayes, B.E. (2005). Butyrate, a small pleiotropic molecule with multiple cellular and molecular actions: Its role as an anti-atherogenic agent. *Recent Research Development in Molecular Cellular Biochemistry*, Vol. 2, pp. 123-151, Research Signpost, ISBN 81-7736-294-1, Kerala, India

Ranganna, K., Yatsu, F.M., & Mathew, O.P. (2006). Insights into the pathogenesis and intervention of atherosclerosis. *Vascular Disease Prevention*, Vol. 3, No. 4, pp. 375-390, ISSN 1567-2700

Ranganna, K., Yatsu, F.M., Hayes, B.E., Milton, S.G., & Jayakumar, A. (2000). Butyrate inhibits proliferation-induced proliferating cell nuclear antigen expression (PCNA) in rat vascular smooth muscle cells. *Molecular cellular Biochemistry*, Vol. 205, No.1-2, (February 2000), pp. 149-161, ISSN 0300-8177

Ranganna, K., Yousefipour, Z., Yatsu, F.M., Milton, S.G., & Hayes, B.E. (2003). Gene expression profile of butyrate-inhibited vascular smooth muscle cell proliferation. *Molecular cellular Biochemistry*, Vol. 254, No. 1-2, (December 2003), pp. 21-36, ISSN 0300-8177

Ranganna, K., Mathew, O.P., Yousefipour, Z., Yatsu, F.M., Hayes, B.E., & Milton, S.G. (2007). Involvement of glutathione/glutathione S-transferase antioxidant system in butyrate-inhibited vascular smooth muscle cell proliferation. *FEBS Journal*, Vol. 274, No. 22, (November 2007), pp. 5962–5978, Online ISSN 1742 4658

Ross R. (1993). The pathogenesis of atherosclerosis: a perspective for the 1990s. *Nature*, Vol. 362, No. 6423, (April 1993), pp. 801-809, ISSN 0028-0836

Ross, R. (1995). Cell biology of atherosclerosis. *Annual Review of Physiology*, Vol. 57, (March 1995), pp. 791-804, ISSN 0066-4278

Sahar, S., Reddy, M.A., Wong, C., Meng, L., Wang, M., & Natarajan, R. (2007). Cooperation of SRC-1 and p300 with NF-kB and CREB in angiotensin II-induced IL-6 expression in vascular smooth muscle cells. *Arteriosclerosis Thrombosis and Vascular Biology*, Vol. 27, No. 7, (July 2007), pp. 1528 –1534, ISSN 1079-5642

Santini, V., Gozzini, A., & Ferrari, G. (2007). Histone deacetylase inhibitors: molecular and biological activity as a premise to clinical application. *Current Drug Metabolism*, Vol. 8, No.4, (May 2007), pp. 383-393, ISSN 1389-2002

Schreiber, S.L., & Bernstein, B.E. (2002). Signaling network model of chromatin. *Cell*, Vol. 111, No. 6, (December 2002), pp. 771-778, ISSN 0092-8674

Sharma, S., Kelly, T.K., & Jones, P.A. (2010). Epigenetics in cancer. *Carcinogenesis*, Vol. 31, No. 1, (January 2010), pp. 27–36, ISSN 0143-3334

Simons, M., Edelman, E.R., & Rosenberg, R.D. (1994). Antisense proliferating cell nuclear antigen oligonucleotides inhibit intimal hyperplasia in a rat carotid artery injury model. *Journal of Clinical Investigations*, Vol. 93, No. 6, (June 1994), pp. 2351-2356, ISSN 0021-9738

Song, S., Kang, S.W., & Choi, C. (2010). Trichostatin A enhances proliferation and migration of vascular smooth muscle cells by downregulating thioredoxin 1. *Cardiovascular Research*, Vol. 85, No. 1, (January 2010), pp. 241-249, ISSN 0008-6363

Steinberg, D., & Witztum, J.L. (2010). History of discovery. Oxidized Low-Density Lipoprotein and Atherosclerosis. *Arteriosclerosis, Thrombosis and Vascular Biology*, Vol. 30, No. 12 (December 2010), pp. 2311-2316, ISSN 1079-5642

Tangirala, R.K., Tsukamoto, K., Chun, S.H., Usher, D., Puré, E., & Rader, D.J. (1999). Regression of atherosclerosis induced by liver-directed gene transfer of apolipoprotein A-1 in mice. *Circulation*, Vol. 100, No. 17, (October 1999), pp. 1816-1822, ISSN 0009-7322

Taverna, S.D., Li, H., Ruthenburg, A.J., Allis, C.D., & Patel, D.J. (2007). How chromatin-binding modules interpret histone modifications: lessons from professional pocket pickers. *Nature Structural and Molecular Biology*, Vol.14, No. 11, (November 2007), pp. 1025–1040, ISSN 1545-9993

Teirstein, P.S., & King, S. (2003). Vascular radiation in a drug-eluting stent world: It's not over till it's over. *Circulation*, Vol. 108, No. 4, (July 2003), pp. 384-385, ISSN 0009-7322

Toshiro, M., Ueno, T., Tanaka, M., Oka, H., Miyamotq, T., Osajima, K., et al. (2005). Antiproliferative action of an angiotensin I-converting enzyme inhibitory peptide, Val-Tyr, *via* an L-type Ca^{2+} channel inhibition in cultured vascular smooth muscle cells. *Hypertension Research*, Vol. 28, No. 6, (June, 2005), pp. 545–552, ISSN 1348-4214

Turner, B.M. (2003). Memorable transcription. *Nature Cell Biology*, Vol. 5, No. 5, (May 2003), pp. 390-393, ISSN 1465-7392

Turunen, M.P., Aavik, E., & Yla-Herttuala, S. (2009). Epigenetics and atherosclerosis. *Biochemical et Biophysical Acta*, Vol. 1790, No. 9, (September 2009), pp. 886-891, ISSN 0006-3002

Tzeng, E., Shears, L.L., & Robbins, P.D, Pitt, B.R., Geller, D.A., Watkins, S.C., et al. (1996). Vascular gene transfer of the human inducible nitric oxide synthase: characterization of activity and effects of myointimal hyperplasia. *Molecular Medicine*, Vol. 2, No. 2, (March 1996), pp. 211-225, ISSN 1076-1551

Van Assche, T., Huygelen, V., & Crabtree, M.J. (2011). Targeting vascular redox biology through antioxidant gene delivery: a historical view and current prospective. *Recent Patents on Cardiovascular Drug Discovery*, Vol. 6, No. 2 , (May 2011), pp. 89-102, ISSN 1574-8901

Vinh, A., Gaspari, T.A., Liu, H.B., Dousha, L.F., Widdop, R.E., & Dear, A.E. (2008). A novel histone deacetylase inhibitor reduces abdominal aortic aneurysm formation in angiotensin II-infused apolipoprotein E-deficient mice. *Journal of Vascular Research*, Vol. 45, No. 2, (March 2008), pp. 143–152, ISSN 1018-1172

Von der Leyen, H.E., & Dzau D.J. (2001). Therapeutic potential of nitric oxide synthase gene manipulation. *Circulation*, Vol. 103, No. 22, (June 2001), pp. 2760-2765, ISSN 0009-7322

Waksman, R., Bhargava, B., White L, Chan, R.C., Mehran, R., Lansky, A.J. et al. (2000). Intracoronary b-radiation therapy inhibits recurrence of in-stent restenosis. *Circulation*, Vol. 101, No. 16, (April 25), pp. 1895-1898, ISSN 0009-7322

Waltregny, D., Gle´nisson, W., Tran, S.L., North, B.J., Verdin, E., Colige, A., etal. (2005). Histone deacetylase HDAC8 associates with smooth muscle α-actin and is essential for smooth muscle cell contractility. *FASEB J.* Vol. 19, No. 8, (June 2005), pp. 966 – 968, ISSN 0892-6638

Wilson, G. J., Polovick, J. E., Huibregtse, B.A., & Poff B. C. (2007). Overlapping paclitaxel-eluting stents: Long-term effects in a porcine coronary artery model. *Cardiovascular Research*, Vol. 76, No. 2, (November 2007), pp. 361 – 372, ISSN 0008-6363

Witztum, J.L. (1997). Immunological response to oxidized LDL. *Atherosclerosis*, Vol. 131, No. 2, (June 1997), pp. S9–S11, ISSN 0021-9150

Xu, X., Ha, C.H., Wong, C., Wang, W., Hausser, A., Pfizenmaier, K., etal. (2007). Angiotensin II stimulates protein kinase D-dependent histone deacetylase 5 phosphorylation and nuclear export lading to vascular smooth muscle cell hypertrophy. *Arteriosclerosis Thrombosis and Vascular Biology*, Vol. 27, No. 11, (November 2007), pp. 2355–2362, ISSN 1079-5642

Yan, Z.Q., Yao, Q.P., Zhang, M.L., Qi, Y.X., Guo, Z.Y., Shen, B.R., et al. (2009). Histone deacetylases modulate vascular smooth muscle cell migration induced by cyclic mechanical strain. *Journal of Biomechanics*, Vol. 42, No. 7, (May 2009), pp. 945–948, ISSN 0021-9290

Zeiffer, U., Schober, A., Lietz, M., Liehn, E.A., Erl, W., Emans, N., et al. (2004). Neointimal smooth muscle cells display a proinflammatory phenotype resulting in increased leukocyte recruitment mediated by P-selectin and chemokines. *Circulation Research*, Vol. 94, No. 6, (April 2004), pp. 776-784, ISSN 0009-7330

Zhou, X., Caligiuri, G., Hamsten, A., Lefvert, A. K., & Hansson, G.K., (2001). LDL immunization induces T-cell-dependent antibody formation and protection against atherosclerosis. *Arteriosclerosis Thrombosis and Vascular Biology*, Vol. 21, No. 1, (January 2001), pp. 108–114, ISSN 1079-5642

8

Molecular Understanding of Endothelial Cell and Blood Interactions with Bacterial Cellulose: Novel Opportunities for Artificial Blood Vessels

Helen Fink[1], Anders Sellborn[2] and Alexandra Krettek[3,4]
[1]Dept of Chemical and Biological Engineering, Chalmers University of Technology
[2]Dept of Surgery, Inst. of Clin. Sciences, Sahlgrenska Acad. at University of Gothenburg
[3]Dept of Intern. Med., Inst. of Medicine, Sahlgrenska Acad. at University of Gothenburg
[4]Nordic School of Public Health
Sweden

1. Introduction

Cardiovascular disease (CVD) is the main cause of death or invalidism in high-income countries today. Moreover, worldwide demographic changes are aiding CVD's rapid progression towards the number one killer in middle- and low-income countries. The World Health Organisation estimates that if current trends are allowed to continue, about 20 million people will die from CVD by 2015. This group of disorders, which affect the heart and blood vessels, includes coronary heart disease, cerebrovascular disease and peripherial arterial disease, deep vein thrombosis and pulmonary embolism.

The main cause of these acute life-threatening conditions is atherosclerosis. Atherosclerotic plaques and restenosis can result in severe occlusions of peripheral and coronary arteries. Current treatments include drug therapy and bypass surgery, and depend on the severity of the disease. All treatments require molecular understanding of the processes that govern atherosclerosis. This is especially important when introducing artificial graft materials *in vivo*.

Generally, the first choice for vascular replacement graft material is the patient's own vessels, i.e., autologous vessels. If these are in shortage supply or do not exhibit sufficient quality due to, e.g., other diseases or previous surgery, artificial alternatives become necessary. Today, clinics use biomaterials such as expanded polytetrafluorethylene (ePTFE) and polyethylene terephtalate fibre (Dacron®) as prosthetic grafts for reconstructive vascular surgery. However, their performance is dismal in small diameter vessels (>6 mm) like coronary arteries and peripheral arteries below the knee, resulting in early thrombosis and intimal hyperplasia. Therefore, about 10% of patients with CVD are left untreated due to the lack of replacement material for small vessels.

Considering the large number of patients who need replacement vessels, the substantial demand for alternative small-caliber grafts is urgent, driving scientists to search for and develop new materials. Recently, this has even led to the use of completely biological vessels. However, the growth of such requires months, rendering them unsuitable for acute situations such as heart infarction, which demand a substitute vessel immediately.

2. What is the ideal vascular graft?

Several issues demand consideration when constructing a vascular graft: the mechanical properties of the graft must resemble those of a native blood vessel, and the graft must be biocompatible with its host. One important factor is compliance, i.e., how well the vessel withstands pressure from the bloodstream and whether it can maintain systemic pressure in the vascular system. Vascular grafts should also be "invisible" to the immune system and possess non-thrombogenic properties.

One interesting option is bacterial cellulose (BC), whose unique properties (strength, good integration into host tissue and flexibility that allows production in various shapes and sizes) make it an exciting candidate for vascular graft material. The most abundant biopolymer on earth, cellulose is insoluble in water and degradable by microbial enzymes. Several organisms such as plants, algae and bacteria can produce BC. Some members of the bacterial genus Acetobacter, especially *Gluconacetobacter xylinum*, synthesize and secrete cellulose extracellularly. The network structure of cellulose fibrils resembles that of collagen in the extracellular matrix (ECM).

This chapter describes how BC interacts with human endothelial cells (EC) and blood. Specifically, we will evaluate whether surface modifications could promote adhesion of EC and also whether BC's thrombogenic properties compare favorably with conventional graft materials. These properties are critical because materials intended as vascular grafts must satisfy many important features, including blood compatibility, cell interactions and mechanical properties.

3. Tissue engineering of blood vessels

Tissue engineering is a relatively new scientific discipline that combines cells, engineering and materials to improve or replace biological functions. Langer and Vacanti, two pioneers in the field, describe tissue engineering as an interdisciplinary area that applies the principles of engineering and life sciences to the development of biological substitutes that restore, maintain or improve tissue formation (Langer & Vacanti, 1993).

The basic concept of tissue engineering includes a physical support (3D-scaffold) composed of synthetic polymers or natural materials (collagen, elastin or fibrin). This support mimics ECM and initially serves as a scaffold or template on which cells can organize and mature *in vitro* prior to implantation at the appropriate location.

Initial research in the mid-20th century focused on developing bioinert materials, eliciting a minimal host response characterized by passive blood transport and minimal interactions with blood and tissues. Although widely available, these industrial materials, including Teflon and silicone, were not developed specifically for medical applications. Later, the production of completely non-reactive substances became unrealistic.

Today, other biomaterials are being developed to stimulate reactions between proteins and cells at the molecular level in a highly precise and controllable manner. The key concept underpinning development of such biomaterials is that the scaffold should contain chemical or structural information that mimicks cell-cell communication and controls tissue formation, such as growth factors, the adhesion peptide Arg–Gly–Asp (RGD) and other molecules that mimic ECM components. RGD is the minimal sequence in basement membrane proteins such as fibronectin, fibrinogen and von Willebrand Factor, all required for cell adhesion (Pierschbacher & Ruoslahti, 1984).

A successful tissue engineered blood vessel must: be biocompatible, i.e., noninflammatory, nontoxic, nonimmunogenic and noncarcinogenic; infection-resistant and nonthrombogenic. It also must have appropriate mechanical properties, e.g., tensile strength, burst strength, good suture retention and compliance, and possess appropriate vasoactive physiological properties, including contraction or relaxation in response to neural or chemical stimuli and more.

The feasibility of constructing and using tissue engineered blood vessels was first demonstrated in landmark studies by L'Heureux (L'Heureux et al., 1998) and Niklason (Niklason et al., 1999). The vessels, which were produced using different in vitro techniques, had very good mechanical properties and functioned well in experimental animals. Although *in vitro* and experimental techniques have been developed since then, no clinical implantations have been made until now.

3.1 Biomaterials/biomaterial scaffolds
Williams defines biomaterial as any natural or man-made material that comprises the whole or part of a living structure or biomedical device that performs, augments, or replaces a natural function (Williams, 1999).

Many different materials have been investigated for biomaterial applications. They can be divided into natural materials, i.e., collagen (Weinberg & Bell, 1986; L'Heureux et al., 1998); fibrin (Cummings et al., 2004; Kumar & Krishnan, 2002); hyaluronic acid (Remuzzi et al., 2004; Turner et al., 2004); silk fibroin (Zhang et al., 2009) and BC (Backdahl et al., 2006; Klemm et al., 2001; Bodin et al., 2007; Fink et al., 2010)) and synthetic polymers, i.e., polyglycolic acid (PGA) (Niklason et al., 1999; McKee et al., 2003), polyethylene terephthalate (PET) (Sharefkin et al., 1983; Herring et al., 1984) and ePTFE (Zilla et al., 1987; Meinhart et al., 2005). The required properties for biomaterials vary with cell type, implantation site and strategy for tissue formation. Common demands for all biomaterials include biocompatibility, e.g., avoiding foreign body reactions, capsule formation and chronic inflammatory reactions. Additionally, materials intended to be in contact with blood require evaluation for thrombogenicity. Mechanical properties are important and depend on the target tissue. Since biomaterials used as vascular grafts must withstand blood pressure, they must be investigated for burst pressure, compliance, suture strength and fatigue before using them as implants.

A recent and popular approach involves electrospinning different materials to create nanofibre constructs. Both electrospun synthetic polymers and native ECM proteins have been used for cell seeding to construct vascular grafts (Hashi et al., 2007; Huang et al., 2001; Boland et al., 2004; Kenawy el et al., 2003).

3.2 Materials for vascular grafts
Jaboulay and Briau performed the first arterial transplantation in 1896, but imperfect anastomoses resulted in thrombosis (Jaboulay & Briau, 1896). Since then, more sophisticated techniques have been developed. The search for arterial vascular grafts began in 1952, when Voorhees discovered Vinyon N (nylon), the first fabric graft (Voorhees et al., 1952). A few years later, DeBakey discovered Dacron® in 1958 (Nose, 2008). Today, arterial and even especially venous autografts are used routinely in surgery, creating bypasses for patients with peripheral or coronary occlusive vascular diseases. However, autograft availability is limited, particularly for arteries.

Dacron® and ePTFE are still widely used as arterial replacements. Despite their success in replacing large diameter (>6 mm) high-flow vessels, these materials show thrombogenicity and compliance mismatch in low-flow or small-diameter vessels. Sophisticated techniques have been evaluated to enhance patency, including chemical modifications, coatings and seeding of the surface with different cells. In contrast to natural materials, synthetics often lack adhesion sites. Although passive materials can reproduce sufficient physiological mechanical strength, proper metabolic function and cellular signalling requires intact cellular machinery.

BC is an attractive material for biomaterial applications. Its structure resembles that of collagen, the component in arteries and veins that gives the blood vessel its strength. BC's manufacturing process allows versatility in shape and size, including tubes. Studies have shown successful growth of cardiac rat-derived myocytes and fibroblasts (Entcheva et al., 2004), rat-derived hepatocytes (Kino et al., 1998; Yang et al., 1994) and osteoprogenitor cells (Takata et al., 2001) from mice on cellulose-based materials. However, these matrices are based not on natural cellulose but rather on derivatives such as cellulose acetate and regenerative cellulose.

Although BC is biocompatible, it generally does not promote cell growth (Watanabe et al., 1993a). Thus, BC must be modified to support EC adherence. Modification of wet state BC is challenging because fibre structure and strength must be maintained. This is especially important for vascular grafts, which must withstand blood pressure.

4. Different approaches to engineered blood vessels

4.1 Collagen-based blood vessel model
Weinberg and colleagues developed a collagen-based blood vessel model (Weinberg et al., 1986). Improvement of the construct's mechanical properties is ongoing due to poor mechanical integrity.

4.2 Cell self-assembly model
The cell self-assembly model is made using intact layers of human vascular cells grown to overconfluence to form visible sheets of cells and ECM (L'Heureux et al., 1993, 1998). A sheet of smooth muscle cells (SMCs) is rolled around a mandrel to form the medial layer. Similarly, a sheet of fibroblasts is rolled over the SMC sheet media, forming an adventitial layer. Finally, ECs seeded onto the lumen of the matured vessel form a confluent monolayer. These constructs withstood more than 2000 mmHg pressure before bursting.

4.3 Cell-seeded polymeric scaffold–hybrid graft
This graft was developed by Niklason (Niklason et al., 1999). Vascular cells were seeded into a biodegradable scaffold (PGA) and cultured for 8 weeks under pulsatile radial stress (165 beats per minute and 5% radial strain). ECs seeded onto the lumen of the construct formed a confluent monolayer. Cultured under pulsatile conditions, the histological structure of the constructs resembled that of native arteries. Due to high collagen content, the constructs had a burst pressure greater than 2000 mmHg and they could contract. *In vivo* studies of tissue engineered blood vessels in Yucatan miniature pigs were promising.

With degradable material such as PGA, it is critical to ensure adequate strength of ECM (collagen, elastin) produced by the vascular cells. Degradation products may be toxic to the

Molecular Understanding of Endothelial Cell and Blood Interactions with Bacterial Cellulose:
Novel Opportunities for Artificial Blood Vessels

165

cells. Non-degradable scaffolds offer durable support, but tissue acceptance is mandatory. Ideally, the scaffold should be compliant, similar to native vessels.

4.4 Acellularized construct
A rolled small intestinal submucosa (SIS) has been used as a small diameter vascular graft. A cell-free, 100-μm-thick collagen layer derived from small intestine, SIS is compliant, making it an interesting candidate for vascular implantation and requiring investigation (Roeder et al., 1999, Huynh et al., 1999).

4.5 Artificial artery generated in the peritoneal cavity
In the peritoneal cavity, artificial arteries are generated on silastic tubes. The arteries are lined by nonthrombogenic, mesothelial (endothelial-like) cells. The feasibility of this approach in humans is a matter of debate.

5. Bacterial synthesized cellulose as biomaterial

Cellulose, the most abundant biopolymer on earth, is insoluble in water and degradable by microbial enzymes. Several organisms, e.g., plants, algae and bacteria can produce cellulose, and the bacteria *Gluconacetobacter xylinum* can synthesize and secret cellulose extracellularly (Brown et al., 1976). BC is composed of linear nanosized fibrils of D-glucose molecules (Ross et al., 1991). The network structure of cellulose fibrils resembles that of collagen in the ECM of native connective tissue (Fig. 1) (Backdahl et al., 2006).

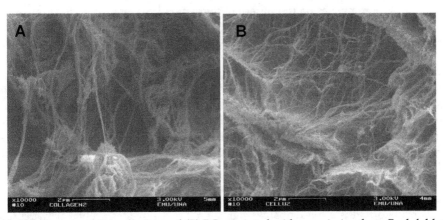

Fig. 1. SEM images of (A) collagen and (B) BC reprinted with permission from Backdahl et al., 2006. Copyright Elsevier 2006.

Although BC is not a hydrogel in the true sense of the meaning, it is often referred to as such because of its high water content, insolubility in water and highly hydrophilic nature. Since BC consists of a highly entangled network of fibrils, it also provides strong mechanical properties that ensure the ability of tissue engineered blood vessels to withstand mechanical forces and prevent rupture. BC can be designed and shaped into three dimensional structures such as tubes or sheets (Backdahl et al., 2006). A major advantage of using BC rather than cellulose produced by any other organism is that BC is completely free of biogenic compounds such as lignin, pectin and arabinan found in, e.g., plant cellulose. During the production process, it is also possible to modify several other properties including pore size, surface properties and layering of the material (Backdahl et al., 2008).

BC is used in various areas including food matrix (nata de coco), dietary fibres, acoustic or filter membranes and ultra-strength paper. In addition, BC has been suggested as a potential material for tissue engineering in several areas, e.g., as scaffold for tissue engineering of cartilage, blood vessels (BASYC®) and successful treatment of second and third degree burns, stomach ulcers and other situations that require a temporary skin substitute (Biofill®, Gengiflex®, XCell®) or to recover periodontal tissue (Gengiflex®) (Czaja et al., 2006; Svensson et al., 2005; Fontana et al., 1990).

5.1 Structure and morphology

Beginning with the water-soluble monosaccharide D-glucose, cellulose synthesis is produced extracellularly as pellicles at the air/liquid interface. Glucan chains of BC are extruded from several enzyme complexes and aggregated by van der Waals forces to form sub-fibrils, approximately 1.5 nm wide. BC sub-fibrils crystallise into microfibrils and then into bundles, which form a dense reticulated structure stabilized by hydrogen bonding. In culture medium, the bundles assemble into ribbons, forming a network of cellulose. This network of cellulose nanofibrils provides BC with high mechanical strength and a water retention capacity of about 99% (Iguchi et al., 2000).

The macroscopic morphology of BC varies with different culture conditions. In static conditions, BC accumulates on the surface of nutrient-rich culture medium, at the oxygen-rich air-liquid interface. Statically cultured BC has lower crystallinity than BC fermented during agitation.

Our molecular studies on EC-blood interactions with BC used BC synthesized by *Gluconacetobacter xylinum* (ATCC 1700178, American Type Culture Collection). Cellulose tubes were grown in corn steep liquid media at 30°C for 7 days. The cellulose was then purified by boiling, first in 0.1 M NaOH at 60°C for 4h and then in Millipore™ water. Finally, the cellulose was sterilised by autoclaving for 20 minutes. Due to the production process, BC consists of two distinctly different layers: one side has a compact network of fibrils with few if any pores, and the other side has a porous network structure. A density gradient arises between the sides.

5.2 Mechanical properties

The optimal scaffold is a biocompatible biomaterial that provides proper mechanical and physical properties, thus promoting cell adhesion and tissue formation. Prior to implantation into animals, BC tubes undergo extensive mechanical testing (burst strength, compliance and tensile strength). Films or sheets of BC show remarkable mechanical strength, due to high crystallinity, high planar orientation of the ribbons, ultrafine structure and a complex network (Iguchi et al., 2000). The mechanical properties of BC tubes are similar to those of pig carotid arteries (Backdahl et al., 2006). BC's compliance curve resembles that of a native artery more than any other synthetic material on the market, which is advantageous. Material density can be altered by varying the culture conditions or by post-culture modifications.

5.3 Biocompatibility

Integration of a material with the host tissue is essential for the success of tissue engineered blood vessels. According to Williams, the biocompatibility of a material is defined as "the ability of a material to perform with an appropriate host response in a specific application" (Williams, 1999). Therefore, an appropriate host response would involve a biomaterial that induces a very low inflammatory and foreign body response in the host tissue.

A study by Helenius et al. showed that BC is well integrated into the host tissue and does not induce inflammatory or foreign body responses (Helenius et al., 2006). They implanted BC pieces subcutaneously in rats and explanted them after 1, 4 and 12 weeks. Incorporation of the implant in the host tissue made it difficult to distinguish a clear interface between the implant and the host tissue (Helenius et al., 2006). These results are supported by another *in vivo* study, where BC tubes were implanted into the carotid arteries in pigs (Wippermann et al., 2009). Therefore, BC clearly has good biocompatibility and shows promising potential as scaffold material.

5.4 Surface modification

One challenge in the field of vascular grafts involves promoting EC attachment and spreading, since many biomaterials similar to BC exhibit limited support for cellular adhesion (Watanabe et al., 1993b). Over the years, many strategies have been developed to modify material surfaces.

To optimize cell-biomaterial interactions, manufacturers coat synthetic scaffolds with cell adhesive proteins such as collagen, fibronectin or laminin (Seeger & Klingman, 1988; Kaehler et al., 1989). However, varying protein composition results in a biofilm with passive protein adsorption, and that composition can modify over time (Vroman, 1987). Additionally, protein adsorption to BC is very low.

Much attention has focused on cell adhesion peptide RGD and its derivatives as possible alternative for stimulating reproducible and predictable cell adhesion (D'Souza et al., 1991; Hersel et al., 2003; Walluscheck et al., 1996; Gabriel et al., 2006). Most RGD modifications occur via covalent binding to the material (Massia & Hubbell, 1990). Although cellulose contains reactive hydroxyl groups that can be chemically modified, these very same hydroxyl groups participate in hydrogen bonding, which holds the cellulose fibre network together. Disruption of these bonds associates with loss of fibre ultrastructure (Sassi & Chanzy, 1995; Sassi et al., 2000). Dry films of BC have been modified with carboxymethyl and acetyl groups (Kim et al., 2002). However, surface modifications to wet state BC remain incompletely understood. Thus, modification of a BC hydrogel is especially challenging, since solvent exchange and cellulose modification typically destroy the hydrogel morphology.

Modification of a BC hydrogel is especially challenging because solvent exchange and cellulose modification typically destroy hydrogel morphology. Thus far, most modifications have been performed on dried BC. Consequently, a new method is needed to increase cell attachment without altering the structure of the BC network.

5.4.1 Xyloglucan

Xyloglucan (XG), the most abundant hemicellulose, is present in the primary wall of many plants. In contrast to cellulose, XG is water-soluble and interacts strongly with cellulose fibres (Hanus & Mazeau, 2006). We have taken advantage of these properties, which provide an elegant means of introducing cell adhesion peptide RGD with XG as a carrier molecule to BC.

BC and cotton linters, as reference material, were modified with XG and XG bearing a GRGDS pentapeptide (Bodin et al., 2007). Compared with organic solvents, modification in the water phase was clearly advantageous for preserving the morphology, as observed with SEM (Fig. 2). XG adsorption increased the wettability only to a minor extent, possibly explaining the decreased or undetectable adsorption of adhesive proteins shown by QCM-D. QCM-D studies further revealed that fibrinogen antibodies do not bind to BC, leading to the conclusion that cell enhancement would result from the presence of RGD epitopes, not from unspecific protein adsorption, e.g., fibronectin, from the cell culture medium. XG also enhances hepatocyte adhesion (Seo et al., 2004), and modification of BC with XG does not adversely affect ECs.

5.4.1.1 Increased cell spreading and adhesion on XGD-modified BC

XG-RGD-modification increased cell adhesion by 20%, and also increased the metabolism of seeded ECs as compared with unmodified BC. In contrast, the proliferation rate was less affected, presumably due to biological variation between cell donors. Our results (Fink et al., 2011a) concur with studies on RGD-grafted regenerated cellulose, which showed that an adhesion peptide enhances adhesion by approximately 20% (Bartouilh de Taillac et al., 2004). Another study showed that cellulose binding proteins bound to different adhesion peptides improve adhesion and spreading of human microvascular cells to cellulose (Andrade et al., 2010). In our study, the absence of serum negatively influenced cell adhesion on unmodified BC but did not act similarly in modified BC, further indicating that increased adhesion is peptide specific.

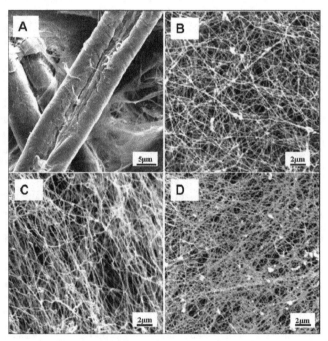

Fig. 2. SEM micrograph of BC morphology of (A) cotton linter, (B) unmodified BC, (C) XG-RGD modified BC and (D) acetone treated BC. Reprinted with permission from Bodin et al., 2007. Copyright American Chemical Society 2007.

Initial cell attachment is crucial to subsequent behaviour such as spreading, proliferation and cell differentiation on substrates. The extent of cell spreading is an important parameter for the biocompatibility of materials. EC adhesion to the ECM proteins is normally followed by cell spreading, a process in which cells reorganize the f-actin cytoskeleton, resulting in flattening and spreading of the cell. These polymerised actin filaments attach the cells to the substrate via focal adhesions. Cells grown on RGD-modified BC spread out, displaying a well-organized actin cytoskeleton with prominent f-actin fibres. They also grow in clusters, which we believe is a step towards achieving a confluent monolayer.

6. Endothelial cells as cellular source for graft lining

The endothelium is composed of a monolayer of squamous epithelial cells that line the inside of blood vessels in a confluent layer, with a total area of 350-1000 m^2 and a weight of 0.5-1.5 kg (Pries et al., 2000; Jaffe, 1987). The morphology of these cells is flat, resembling a cobblestone pattern. This morphology is essential to maintaining good blood flow without turbulence. ECs function not only as a physiological barrier, separating the blood from surrounding tissues, but also as a dynamic layer of cells that displays antithrombotic properties in its resting state. This is achieved by physically preventing elements in the blood from contacting prothrombotic elements in the subendothelium and by active synthesis of various mediators. Endothelial functions help maintain blood vessel function. The endothelium upholds delicate balances in the vasculature, i.e., vasoconstriction/vasodilatation, anticoagulant/procoagulant properties, blood cell adherence/nonadherence and growth promotion/inhibition. It regulates vascular tone, maintains hemostasis, controls vascular structure and mediates inflammatory and immunological responses.

The endothelium responds to inflammatory conditions by regulating its own permeability and releasing a variety of substances. It mediates inflammation with pro-inflammatory mediators including cytokines such as the interleukins (IL) (e.g., IL-1β, IL-6, IL-8), platelet-activating factor (PAF) and also by expressing endothelial cell leukocyte adhesion molecule-1 (ELAM-1) and intercellular adhesion molecule 1 (ICAM-1), inflammatory mediators that control the interaction between EC and circulating blood cells and leukocytes, leading to extravasation of leukocytes.

During an inflammatory response, adhesion molecule P-selectin is expressed on ECs after exposure to leukotrine B4 or histamine, which are produced by mast cells. Tumor necrosis factor alpha (TNF-α) and lipopolysaccharides (LPS) induce P-selectin expression and the synthesis of E-selectin, another selectin that appears a few hours after the inflammatory process begins. Because the interactions between these selectins and their corresponding glycoprotein ligands (sialyl-Lewis^x moiety) on leukocytes are relatively weak and reversible, leukocytes are unable to attach firmly to the endothelium. Instead, they "roll" along the surface of the vessel wall. The interactions are enhanced as other integrins are induced on the endothelium.

Leukocyte integrins LFA-1 and Mac-1 normally adhere only weakly to leukocytes. On the other hand, IL-8 and other chemokines bound to the endothelial surface trigger a conformational change in LFA-1 and Mac-1 on the rolling leukocytes, increasing adhesiveness and consequently firmly anchoring the leukocytes to the endothelium. Rolling is arrested and the leukocytes squeeze between the ECs into the subendothelial tissue, a process known as diapedesis.

6.1 Angiogenesis and vessel remodeling

ECs regulate vessel structure by producing both growth promoting and growth inhibiting factors. SMC growth is stimulated by platelet-derived growth factor (PDGF), fibroblast growth factor (FGF), transforming growth factor alpha (TGF-α), endothelin and angiotensin II. Growth is inhibited by nitric oxide (NO), prostacylin (PGI$_2$), some FGFs, insulin-like growth factor 1 (IGF-1) and thrombospondin.

Angiogenesis is regulated by a variety of growth factors. Hypoxia and inflammatory cytokines such as FGF increase vascular endothelial growth factor-A (VEGF-A) levels through autocrine and paracrine mechanisms. VEGF-A, an endothelial-specific growth factor that consists of a heparin-binding homodimer, is a major regulator of EC function and angiogenesis. VEGF-A activates several EC functions, e.g., proliferation, migration and NO-release, processes that participate importantly in new blood vessel formation. VEGF-A also increases vessel wall permeability. Both VEGF and FGF induce EC production of proteases such as matrix metalloproteinases (MMPs) and plasminogen activator (PA). At least twenty MMPs participate in angiogenesis (Kroll & Waltenberger, 2000; Lamalice et al., 2007).

Proteases digest the basement membrane, allowing ECs to invade surrounding tissue, where they proliferate and migrate to form a sprout. The sprout elongates and the ECs differentiate to form a lumen. ECs in the newly formed vessel produce PDGF-BB, which attracts mural cells (pericytes to capillaries/SMC to larger arteries and veins) and stabilises the vessel. Expressed on ECs, heparin sulphate proteoglycans and their glycosaminoglycans (GAG) side-chains play an important role in angiogenesis because they bind circulating growth factors like VEGF (Kroll & Waltenberger, 2000).

6.2 Regulation of vascular tone

ECs regulate vessel tone and, consequently, local blood flow by managing the communication between the blood and the underlying SMCs, and by releasing substances that influence SMCs to relax or contract. In addition, ECs synthesise both vasodilating and vasoconstricting agents.

Vasodilatation is mediated through PGI$_2$ and (NO/endothelium-derived relaxing factor (EDRF) and endothelium-derived hyperpolarizing factor (EDHF), where NO plays a central role. Vasoconstricting agents released by ECs include endothelin, angiotensin II and thromboxane A$_2$ (TXA$_2$).

Shear stress, bradykinin, thrombin, serotonin and various drugs stimulate ECs to release prostacyklin, thus stimulating adenylate cyclase, which increases cyclic adenosine monophosphate (cAMP) in SMCs. NO is synthesized from L-arginine by NO synthase and diffuses to SMCs, where it activates guanylate cyclase to produce cyclic guanosine monophosphate (cGMP). This leads to decreased intracellular calcium and muscle relaxation. Sensing mechanical changes in the environment, f-actin mediates mechanical induction of NO, leading to signal transduction into the cell.

The eNOS gene contains a shear stress regulatory element (SSRE) that increases or decreases eNOS activity (Balligand et al., 2009). Acetylcholine stimulation of M1 muscarinic receptors releases endothelium-derived hyperpolarizing factor (EDHF), changing membrane potential (Pagliaro et al., 2000). Endothelin consists of three isoforms, ET-1, ET-2 and ET-3. ECs produce endothelin-1, the most potent mediator of vasoconstriction. Two endothelin receptors are found in the vasculature: ET$_A$ on SMCs and ET$_B$ on ECs. Binding of endothelin-

Molecular Understanding of Endothelial Cell and Blood Interactions with Bacterial Cellulose:
Novel Opportunities for Artificial Blood Vessels

171

1 to the ET_A-receptor results in signal transduction and smooth muscle relaxation. On the other hand, activation of ET_B on ECs stimulates NO and PGI_2 production. In contrast, angotensin II is a much weaker vasoconstrictor. Renin cleaves angiotensinogen to angiotensin I, which is then converted to angiotensin by endothelial angiotensin-converting enzyme (ACE) (Nordt & Bode, 2000).

7. Blood compatibility of biomaterials is a challenge

A nonthrombogenic surface is the key to a successful vascular graft. Non-thrombogenicity can be achieved by various surface modifications. Since ECs could provide a nonthrombogenic surface, intense investigation has focussed on endothelialisation in this context. In our studies, we used ECs passage 4 from non-diseased human saphenous veins, by-products of coronary bypass surgery.

The thrombogenicity of a biomaterial is an essential factor for any material that will be in contact with blood. Although the thrombogenic property of cellulose has been extensively researched as it has been used for haemodialysis membranes (Fushimi et al., 1998; Mao et al., 2004), the thrombogenicity of BC remains undetermined because it is a relatively new material for vessel grafts. Therefore, one of our studies focussed on delineating the blood compatibility of BC in comparison with ePTFE and PET vascular grafts, which are both used clinically as graft material (Fink et al., 2011b).

The endothelium's most important function in relation to biomaterials is hemostatic control. Under normal physiological conditions, ECs express thrombo-resistant molecules, but they must be able to switch to a procoagulant state upon injury to initiate coagulation and clot formation. Since blood is transported under high pressure, minimization of blood loss requires a rapid response. Some molecules are continuously secreted by ECs while others are only produced upon stimulation. Molecules can be expressed on the surface or secreted into the blood stream. The different endothelial anti- and procoagulant factors are discussed below in their biological context.

7.1 Primary hemostasis – Platelet adhesion, activation and aggregation

Prostacylin I_2 (PGI_2), nitric oxide (NO) and adenosine diphosphatase (ADPase) suppress platelet activation, aggregation and platelet-wall-interaction. Both NO and PGI_2 are secreted and act in a paracrine manner, whereas ADPase is expressed on the EC surface. Platelet inhibition by PGI_2 is mediated through a guanosine nucleotide binding receptor. This receptor-mediated signal transduction increases cAMP levels and inhibits platelet activation and the release of proaggregatory compounds such as TXA_2 (Moncada, 1982). PGI_2 production is stimulated by diverse agonists such as thrombin, histamine and bradykinin, and synthesised via arachidonic acid (AA) and prostaglandin (PGG_2) (Wu, 1995).

ECs produce EDRFs, which are responsible for acetylcholine-induced vasorelaxation. The most important EDRF is NO, which synthesises nitric oxide synthase (NOS) by converting L-arginine. NO is a small molecule, so it diffuses easily. When NO enters platelets, it inhibits their adhesion and activation via guanylyl cyclise (Radomski et al., 1987c). PGI_2 and NO have synergistic effects on inhibition of platelet adhesion, activation and aggregation and also reverse platelet aggregation (Radomski et al., 1987a; b)

7.2 Secondary hemostasis – Coagulation

The endothelium physically separates coagulation factor VIIa from tissue factor (TF) and prevents platelet exposure to collagen and von Willebrandt factor (vWF) (Fig. 3).

Thrombomodulin (TM) is expressed on the surface of ECs. Thrombin binds to TM, thereby undergoing a conformational change that results in enhanced affinity for protein C. Thrombin is the only enzyme capable of activating protein C. Activated protein C cleaves and inactivates clotting factors Va and VIIIa (Esmon, 1993). The thrombin-TM complex, effectively removes thrombin from the blood and internalises it, leading to its degradation. The TM molecule can also bind FXa, thus inhibiting prothrombin activation (Thompson & Salem, 1986). Protein S, also synthesised by ECs, binds to the endothelial surface and protein Ca to form a complex, thus enhancing FVa and FVIIIa inhibition (Fig. 3).

The endothelium expresses heparin sulphate proteoglycans with anticoagulant activity on its surface. Heparin is a cofactor for antithrombin III, a plasma protein present that can inhibit thrombin, IXa, FXa and XIIa. The complex binding of thrombin to antithrombin III occurs slowly. This process is accelerated by the interaction with heparin, which has many binding sites for antithrombin, and serves to localise and increase its activity more than a thousand-fold. The β-isoform of antithrombin is more highly effective than the α-isoform. Moreover, the β-isoformis effectively inhibits thrombin-induced SMC proliferation (Swedenborg, 1998). Synthesised in the liver and also by ECs, tissue factor pathway inhibitor (TFPI) forms a complex with Xa and inactivates the VIIa-tissue factor complex by binding to it.

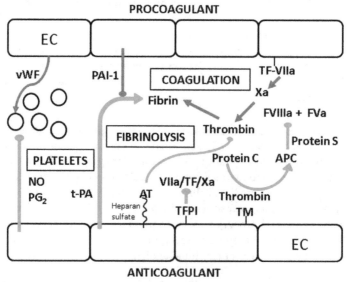

Fig. 3. Schematic illustration of the regulation of coagulation by ECs.

7.2.1 Procoagulation factor

The endothelium also participates importantly in the initiation of coagulation, which arrests bleeding. It expresses a variety of procoagulant factors, including vWF, coagulation factors V and VII, TF and high molecular weight kininogen (HMWK).

ECs synthesise vWF, a platelet adhesion molecule that secretes following stimulation by thrombin, and stores it in vesicles (Weibel-Palade bodies). vWF possesses binding sites for coagulation factor VIII, collagen (exposed after injury) and platelets (GPIb- XI-V), and acts as a bridging molecule in platelet aggregation and activation (Ruggeri, 1994). Importantly, the absence of vWF leads to severe bleeding disorders.

ECs also secrete TF, which is found mainly in the subendothelium at sites not normally exposed to the bloodstream. The basal production of TF is low in comparison with the underlying SMCs and fibroblasts, but it can increase 10- to 40-fold upon stimulation. In addition, ECs have binding sites for factor VII, IX, IXa, X and Xa. Binding to factor IXa inhibits EC decay in the presence of factors VIII and X, which provide an additional feedback mechanism for cell-bound procoagulant activity (Jaffe, 1987; Vane et al., 1990).

7.2.2 Fibrinolysis

The endothelium also helps regulated fibrinolysis (Fig. 3). The degradation of fibrin requires plasmin. Plasminogen binds to the cell surface and facilitates plasmin conversion by two PAs, tissue type plasminogen activator (tPA) and urokinase (uPA) (van Hinsbergh). Physiologically, the most important PA in vascular fibrinolysis is tPA. Indeed, tPA enhances the conversion of plasminogen 100-fold when it binds to fibrin. The release of tPA is either constitutively or pathway-mediated. Thrombin, FVa, bradykinin, PAF and shear stress all induce the synthesis and release of tPA from ECs (Emeis, 1992; Giles et al., 1990; Brown et al., 1999). When tPA binds to the EC surface, it is protected from degradation by the two PA inhibitors (PAI), PAI-1 and PAI-2, which are also released by ECs. PAI-1 requires vitronectin, present in ECM, to maintain its activity; it is the main inhibitor to tPA. Recombinant t-PA (rt-PA) is the most frequently used substance for inducing thrombolysis by pharmacological means (Noble et al., 1995; Bennett et al., 1991).

7.2.3 Biomaterial-induced coagulation

Evaluation of coagulation induced by biomaterials is mostly studied in terms of platelet adhesion, partial thromboplastin time (PTT), protein adsorption by QCM-D or ellipsometry (Liu et al., 2009; Mao et al., 2004;van Oeveren et al., 2002; Keuren et al., 2003). The QCM-D method is surface-sensitive, but the distance from the surface to where measurement is possible is limited. Currently, it is not possible to attach BC to quartz crystals. Therefore, cellulose other than BC must be used. However, this material could be used for QCM-D measurements as a model surface, complementing other studies. Because ellipsometry is an optical method, it is not possible to use native BC for this assay either. Automated calibrated thrombin generation is very sensitive and has become a widespread method for quantitative analysis of coagulation kinetics in blood plasma (van Oeveren et al., 2002; Gerotziafas et al., 2005; Hemker et al., 2003). Thrombin generation is also considered the most sensitive method to assay thrombogenicity.

Since BC is used in a wet state, finding appropriate analysis techniques has been challenging. To our knowledge, ours is the first study to investigate the thrombogenic properties of BC compared with other graft materials (Fink et al., 2011b). We also developed a modified automated calibrated thrombin generation assay (Fink et al., 2010). This makes it possible to follow thrombin generation, in the presence of a material, in real time rather than using an endpoint assay. Our assay has led to new insights into the kinetics of thrombin generation induced by a material surface, which otherwise would have been missed.

Most methods that study the coagulation process measure coagulation in the bulk without regards to where it began or the kinetics describing the propagation from the initiation point. Our method (Fink et al., 2011b) makes it possible to visualize the exact initiation point of coagulation and determine how coagulation propagates (Kantlehner et al., 2000). The captured images are used to calculate the coagulation time of the plasma at the surface (surface coagulation time) and into the bulk (propagation). Such factors are highly relevant to the study of material interactions with blood.

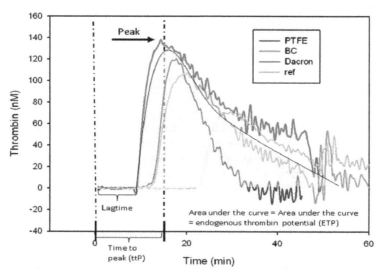

Fig. 4. Thrombogram generated from thrombin generation assay displaying lagtime, time to peak (ttPeak), peak and endogenous thrombin potential (ETP).

We measured the levels of thrombin and factor XIIa using calibrated automated thrombography, which displays the concentration of thrombin and factor XIIa, respectively, in clotting plasma with or without platelets (platelet-rich plasma/platelet-free plasma, PRP/PFP). The splitting of a fluorogenic substrate is monitored for either thrombin or factor XIIa and compared with a known thrombin or factor XIIa activity, respectively, in a parallel non-clotting sample. To evaluate thrombin and factor XIIa generation exclusively induced by the biomaterial surfaces, we fixed material samples with heparinised O-rings and analysed them by calculating the average rate of fluorescence increase over a period of 60 min.

7.2.3.1 Biomaterial induced coagulation of biological cellulose

We compared biomaterial-induced coagulation of BC with clinically used graft materials, i.e., ePTFE and PET. In addition, we visualised coagulation propagation at the material surfaces and into the plasma bulk.

Thrombin generation experiments revealed dramatic differences between the tested materials (Fink et al., 2010). Both ePTFE and BC generate longer lagtimes and time to Peak (ttPeak) values than PET (Fig. 4). Furthermore, BC generates the lowest 'Peak', indicating a

Molecular Understanding of Endothelial Cell and Blood Interactions with Bacterial Cellulose:
Novel Opportunities for Artificial Blood Vessels

175

slower coagulation process at the surface. These results are also supported by the measurements of factor XIIa generation and analysis of surface coagulation times, where BC had the lowest FIIa generation and slowest propagation of coagulation into the bulk (Fig. 5). Compared with PET, thrombin generation in the whole blood Chandler-Loop system depicted the same response, yielding decreased accumulation of thrombin-antithrombin III complex (TAT) on both BC and ePTFE. Since the measurements are performed after one hour and not continuously, the difference in coagulation speed cannot be observed. On the other hand, this assay is performed in whole blood during flow conditions that more closely resemble an *in vivo* situation compared to measurements in platelet-free plasma during static conditions. It is interesting and promising that these two systems show similar results.

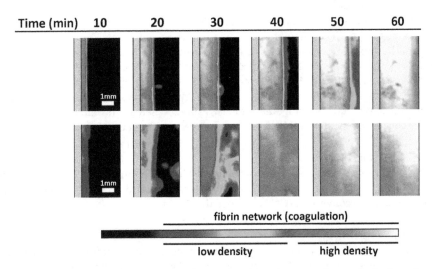

Fig. 5. Representative time-lapse images from a comparative experiment in the imaging of coagulation setup. Graft material samples are attached along the left wall in the images. The colour represents the density of the formed fibrin network (Courtesy of Lars Faxälv, PhD).

Hypothetically, the slower coagulation process on BC (Fig. 5) could be an advantage when blood contacts biomaterial applications, because it would provide time for the blood flow to divert and dilute activated coagulation products. The whole blood model also shows that 4 mm BC tubes perform well regarding anti-thrombogenic properties and perform better compared with ePTFE than 6 mm tubes. Measurements of thrombin generation correlate very well with the XIIa generation assay and visualisation of propagation. Together these methods potentially could provide fast screening methods for evaluating the thrombogenicity of biomaterials.

The amount of TAT generated depends on blood velocity (e.g., shear rate) in the loop system. Higher velocities associate with increased TAT generation. Shear rates are higher in the 4 mm loop system compared with the 6 mm system, and the narrower material also exhibits greater coagulation activation. Interestingly, however, platelet consumption does not increase, suggesting platelet activation. The amount of TAT generated on ePTFE increased 18-fold on 4 mm tubes as compared with 6 mm tubes, but we detected only a 3-fold increase for BC tubes. In comparison with the other tested materials, the platelet consumption of BC is remarkably low, especially compared with heparinised polyvinyl chloride (PVC), which is known to have low thrombogenic properties (Johnell et al., 2005). In addition, cellulose showed no visible sign of clotting following one hour of incubation with whole blood containing only small amounts of soluble heparin.

7.3 Complement system

The immune complement system (CS) is part of the innate immune system. Its main task is to protect the body from pathogenic agents like bacteria, viruses and fungi. On contact with a foreign surface, e.g., a bacterial surface, the CS activates in a cascade that either destroys the bacterial surface or releases bioactive degradation products, or both, causing inflammatory reactions in the surrounding tissue.

Consisting of more than 30 different cell-bound and soluble proteins that circulate as inactive zymogens under nonpathological conditions, the immune CS is present in blood and serum. Its most important factor is complement factor 3 (C3). Cleavage of C3 by C3 convertase creates C3a and C3b, causing a cascade of further cleavage and activation events. Three different pathways lead to the creation of C3 convertase: the classical pathway, the alternative pathway and the mannose-binding lectin pathway. The classical complement pathway typically requires antibodies for activation, whereas the alternative and lectin pathways can be activated by C3 hydrolysis or antigens without the presence of antibody.

7.3.1 Classical pathway

Classical convertase is initiated when antibodies bind to a surface such as a bacterium. When factor C1 binds to an antibody, it cleaves is cleaved and binds to additional factors forming the classical convertase (C4b2a) (Kinoshita, 1991).

7.3.2 Alternative pathway

The alternative pathway is triggered by either spontaneous C3 hydrolysis, which forms C3a and C3b, or covalent binding of C3b from the classical and lectin pathways to a surface. The C3b molecule is capable of covalently binding to a pathogenic membrane surface in its vicinity. If there is no pathogen in the blood, the C3a and C3b protein fragments will deactivate when they rejoin with each other. Upon binding with a cellular membrane, C3b is binds to factor Ba and P, forming the alternative pathway C3-convertase (C3bBbP). A characteristic feature of the alternative pathway is a feedback mechanism that leads to accelerated C3 activation. Such mechanisms are not present in the classical pathway (Medicus et al., 1976; Rother et al., 1998).

7.3.3 Mannose-binding lectin pathway

A variant of the classical pathway, the Mannose-binding lectin pathway does not require antibodies. Activation of this pathway occurs when mannose-binding lectin (MBL) binds to mannose residues on the pathogen surface. Subsequently, the MBL complex can split C4 and C2, generating C3-convertase, as in the classical pathway (Petersen et al., 2001). This pathway will not be discussed further in this chapter.

The convertases from both the classical and alternative pathways cleave C5 into C5a and C5b. The C5b molecule associates with C6, C7, C8, and C9, forming the C5b-9 membrane attack complex (MAC), which is inserted into the cell membrane and initiates cell lysis. The C5b-9, also called the terminal complement complex (TCC), may exist as a soluble active form denoted sC5b-9. This soluble form can be measured to assess complement activation . The C5a and C3a fragments are anaphylatoxins that participate in the recruitment of inflammatory cells and trigger mast cell degranulation. Therefore, these anaphylatoxins participate in many forms of acute and chronic inflammation including sepsis (Guo et al., 2004; Ward, 2008).

7.3.4 Complement activation

Extracorporal treatments such as haemodialysis and cardiopulmonary bypass activate the CS. Contact between blood and biomaterials may generate degradation fragments of complement C3a and C5a and soluble C5b-9. These fragments result in chemotaxis of leukocytes, cytokine release and generation of prostaglandins, resulting in a life-threatening condition termed "whole body" inflammation. Biomaterial induced CS is activated by both the classical and alternative pathways (Nilsson et al., 2007).

The Chandler-Loop system was also used to assess CS activation. The complement activation parameters (C3a and C5b-9) were much higher for BC compared with the other materials, for both 4 and 6 mm tubes. Cellulose is known to induce complement activation in hemodialysis membranes (Frank et al., 2001). The mechanisms underlying these results for BC are still unclear and require further investigation. Bacterial fragments could still be present in the material. However, endotoxin values are well within the limit for cardiovascular devices. It is also possible that exposed hydroxyl groups induce complement activation through the alternative pathway (Arima et al., 2009; Toda et al., 2008). The physiological significance *in vivo* of this complement activation remains undetermined. Interestingly, platelet activation is low even when complement activation is high. According to the literature, platelet consumption and complement activation are closely related (Fushimi et al., 1998; Hamad et al., 2008; Peerschke et al., 2006; Gyongyossy-Issa et al., 1994).

8. What are the future therapeutic possibilities?

This chapter has presented possible approaches to modifying BC that enhance EC growth *in vitro*. The XG method, an easy one-step procedure carried out in water, is an elegant technique for modifying BC to promote EC. Its advantage is the preservation of the fibre structure, thus maintaining its strength. The modification of BC with the XG technique is far from limited to the RGD peptide. Different peptide sequences or other active groups and growth factors could be attached to the XG molecule. Platelets could potentially adhere to exposed RGD peptides. Therefore, other peptides, more specific to ECs, or different combinations of peptides should be explored.

Measurements of thrombin generation correlated well with the XIIa generation assay and visualisation of the propagation of coagulation. Together, these methods could offer potential fast screening methods for evaluating the thrombogenicity of biomaterials and future surface modifications.

BC could be used for vascular grafts in two different approaches: (i) implantation as a tube without cells or (ii) seeding prior to implantation. The ideal BC modification would provide an initial nonthrombogenic surface and promote long-term endothelialisation. Future modifications of BC could include heparinisation or combinations of surface modifications, e.g., different peptides or coatings. Heparin is a potent antithrombotic agent that functions by binding antithrombin. In recent years, heparinised ePTFE grafts (Propaten®) have been developed (Losel-Sadee & Alefelder, 2009). Although encouraging outcomes for below-knee bypass are reported, the compliance mismatch of ePTFE grafts still remains. However, this is an exciting modification and preliminary studies on heparinised BC tubes show considerably lower amounts of thrombin on the hep-BC surface.

Our studies show that modification of BC with the adhesion-promoting peptide RGD results in increased EC adhesion, metabolism and spreading. Furthermore, BC induces slower coagulation than clinically available materials such as Gore-Tex® and Dacron® and induces the least contact activation as evaluated by Factor XIIa generation. In addition, BC consumes low quantities of platelets and generates low thrombin values as compared with Dacron® and Gore-Tex®.

9. Conclusion

Our work demonstrates that it is possible to introduce an adhesion peptide to BC that enhances EC adhesion without altering the fibre network or mechanical properties. The anti-thrombogenic properties of BC, especially 4 mm tubes, are promising as compared with conventional graft materials. Therefore, BC emerges as a promising, novel vascular graft material for small-caliber grafts. Molecular studies confirm that BC exhibits low thrombogenicity and extensive EC adhesion, which are beneficial when introducing artificial materials *in vivo* during by-pass surgery. Together with the modification methods presented in this chapter, BC has the potential to become a material for artificial vessels, thus underlining the importance of increasing molecular understanding of EC and BC interactions to create novel opportunities for artificial blood vessels.

10. Acknowledgements

The Authors thank Karen Williams for editorial expertise.

11. References

Andrade, F. K., et al. 2010. Improving bacterial cellulose for blood vessel replacement: Functionalization with a chimeric protein containing a cellulose-binding module and an adhesion peptide. *Acta Biomater*, 6, 4034-41.

Arima, Y., et al. 2009. Complement Activation by Polymers Carrying Hydroxyl Groups. *ACS Applied Materials & Interfaces*.

Backdahl, H., et al. 2008. Engineering microporosity in bacterial cellulose scaffolds. *J Tissue Eng Regen Med*, 2, 320-30.

Backdahl, H., et al. 2006. Mechanical properties of bacterial cellulose and interactions with smooth muscle cells. *Biomaterials*, 27, 2141-9.

Balligand, J. L., et al. 2009. eNOS activation by physical forces: from short-term regulation of contraction to chronic remodeling of cardiovascular tissues. *Physiol Rev*, 89, 481-534.

Molecular Understanding of Endothelial Cell and Blood Interactions with Bacterial Cellulose:
Novel Opportunities for Artificial Blood Vessels

179

Bartouilh De Taillac, L., et al. 2004. Grafting of RGD peptides to cellulose to enhance human osteoprogenitor cells adhesion and proliferation. *Composites Science and Technology,* 64, 827-837.

Bennett, W. F., et al. 1991. High resolution analysis of functional determinants on human tissue-type plasminogen activator. *J Biol Chem,* 266, 5191-201.

Bodin, A., et al. 2007. Modification of nanocellulose with a xyloglucan-RGD conjugate enhances adhesion and proliferation of endothelial cells: Implications for tissue engineering. *Biomacromolecules,* 8, 3697-3704.

Boland, E. D., et al. 2004. Electrospinning collagen and elastin: preliminary vascular tissue engineering. *Front Biosci,* 9, 1422-32.

Brown, N. J., et al. 1999. Bradykinin stimulates tissue plasminogen activator release in human vasculature. *Hypertension,* 33, 1431-5.

Brown, R. M., Jr., et al. 1976. Cellulose biosynthesis in Acetobacter xylinum: visualization of the site of synthesis and direct measurement of the in vivo process. *Proc Natl Acad Sci U S A,* 73, 4565-9.

Cummings, C. L., et al. 2004. Properties of engineered vascular constructs made from collagen, fibrin, and collagen-fibrin mixtures. *Biomaterials,* 25, 3699-706.

Czaja, W., et al. 2006. Microbial cellulose--the natural power to heal wounds. *Biomaterials,* 27, 145-151.

D'Souza, S. E., et al. 1991. Arginyl-glycyl-aspartic acid (RGD): a cell adhesion motif. *Trends Biochem Sci,* 16, 246-50.

Emeis, J. J. 1992. Regulation of the acute release of tissue-type plasminogen activator from the endothelium by coagulation activation products. *Ann N Y Acad Sci,* 667, 249-58.

Entcheva, E., et al. 2004. Functional cardiac cell constructs on cellulose-based scaffolding. *Biomaterials,* 25, 5753-62.

Esmon, C. T. 1993. Molecular events that control the protein C anticoagulant pathway. *Thromb Haemost,* 70, 29-35.

Fink, H., et al. 2010. Real-time measurements of coagulation on bacterial cellulose and conventional vascular graft materials. *Acta Biomaterialia,* 6, 1125-1130.

Fink, H., et al. 2011a. Bacterial cellulose modified with xyloglucan bearing the adhesion peptide RGD promotes endothelial cell adhesion and metabolism—a promising modification for vascular grafts. Journal of Tissue Engineering and Regenerative Medicine, 5, 454-463.

Fink, H., et al. 2011b. An in vitro study of blood compatibility of vascular grafts made of bacterial cellulose in comparison with conventionally-used graft materials. *Journal of Biomedical Materials Research Part A,* 97A, 52-58.

Fontana, J., et al. 1990. Acetobacter cellulose pellicle as a temporary skin substitute. *Applied Biochemistry and Biotechnology,* 24-25, 253-264.

Frank, R. D., et al. 2001. Role of contact system activation in hemodialyzer-induced thrombogenicity. *Kidney Int,* 60, 1972-81.

Fushimi, F., et al. 1998. Platelet adhesion, contact phase coagulation activation, and C5a generation of polyethylene glycol acid-grafted high flux cellulosic membrane with varieties of grafting amounts. *Artif Organs,* 22, 821-6.

Gabriel, M., et al. 2006. Direct grafting of RGD-motif-containing peptide on the surface of polycaprolactone films. *J Biomater Sci Polym Ed*, 17, 567-77.

Gerotziafas, G. T., et al. 2005. Towards a standardization of thrombin generation assessment: the influence of tissue factor, platelets and phospholipids concentration on the normal values of Thrombogram-Thrombinoscope assay. *Thromb J*, 3, 16.

Giles, A. R., et al. 1990. The fibrinolytic potential of the normal primate following the generation of thrombin in vivo. *Thromb Haemost*, 63, 476-81.

Guo, R. F., et al. 2004. Role of C5a-C5aR interaction in sepsis. *Shock*, 21, 1-7.

Gyongyossy-Issa, M. I., et al. 1994. Complement activation in platelet concentrates is surface-dependent and modulated by the platelets. *J Lab Clin Med*, 123, 859-68.

Hamad, O. A., et al. 2008. Complement activation triggered by chondroitin sulfate released by thrombin receptor-activated platelets. *J Thromb Haemost*, 6, 1413-21.

Hanus, J. & Mazeau, K. 2006. The xyloglucan-cellulose assembly at the atomic scale. *Biopolymers*, 82, 59-73.

Hashi, C. K., et al. 2007. Antithrombogenic property of bone marrow mesenchymal stem cells in nanofibrous vascular grafts. *Proc Natl Acad Sci U S A*, 104, 11915-20.

Helenius, G., et al. 2006. In vivo biocompatibility of bacterial cellulose. *J Biomed Mater Res A*, 76, 431-8.

Hemker, H. C., et al. 2003. Calibrated automated thrombin generation measurement in clotting plasma. *Pathophysiol Haemost Thromb*, 33, 4-15.

Herring, M., et al. 1984. Endothelial seeding of Dacron and polytetrafluoroethylene grafts: the cellular events of healing. *Surgery*, 96, 745-55.

Hersel, U., et al. 2003. RGD modified polymers: biomaterials for stimulated cell adhesion and beyond. *Biomaterials*, 24, 4385-415.

Huang, L., et al. 2001. Engineered collagen-PEO nanofibers and fabrics. *J Biomater Sci Polym Ed*, 12, 979-93.

Iguchi, M., et al. 2000. Bacterial cellulose — a masterpiece of nature's arts. *Journal of Materials Science*, 35, 261-270.

Jaboulay, M. & Briau, E. 1896. Recherches experimentales sur la suture et al greffe arterielle. *Lyon Med*, 81, 97.

Jaffe, E. A. 1987. Cell biology of endothelial cells. *Hum Pathol*, 18, 234-9.

Johnell, M., et al. 2005. The influence of different heparin surface concentrations and antithrombin-binding capacity on inflammation and coagulation. *Biomaterials*, 26, 1731-9.

Kaehler, J., et al. 1989. Precoating substrate and surface configuration determine adherence and spreading of seeded endothelial cells on polytetrafluoroethylene grafts. *J Vasc Surg*, 9, 535-41.

Kantlehner, M., et al. 2000. Surface coating with cyclic RGD peptides stimulates osteoblast adhesion and proliferation as well as bone formation. *Chembiochem*, 1, 107-14.

Molecular Understanding of Endothelial Cell and Blood Interactions with Bacterial Cellulose:
Novel Opportunities for Artificial Blood Vessels

181

Kenawy El, R., et al. 2003. Electrospinning of poly(ethylene-co-vinyl alcohol) fibers. *Biomaterials*, 24, 907-13.

Keuren, J. F. W., et al. 2003. Thrombogenicity of polysaccharide-coated surfaces. *Biomaterials*, 24, 1917-1924.

Kim, D.-Y., et al. 2002. Surface acetylation of bacterial cellulose. *Cellulose*, 9, 361-367.

Kino, Y., et al. 1998. Multiporous cellulose microcarrier for the development of a hybrid artificial liver using isolated hepatocytes. *J Surg Res*, 79, 71-6.

Kinoshita, T. 1991. Biology of complement: the overture. *Immunol Today*, 12, 291-5.

Klemm, D., et al. 2001. Bacterial synthesized cellulose -- artificial blood vessels for microsurgery. *Progress in Polymer Science*, 26, 1561-1603.

Kroll, J. & Waltenberger, J. 2000. [Regulation of the endothelial function and angiogenesis by vascular endothelial growth factor-A (VEGF-A]. *Z Kardiol*, 89, 206-18.

Kumar, T. R. & Krishnan, L. K. 2002. A stable matrix for generation of tissue-engineered nonthrombogenic vascular grafts. *Tissue Eng*, 8, 763-70.

L'Heureux, N., et al. 1998. A completely biological tissue-engineered human blood vessel. *FASEB J*, 12, 47-56.

Lamalice, L., et al. 2007. Endothelial cell migration during angiogenesis. *Circ Res*, 100, 782-94.

Langer, R. & Vacanti, J. P. 1993. Tissue engineering. *Science*, 260, 920-6.

Liu, P. S., et al. 2009. Grafting of zwitterion from cellulose membranes via ATRP for improving blood compatibility. *Biomacromolecules*, 10, 2809-16.

Losel-Sadee, H. & Alefelder, C. 2009. Heparin-bonded expanded polytetrafluoroethylene graft for infragenicular bypass: five-year results. *J Cardiovasc Surg (Torino)*, 50, 339-43.

Mao, C., et al. 2004. Various approaches to modify biomaterial surfaces for improving hemocompatibility. *Advances in Colloid and Interface Science*, 110, 5-17.

Massia, S. P. & Hubbell, J. A. 1990. Covalent surface immobilization of Arg-Gly-Asp- and Tyr-Ile-Gly-Ser-Arg-containing peptides to obtain well-defined cell-adhesive substrates. *Anal Biochem*, 187, 292-301.

Mckee, J. A., et al. 2003. Human arteries engineered in vitro. *EMBO Rep*, 4, 633-8.

Medicus, R. G., et al. 1976. Alternative pathway of complement: recruitment of precursor properdin by the labile C3/C5 convertase and the potentiation of the pathway. *J Exp Med*, 144, 1076-93.

Meinhart, J. G., et al. 2005. Enhanced endothelial cell retention on shear-stressed synthetic vascular grafts precoated with RGD-cross-linked fibrin. *Tissue Eng*, 11, 887-95.

Moncada, S. 1982. Prostacyclin and arterial wall biology. *Arteriosclerosis*, 2, 193-207.

Niklason, L. E., et al. 1999. Functional Arteries Grown in Vitro. *Science*, 284, 489-493.

Nilsson, B., et al. 2007. The role of complement in biomaterial-induced inflammation. *Mol Immunol*, 44, 82-94.

Noble, S., et al. 1995. Enoxaparin. A reappraisal of its pharmacology and clinical applications in the prevention and treatment of thromboembolic disease. *Drugs*, 49, 388-410.

Nordt, T. K. & Bode, C. 2000. [Endothelium and endogenous fibrinolysis]. *Z Kardiol*, 89, 219-26.

Nose, Y. 2008. Dr. Michael E. DeBakey and his contributions in the field of artificial organs. September 7, 1908-July 11, 2008. *Artif Organs*, 32, 661-6.

Pagliaro, P., et al. 2000. The endothelium-derived hyperpolarizing factor: does it play a role in vivo and is it involved in the regulation of vascular tone only? *Ital Heart J*, 1, 264-8.

Peerschke, E. I., et al. 2006. Blood platelets activate the classical pathway of human complement. *J Thromb Haemost*, 4, 2035-42.

Petersen, S. V., et al. 2001. The mannan-binding lectin pathway of complement activation: biology and disease association. *Mol Immunol*, 38, 133-49.

Pierschbacher, M. D. & Ruoslahti, E. 1984. Cell attachment activity of fibronectin can be duplicated by small synthetic fragments of the molecule. *Nature*, 309, 30-3.

Pries, A. R., et al. 2000. The endothelial surface layer. *Pflügers Archiv European Journal of Physiology*, 440, 653-666.

Radomski, M. W., et al. 1987a. The anti-aggregating properties of vascular endothelium: interactions between prostacyclin and nitric oxide. *Br J Pharmacol*, 92, 639-46.

Radomski, M. W., et al. 1987b. Comparative pharmacology of endothelium-derived relaxing factor, nitric oxide and prostacyclin in platelets. *Br J Pharmacol*, 92, 181-7.

Radomski, M. W., et al. 1987c. The role of nitric oxide and cGMP in platelet adhesion to vascular endothelium. *Biochem Biophys Res Commun*, 148, 1482-9.

Remuzzi, A., et al. 2004. Vascular smooth muscle cells on hyaluronic acid: culture and mechanical characterization of an engineered vascular construct. *Tissue Eng*, 10, 699-710.

Ross, P., et al. 1991. Cellulose biosynthesis and function in bacteria. *Microbiol Rev*, 55, 35-58.

Rother, K., et al. 1998. *The complement system*, Berlin, Springer.

Ruggeri, Z. M. 1994. Glycoprotein Ib and von Willebrand factor in the process of thrombus formation. *Ann N Y Acad Sci*, 714, 200-10.

Sassi, J.-F. & Chanzy, H. 1995. Ultrastructural aspects of the acetylation of cellulose. *Cellulose*, 2, 111-127.

Sassi, J.-F., et al. 2000. Relative susceptibility of the Iα and Iβ phases of cellulose towards acetylation. *Cellulose*, 7, 119-132.

Seeger, J. M. & Klingman, N. 1988. Improved in vivo endothelialization of prosthetic grafts by surface modification with fibronectin. *J Vasc Surg*, 8, 476-82.

Seo, S. J., et al. 2004. Xyloglucan as a synthetic extracellular matrix for hepatocyte attachment. *J Biomater Sci Polym Ed*, 15, 1375-87.

Sharefkin, J. B., et al. 1983. Seeding of Dacron vascular prostheses with endothelium of aortic origin. *J Surg Res*, 34, 33-43.

Molecular Understanding of Endothelial Cell and Blood Interactions with Bacterial Cellulose:
Novel Opportunities for Artificial Blood Vessels

183

Swedenborg, J. 1998. The mechanisms of action of alpha- and beta-isoforms of antithrombin. *Blood Coagul Fibrinolysis,* 9 Suppl 3, S7-10.

Svensson, A., et al. 2005. Bacterial cellulose as a potential scaffold for tissue engineering of cartilage. *Biomaterials,* 26, 419-431.

Takata, T., et al. 2001. Migration of osteoblastic cells on various guided bone regeneration membranes. *Clin Oral Implants Res,* 12, 332-8.

Thompson, E. A. & Salem, H. H. 1986. Inhibition by human thrombomodulin of factor Xa-mediated cleavage of prothrombin. *J Clin Invest,* 78, 13-7.

Toda, M., et al. 2008. Complement activation on surfaces carrying amino groups. *Biomaterials,* 29, 407-417.

Turner, N. J., et al. 2004. A novel hyaluronan-based biomaterial (Hyaff-11) as a scaffold for endothelial cells in tissue engineered vascular grafts. *Biomaterials,* 25, 5955-64.

Walluscheck, K. P., et al. 1996. Endothelial cell seeding of de-endothelialised human arteries: improvement by adhesion molecule induction and flow-seeding technology. *Eur J Vasc Endovasc Surg,* 12, 46-53.

Van Hinsbergh, V. W. Regulation of the synthesis and secretion of plasminogen activators by endothelial cells.

Van Oeveren, W., et al. 2002. Comparison of coagulation activity tests in vitro for selected biomaterials. *Artif Organs,* 26, 506-11.

Van Oeveren, W., et al. 2002. Comparison of Coagulation Activity Tests In Vitro for Selected Biomaterials. *Artificial Organs,* 26, 506-511.

Vane, J. R., et al. 1990. Regulatory functions of the vascular endothelium. *N Engl J Med,* 323, 27-36.

Ward, P. A. 2008. Sepsis, apoptosis and complement. *Biochem Pharmacol,* 76, 1383-8.

Watanabe, K., et al. 1993a. A new bacterial cellulose substrate for mammalian cell culture. *Cytotechnology,* 13, 107-114.

Watanabe, K., et al. 1993b. A new bacterial cellulose substrate for mammalian cell culture. *Cytotechnology* 13, 107-114.

Weinberg, C. B. & Bell, E. 1986. A blood vessel model constructed from collagen and cultured vascular cells. *Science,* 231, 397-400.

Williams, D. F. 1999. *The Williams dictionary of biomaterials,* Liverpool, Liverpool Univ. Press.

Wippermann, J., et al. 2009. Preliminary results of small arterial substitute performed with a new cylindrical biomaterial composed of bacterial cellulose. *Eur J Vasc Endovasc Surg,* 37, 592-6.

Voorhees, A. B., Jr., et al. 1952. The use of tubes constructed from vinyon "N" cloth in bridging arterial defects. *Ann Surg,* 135, 332-6.

Vroman, L. 1987. Methods of investigating protein interactions on artificial and natural surfaces. *Ann N Y Acad Sci,* 516, 300-5.

Wu, K. K. 1995. Molecular regulation and augmentation of prostacyclin biosynthesis. *Agents Actions Suppl,* 45, 11-7.

Yang, M. B., et al. 1994. Hollow fibers for hepatocyte encapsulation and transplantation: studies of survival and function in rats. *Cell Transplant,* 3, 373-85.

Zhang, X., et al. 2009. Dynamic culture conditions to generate silk-based tissue-engineered vascular grafts. *Biomaterials,* 30, 3213-23.

Zilla, P., et al. 1987. Endothelial cell seeding of polytetrafluoroethylene vascular grafts in humans: a preliminary report. *J Vasc Surg,* 6, 535-41.

Permissions

The contributors of this book come from diverse backgrounds, making this book a truly international effort. This book will bring forth new frontiers with its revolutionizing research information and detailed analysis of the nascent developments around the world.

We would like to thank Dr. Sampath Parthasarathy, for lending his expertise to make the book truly unique. He has played a crucial role in the development of this book. Without his invaluable contribution this book wouldn't have been possible. He has made vital efforts to compile up to date information on the varied aspects of this subject to make this book a valuable addition to the collection of many professionals and students.

This book was conceptualized with the vision of imparting up-to-date information and advanced data in this field. To ensure the same, a matchless editorial board was set up. Every individual on the board went through rigorous rounds of assessment to prove their worth. After which they invested a large part of their time researching and compiling the most relevant data for our readers. Conferences and sessions were held from time to time between the editorial board and the contributing authors to present the data in the most comprehensible form. The editorial team has worked tirelessly to provide valuable and valid information to help people across the globe.

Every chapter published in this book has been scrutinized by our experts. Their significance has been extensively debated. The topics covered herein carry significant findings which will fuel the growth of the discipline. They may even be implemented as practical applications or may be referred to as a beginning point for another development. Chapters in this book were first published by InTech; hereby published with permission under the Creative Commons Attribution License or equivalent.

The editorial board has been involved in producing this book since its inception. They have spent rigorous hours researching and exploring the diverse topics which have resulted in the successful publishing of this book. They have passed on their knowledge of decades through this book. To expedite this challenging task, the publisher supported the team at every step. A small team of assistant editors was also appointed to further simplify the editing procedure and attain best results for the readers.

Our editorial team has been hand-picked from every corner of the world. Their multi-ethnicity adds dynamic inputs to the discussions which result in innovative

outcomes. These outcomes are then further discussed with the researchers and contributors who give their valuable feedback and opinion regarding the same. The feedback is then collaborated with the researches and they are edited in a comprehensive manner to aid the understanding of the subject.

Apart from the editorial board, the designing team has also invested a significant amount of their time in understanding the subject and creating the most relevant covers. They scrutinized every image to scout for the most suitable representation of the subject and create an appropriate cover for the book.

The publishing team has been involved in this book since its early stages. They were actively engaged in every process, be it collecting the data, connecting with the contributors or procuring relevant information. The team has been an ardent support to the editorial, designing and production team. Their endless efforts to recruit the best for this project, has resulted in the accomplishment of this book. They are a veteran in the field of academics and their pool of knowledge is as vast as their experience in printing. Their expertise and guidance has proved useful at every step. Their uncompromising quality standards have made this book an exceptional effort. Their encouragement from time to time has been an inspiration for everyone.

The publisher and the editorial board hope that this book will prove to be a valuable piece of knowledge for researchers, students, practitioners and scholars across the globe.

List of Contributors

L. R. Ritter
Department of Mathematics, Southern Polytechnic State University, USA

Akif Ibragimov
Department of Mathematics & Statistics, Texas Tech University, USA

Jay R. Walton
Department of Mathematics, Texas A & M University, USA

Catherine J. McNeal
Department of Internal Medicine, Division of Cardiology and Department of Pediatrics, Division of Endocrinology, Scott & White Hospital, USA

J. L. Anderson, S. C. Smith and R. L. Taylor, Jr.
University of New Hampshire, Durham, USA

Jacek Jawien
Jagiellonian University School of Medicine, Chair of Pharmacology, Krakow, Poland

Lawrence M. Agius
Department of Pathology, Mater Dei Hospital, Tal-Qroqq, University of Malta Medical School, Msida, Malta

Luigi Fabrizio Rodella and Rita Rezzani
Anatomy Section, Department of Biomedical Sciences and Biotechnology, University of Brescia, Italy

Almudena Ortega, Lourdes M. Varela, Beatriz Bermudez, Sergio Lopez, Francisco J.G. Muriana and Rocio Abia
Laboratory of Cellular and Molecular Nutrition, Instituto de la Grasa, Consejo Superior de Investigaciones Científicas, Sevilla, Spain

Kasturi Ranganna and Omana P. Mathew
Texas Southern University, Department of Pharmaceutical Sciences, USA

Frank M. Yatsu
University of Texas Health Science Center at Houston, Texas, Department of Neurology, USA

Helen Fink
Dept. of Chemical and Biological Engineering, Chalmers University of Technology, Sweden

Anders Sellborn
Dept. of Surgery, Inst. of Clin. Sciences, Sahlgrenska Acad. at University of Gothenburg, Sweden

Alexandra Krettek
Dept. of Intern. Med., Inst. of Medicine, Sahlgrenska Acad. at University of Gothenburg, Sweden Nordic School of Public Health, Sweden